Case Studies in
Abnormal Psychology

THIRD EDITION

Ethan E. Gorenstein

Behavioral Medicine Program
Department of Psychiatry
Columbia University Medical Center

Ronald J. Comer

Department of Psychology
Princeton University

Contributions by:
M. Zachary Rosenthal

Department of Psychology and Neuroscience
Duke University

 worth publishers
Macmillan Learning
New York

Executive Vice President & General Manager: Charles Linsmeier
Vice President, Social Sciences and High School: Shani Fisher
Executive Program Manager: Daniel DeBonis
Associate Developmental Editor: Nick Rizzuti
Executive Marketing Manager: Katherine Nurre
Marketing Assistant: Steven Huang
Senior Media Editor: Stefani Wallace
Media Project Manager: Jason Perkins
Senior Director, Content Management Enhancement: Tracey Kuehn
Senior Managing Editor: Lisa Kinne
Senior Workflow Project Supervisor: Paul W. Rohloff
Director of Design, Content Management: Diana Blume
Senior Design Services Manager: Natasha Wolfe
Cover Design Manager: John Callahan
Art Manager: Matt McAdams
Senior Project Manager: Arindam Bose, Lumina Datamatics, Inc.
Composition: Lumina Datamatics, Inc.
Printing and Binding: LSC Communications
Cover Image: Matt Manley

Library of Congress Control Number: 2022930695

ISBN-13: 978-1-319-33341-6
ISBN-10: 1-319-33341-9
International Edition: ISBN-13: 978-1-319-46666-4

Printed in the United States of America
1 2 3 4 5 6   27 26 25 24 23 22

Worth Publishers
120 Broadway
New York, NY 10271
www.macmillanlearning.com

For Margee, Eleazer, and Julian
—E. E. G.

For my wonderful wife Marlene
—R. J. C.

CONTENTS

In *Case Studies in Abnormal Psychology,* Third Edition, we have sought to provide clinical richness and a sense of genuine humanity across all cases and, in addition, to link the clinical material to current theories and research. In our previous editions and this one, our approach helps readers to appreciate the different perspectives of clients, friends, relatives, and therapists; reveals the nitty-gritty details of treatment programs; underscores relevant theories and studies; and challenges readers to apply their clinical insights, think critically, and make clinical decisions. We believe that *Case Studies in Abnormal Psychology,* Third Edition, can stimulate a deeper understanding of abnormal psychology by its use of the following features that set it apart from other clinical case books:

1. **New cases and case material:** A number of exciting new cases have been added to this third edition. In addition, the cases retained from the earlier editions have been carefully updated to reflect the clinical field's growing insights, new research findings, and DSM-5-TR-based diagnostic changes.

2. **Multiple individual perspectives:** In addition to in-depth descriptions of clinical symptoms, histories, and treatments, each of our cases looks at a disorder from the point of view of the client, the therapist, and a friend or relative. These different points of view demonstrate that a given disorder affects multiple persons, and they help readers empathize with the concerns and dilemmas of both clients and those with whom they interact.

3. **In-depth treatment presentations:** Extra attention is paid to treatment in this book, particularly to the interaction between client and therapist. Our detailed treatment discussions help readers fully appreciate how theories of treatment are translated into actual procedures and how individuals with particular problems respond to a clinician's efforts.

4. **Research-based treatments, integrated approaches:** The treatments described throughout the book represent approaches that are well supported

by empirical research. In most of the cases, the treatment is actually an integration of several approaches, again reflecting current trends and findings in clinical research. Readers will find each of the major models of treatment represented appropriately, respectfully, and without bias.

5. **Interwoven clinical material, theory, and research:** Each case weaves together clinical material, theoretical perspectives, and empirical findings so that readers can appreciate not only the fascinating clinical details but also what they mean. Similarly, they can recognize not only what and how treatment techniques are applied but why such techniques are chosen.

6. **Enhanced diversity and multicultural coverage:** Consistent with the clinical field's ever-growing appreciation of the impact of ethnicity, race, poverty, gender, gender identity, sexual orientation, immigration status, and other cultural factors on psychological functioning, this edition greatly expands its presentations of diversity—featuring a wide array of diverse clients and diverse practitioners. Our cases truly reflect the many faces of the clinical field and of society.

7. *Margin Notes:* **Special pedagogical tools:** An array of pedagogical tools throughout the book helps students process and retain the material, appreciate subtle clinical issues, and apply critical thinking. For example, almost every page of the book features *margin notes* that contain important clinical and research points as well as other food for thought, each introduced at precisely the right moment. Similarly, each case is accompanied by numerous review questions for the reader to answer.

8. *"You Decide":* **Interactive reading and applications:** Three cases in the book, each entitled "You Decide," are presented without diagnosis or treatment so that readers can be challenged to identify the disorder on display, make a diagnosis, suggest appropriate therapies, and consider provocative questions. By taking the perspective of the therapist, readers learn to think actively about the cases and apply their clinical knowledge and insights. These special cases are each followed by a corresponding *case appendix* that reveals the probable diagnosis for the individual in the case, common treatment approaches, and important clinical information about the disorder under examination.

9. **Diagnostic checklists:** Each case is accompanied by a checklist of diagnostic criteria for arriving at the diagnosis in question. The checklists are based on information from DSM-5-TR.

10. **Fully up-to-date material and references:** The theories and treatment approaches that are described reflect the most current writings and research literature. Similarly, the third edition's numerous margin notes are fully up to date.

11. **Modern-day focus:** We live in a world of new and unique challenges—marked by ever-growing digital innovations, important social changes, once-unthinkable

medical challenges, unsettling societal events, profound pressures (especially on underprivileged persons), and more. To set an accurate context for our cases and help the cases "speak" to readers and their experiences, we have consistently incorporated *today's* world into the case book.

12. **Real clinical material:** The cases presented in this book are based on real cases, as are the treatments and outcomes. They are taken from our own clinical experiences and from those of respected colleagues who have shared their clinical cases with us.

13. **Readability and compassion:** We have worked diligently throughout this book to bring clinical matters to life and ensure that readers walk away with the same feelings of deep concern, passion, fascination, wonder, and even frustration that we experience in our work every day. It is our fervent hope that the cases in this edition, like those in the earlier editions, will inspire empathy for clients, their relatives, their friends, and their therapists.

A number of people helped to bring this project to fruition. We are particularly indebted to the remarkable Zach Rosenthal of Duke University, whose expertise, insights, creativity, and writing skills are on display throughout every page of this new edition. From Zach's superb work helping to update and modernize every case in the book to his development of several new cases, we simply could not have achieved an edition of this quality without him. We are also grateful to Danae Hudson and Brooke Whisenhunt, each of Missouri State University, for their outstanding contributions to the second edition of the book—work that continues to permeate this new edition.

Finally, we are indebted to the extraordinary people at Worth Publishers, whose talents and commitment to the education of readers were on display at every turn in this edition of *Case Studies in Abnormal Psychology*. The list of such people is a long one, but let us mention two individuals in particular. First and foremost is Nick Rizzuti, associate developmental editor, who so very skillfully and caringly guided this project—step by step by step—to its successful outcome. We are certain that many more wonderful publishing achievements lie ahead for Nick. In addition, there is Dan DeBonis, executive program manager, whose special mixture of energy, vision, charm, and know-how is a regular treat and a constant formula for publishing success. Nick, Dan, and all the other professionals at Worth have been wonderful, and we deeply appreciate their invaluable contributions.

Ethan E. Gorenstein
Ronald J. Comer
March 2022

CASE 1

Panic Disorder

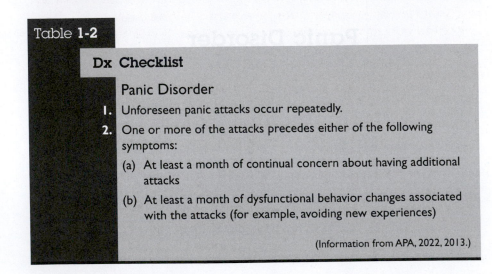

Table 1-1

Dx Checklist

Panic Attack

1. Persons experience a sudden outburst of profound fear or discomfort that rises and peaks within minutes.

2. The attack includes at least four of the following:

    (a) Increased heart rate or palpitations

    (b) Perspiration

    (c) Trembling

    (d) Shortness of breath

    (e) Choking sensations

    (f) Discomfort or pain in the chest

    (g) Nausea or other abdominal upset

    (h) Dizziness or lightheadedness

    (i) Feeling significantly chilled or hot

    (j) Sensations of tingling or numbness

    (k) Sense of unreality or separation from the self or others

    (l) Dread of losing control

    (m) Dread of dying

(Information from APA, 2022, 2013.)

Table 1-2

Dx Checklist

Panic Disorder

1. Unforeseen panic attacks occur repeatedly.

2. One or more of the attacks precedes either of the following symptoms:

    (a) At least a month of continual concern about having additional attacks

    (b) At least a month of dysfunctional behavior changes associated with the attacks (for example, avoiding new experiences)

(Information from APA, 2022, 2013.)

Table 1-3

Dx Checklist

Agoraphobia

1. Pronounced, disproportionate, and repeated fear about being in at least two of the following situations: • Public transportation (e.g., auto or plane travel) • Parking lots, bridges, or other open spaces • Shops, theaters, or other confined places • Lines or crowds • Away from home unaccompanied.

2. Fear of such agoraphobic situations derives from a concern that it would be hard to escape or get help if panic, embarrassment, or disabling symptoms were to occur.

3. Avoidance of the agoraphobic situations

4. Symptoms usually continue for at least 6 months.

5. Significant distress or impairment.

(Information from APA, 2022, 2013.)

José was alone waiting to be checked in to the emergency room, fearing he was having a heart attack. He closed his eyes, inhaling and exhaling, desperate for an impossibly deliberate rhythm. He tried to remember what his therapist had told him about how to cope with panic attacks. But it was hard to do. His mind raced. He couldn't focus. Every time he tried to recall the techniques he had learned—the questions to ask himself, the way to pace his breath—his mind returned to the same terrifying place. What if this is it? What if I am dying?

José had worked hard to build a prosperous life for himself and his family. He had come to the United States from Mexico with his parents when he was 4 years old. His father was a heavy machinery mechanic. For years, he watched his father come home fatigued and sore from back breaking work 6 days a week. Indeed, he was quite preoccupied with worries about his father's health. He hated seeing him so tired all the time, and he felt sorrow for the pain his father felt. But mostly, he worried that his father would not come home one day: a welding accident could cause an explosion; he could be electrocuted fixing a circuit; someone could turn on a mixer without warning while he was inside it, 2-ton steel blades slicing him into pieces. Any of these things could happen, he told himself.

José's mother raised him and his siblings to be devout Catholics deeply committed to their faith, family, and the pursuit of financial fortune. The goal, as she reminded José every time his father had to go to the doctor to be evaluated for pain or another injury, was to get a formal education and earn enough money to

Panic disorder is at least twice as common among women as men.

have a good, salaried job, one with insurance and retirement benefits—one that would allow José to be home at nights and weekends with his own family.

Motivated by his mother's teachings and wanting to make his parents' sacrifices worthwhile, José was a diligent student. He graduated from high school with a 3.0 grade point average and a strong work ethic. He enlisted in the Navy and, to no one's surprise, trained as a mechanic on heavy machines. He served for the minimum number of years, seeing no tours of duty and spending endless days and nights underwater on training missions and simulations. Although he made friends easily and there were other Mexican Americans around him, José never felt totally comfortable in the Navy. This was a familiar feeling. In elementary school José was always picked last for sports teams (except for soccer, of course). In middle and high school his closest friends became more and more homogenously Hispanic. They seemed to understand him better, and he felt more natural with them. When he entered the Navy, he was anxious to be included, anxious about not being the only one with brown skin. When he was in basic training and saw how many others around him were Black, Hispanic, or biracial, he was relieved. But over time his relief gave way to the unease and resentment that followed the racial and ethnic slurs, the jabs and the jokes about being a Mexican. Later, he would look back and recognize that he experienced a steady stream of what are now called microaggressions: subtle things people would say or do, or sometimes not say or not do, and ways he was singled out or treated slightly differently, all of which could reasonably be attributed to his being Mexican American.

José had never used illegal drugs. He was adamantly against it. In high school he drank beer a couple of times but never did any of the heavy binge drinking he knew some of the kids were doing. He did like the way alcohol made him feel. It calmed him a bit and made him feel more comfortable, more loose, and less worried. But he never liked the taste of beer. Later, during his time in the Navy, he took a liking to bourbon and Coke. This became his go-to drink for a night on the town with his Navy buddies or friends from work, and he started keeping a bottle of bourbon in his house. He found the occasional drink would help him wind down before bed.

After his service in the Navy, José enrolled in school to become an engineer. He was eager to learn, disciplined, and dating a young woman named Tita who would later become his wife. School came somewhat easy for José, and after several years he had a 3.6 GPA, a well-paying job at a large manufacturing company, and a clear vision for his future. He would marry Tita soon after graduating college and starting his first full-time gig as an engineer. The pay was good, Tita was newly employed and earning even more than José, and they were ready to begin having children and looking for a home to buy. It was all coming together.

Now, at age 36, José and Tita had two young children and a house they owned in a middle-class suburb. José worked as a mechanical engineer, and his wife was a

---

Microaggressions are commonly experienced by individuals in ethnic, racial, and sexual minority populations. Although studies using cross-sectional approaches have found correlations between microaggressions and adverse mental health outcomes, the long-term effects of microaggressions have not been well studied (Lilienfeld, 2017).

labor and delivery nurse. They went to church every week and took their kids to gymnastics and baseball practice. In the evenings the kids played in the cul-de-sac with their neighborhood friends, while José and his wife nervously talked to the neighbors about this and that mundane topic, all the time with one set of eyes vigilant to make sure none of the children got hurt (José was terrified that they could be run over by one of the delivery vans that darted through their narrow suburban streets). They even had a new dog, a designer mutt called a Labradoodle, and, yes, they had a picket fence too. Ironically, this symbol of suburban prosperity was also a source of distress for José: The gate squeaked when the westerly winds blew and, like flipping a light switch, this squeaking would set José worrying that someone was breaking into his house. No one ever did, but this did not stop his brain from sounding the alarm bells each time. He was an extremely intelligent person, but his brain never seemed to learn that the squeaking shrill sounds were never followed by anything other than those westerly winds. He knew this logically, but he nevertheless couldn't turn his brain's threat detection system off. After all, he had so much to lose, so much he had worked for, and although he never would talk about it, José worried that it could all go away quickly. Intruders, a fire, tornadoes, losing their jobs, whatever it could be, José knew that it could all be gone one day.

He often thought about his high school girlfriend, whom he had admired for her intelligence and drive. She had dreamed of becoming a teacher, and between her straight A's, her love of reading, and her ability to explain complicated things quickly and gracefully, José was certain she would achieve her goals. But one day, home from college, she was tragically killed in a car accident caused by a careless driver, a life of great purpose and meaning lost because of a random event completely beyond her control.

José was devastated when he heard from his friends what happened. He couldn't believe it. She was supposed to have the life she dreamed of. There was never any doubt she would. Yet, in an unlucky instant, she was gone. José vowed to let this motivate him to succeed. He swore to work hard and appreciate everything he had. He kept a picture of her in his home to remind himself to have gratitude each day. Indeed, he was lucky. He was aware that life could have turned out much differently for him, and he often told himself as much to try to feel better.

José had never been depressed. He was more of a worrier. If it wasn't one thing it was another. Kids, marriage, work, the usual life stressors for someone his age. But mostly, José worried that everything he and his family had worked so hard to have could be taken from him in a flash. José thought he *should* feel happy most days, so why was he always feeling so worried? Why did he have moments when he would suddenly become overwhelmed with anxiety? Why did his body sometimes, out of the blue, begin to sweat profusely, his face becoming red, his breath shallow and quick? He feared he would have a heart attack, that everything he had would be taken from him, as it had been from his high school girlfriend. What *was* wrong with him?

José The Attack

José and Tita were returning home from a trip to Miami when he had his first panic attack. After their plane took off from the Miami airport and José settled back in his seat, he noticed that it was getting difficult to breathe. It felt as if all the air had been sucked out of the plane. As José's breathing became increasingly labored, he began staring at the plane's sealed door, contemplating the fresh air on the other side. Then, suddenly, he had another thought, which frightened him. He wondered if he might feel so deprived of oxygen that he would be tempted to make a mad dash for the door and open it in midflight. He struggled to banish this vision from his brain, but soon he became aware of his heart racing furiously. The pounding became almost unbearable. He could feel every beat. The beating grew so strong that he thought he could actually hear it.

José looked over at his wife, Tita, in the seat next to his. She was peacefully immersed in a magazine, oblivious to his condition. He stared at her, wondering what he must look like in such a state. Tita glanced up for a moment, gave José a tender and loving smile, like she had so many times before, and then went back to her reading. She obviously didn't have a clue as to what he was going through. José felt as if he were about to die or lose his mind—he couldn't tell which at this point—and she continued reading as if nothing were happening. Finally José had to say something. Leaning in close to her ear so one else could hear him, he asked Tita if the air in the plane felt hot and stuffy to her. She didn't think so but suggested that her husband open the valve overhead if he felt uncomfortable. He did so but felt only slightly better.

The rest of the plane ride was sheer torture. José spent the entire time trying to escape from the panicky sensations inside him. He tried to get the cool air to flow directly onto his face from the valve above. He tried to distract himself with the in-flight magazine, but, seeing an ad for America's Best Heart Doctors, all he could focus on was the beating of his heart. It was maddening. Nothing worked. As soon as the flight attendant brought the beverage cart to his aisle, he ordered a bourbon and Coke. No bourbon, she told him. But they did have rum. He ordered two bottles of rum and two Cokes. She returned with his drinks, and quickly, while Tita was not looking, he drank the first bottle like it was a shot. He breathed in and out, then poured the next one into a cup half-filled with Coke. He drank the second one quickly and started to feel a bit better. Although he kept wondering whether something terribly bad had happened to him, and he felt embarrassed about it all, he realized that the worst was behind him. Whatever had kick-started his heart had passed. The plane would soon be landing and he knew he would

<aside>Panic disorder usually begins between late adolescence and early adulthood (APA, 2022, 2013; ADAA, 2020; NIMH, 2020a).</aside>

be able to get some fresh air. When the plane ended its taxiing to the jetway and the passengers were finally permitted to disembark, José couldn't get to the door fast enough. As he emerged from the plane, he felt released from a horrible confinement.

After arriving home, José felt better. He was still shaky, but he said nothing to Tita, who had been safely asleep and unaware of what had happened when he drank his way through the first panic attack of his life. José slept well that night, and by the next morning felt like his old self. He decided to put the whole episode behind him.

José continued to feel fine for the next few days. Then one night he awoke at 2:00 A.M. in a cold sweat. His heart felt as though it were about to leap out of his chest; his lungs seemed incapable of drawing any oxygen from the air. His first thought was to open the bedroom window to make it easier for him to breathe. But as José got out of bed, he suddenly drew back in alarm. He recalled the airplane door and what had seemed like an almost uncontrollable urge to force it open in midflight. He wondered if this meant he had an unconscious desire to attempt suicide. José concluded he should stay away from the window. Instead, he sat motionless on the edge of the bed while his thoughts raced along with his heart toward some unreachable finish line. He was frightened and confused. What was going on? Was he experiencing the same thing that had terrified him on the plane, but now it was happening in his house? The commotion he made was enough to awaken Tita. She asked him what was wrong, and he told her his physical symptoms: He couldn't breathe, and his heart was pounding so hard that his chest ached painfully. Tita immediately concluded that her husband was having a heart attack and called an ambulance.

> Many people (and their physicians) mistake their first panic attack for a general medical problem.

The paramedics arrived, administered oxygen, and rushed him to the emergency room. By the time the patient got there, however, he was feeling much better. A cardiologist examined him, performed a battery of tests, and eventually informed José that he had not had a heart attack. In fact, there was nothing obviously wrong with him. The doctor told him he could go home, that the episodes were probably "just anxiety attacks."

José felt relieved that his heart seemed to be okay but was confused as to exactly what was wrong with him. He wanted nothing more than to forget the whole matter. However, as time passed, that became increasingly difficult. In fact, over the course of the next few weeks, he had two more attacks in the middle of the night. In both cases, he just lay in bed motionless, praying that the symptoms would go away.

Then there was a new development. One morning, José was walking down a busy street in his neighborhood, on a routine trip to the store, when he was overcome by the same symptoms he had previously had at night. Out of the blue, his heart started pounding, his breathing became labored, and he felt dizzy; also, he couldn't stop trembling. He looked around for a safe haven—a store or restaurant where he could sit down—but he felt as if he were in a kind of dream world. Everything around him—the people, the traffic, the stores—seemed unreal. He felt bombarded by sights and sounds and found it impossible to focus on anything. The overwhelmed man then recalled the cardiologist's mention of the term *anxiety attack* and came to the sickening realization that the doctor must have detected that he had mental problems. José feared that he was on the verge of a nervous breakdown.

He was several blocks from home but discovered, to his relief, that he could make his way back to the house with less difficulty than he anticipated. Once inside, José sat down on the living room sofa and closed his eyes. He felt certain he was losing his mind; it was just a matter of time before the next attack sent him off the deep end. As he became caught up in his private terror, he heard a sound at the front door. It was Tita returning home from work.

Once again, Tita appeared to have no inkling that anything was amiss. She cheerfully related the details of her day: the way her coworkers argued, the new protocols being bandied about by her supervisor, and so on. José could barely follow what she was saying, further proof, in his mind, that he was rapidly losing his grip. Finally, his wife suggested that they go out for a walk. At this, he realized that the very thought of leaving the house was terrifying to him. What if he had an attack in the middle of the street and could no longer function, physically or mentally? He felt as if he had a time bomb inside him. In response to her suggestion, he simply broke down in tears.

She begged her husband to tell her what was wrong. José confessed that he had just had another one of his attacks, this time on the way to the store, and that this one was so bad he was forced to return home. Now he dreaded going outside. He asked her if she could get him something to drink, perhaps some water.

Tita could see that José was extremely upset, but at the same time she was puzzled. There didn't seem to be anything wrong with him. He was in no obvious physical pain, and he appeared vigorous and alert. She poured him a glass of cold water and insisted they talk to their priest and he call his mother. She also suggested he make an appointment with his primary care physician. They needed to understand why he was having these nervous attacks.

In the week before the appointment, José made a few tentative forays around the neighborhood with Tita and their dog, Rocky. He felt some symptoms while outside but did not have as intense an attack as he had that one time when he was alone. His nighttime episodes increased in frequency, however—to the point that he could count on waking up with an attack almost every time he went to bed.

The Primary Care Doctor with a New Reality

At the doctor's office, José recounted his repeated attacks of racing heart, breathlessness, and tremulousness. He didn't know quite how to describe his fear of losing his mind, nor did he really want to, so he left that part out. He did convey, however, that he had now become so apprehensive about the attacks that he was reluctant to venture outside for fear of being overwhelmed. In describing his symptoms, José noticed that he was actually starting to have some of them.

As he continued, his doctor became increasingly confident that the patient had panic disorder. The doctor marveled to himself at how far medicine had come since he started practicing. Years ago, a patient like José would have been hospitalized for weeks with a suspected heart problem and subjected to dozens of tests. If no major disease turned up, he would be released, but even then the suspicion would linger that he was on the verge of a major cardiac problem, and the patient would be advised to cut back on his activities and keep on the lookout for further symptoms. Far from being reassured, the person would feel like a ticking time bomb.

Now physicians were aware of the power of panic attacks and of how their symptoms mimicked those of a heart attack. As soon as cardiac and other physical conditions were ruled out, practitioners usually turned their attention to the possibility of panic attacks. Indeed, José's was the fourth case of probable panic disorder that the doctor had seen this month alone. Even more gratifying, effective treatments for panic disorder were available, with many patients benefiting from cognitive and behavioral interventions, and these approaches had been adapted culturally for work with Hispanic individuals (Bernal et al., 2018). Now he could offer patients two forms of good news: first, that their heart was fine; and second, that their condition was fully treatable.

After examining José, the doctor informed him that other than a slightly elevated heart rate, everything seemed normal. He told his patient that his symptoms were by no means imaginary; rather, he had a well-known condition known as panic disorder. The doctor also asked José about drug and alcohol use. José proudly declared that he had never used drugs before. He also acknowledged that maybe he drank more alcohol than he should, but that things had been stressful lately. When pressed, José admitted to drinking one drink per day, on average. The doctor didn't seem too worried, but José knew that he was not exactly telling the whole truth. The truth was that José *used* to drink one drink per day, but that was a long time ago. Since starting his job after college, José had gradually started to drink more like one to two drinks per day, typically at night, after Tita went up to get ready for sleep. He had also gone out with his old Navy buddies a couple of times in the past year and had a lot to drink. But these were always for good reasons, he figured. When his friend Pete turned 35, they bar hopped all night long.

Around 3% of people in the United States have panic disorder in a given year; 5% develop the disorder at some point in their lives (ADAA, 2020; NIMH, 2020a; Roy-Byrne, 2020).

Today's physicians must also be careful to consider possible medical explanations before making a diagnosis of panic disorder. Certain medical problems, such as thyroid disease, seizure disorders, cardiac arrhythmias, and mitral valve prolapse (a cardiac malfunction marked by periodic episodes of palpitations) can cause panic attacks. Medical tests can rule out such causes.

When it was his own birthday, he and the guys celebrated hard, a night he hardly remembers from all the boozing. So when the doctor asked him about his alcohol use, he knew he was only telling a half-truth about how much he drank. Still, the doctor didn't say much about it and moved on to other questions. At the end of the appointment, the doctor referred José to Louisa Villanueva, LCSW, a clinical social worker in a nearby community agency that specialized in working with Hispanic patients and immigrants with behavioral health problems.

José was encouraged by his doctor. He left the clinic believing he could be helped, but he felt uncomfortable about meeting with the social worker. He had never seen any kind of mental health professional for anything in his life. He worried that this meant he was going to be viewed by the social worker, and maybe others, as someone who was crazy, insane, or had some kind of disease. Although reassured that his heart was healthy, this newfound reality—that he would need to talk to someone about his panic attack symptoms—was making him feel embarrassed, anxious, and fearful.

When they returned home, Tita urged José to call Ms. Villanueva's clinic, but he continued to put it off for a few more days. Tita, growing increasingly impatient, said she would call herself to arrange the appointment, and José reluctantly agreed. This all was very upsetting to him, so he went to the kitchen and poured himself a rum and Coke.

José in Treatment Regaining Control over His Life

Arriving at Ms. Villanueva's office, José felt a strong combination of hope and shame. He sat in the waiting room and put his head down, pretending to look at something important in his phone, his thumb scrolling erratically over the screen. Eventually he heard Ms. Villanueva call his name, and they walked silently back to her office. She had kind eyes and a gentle demeanor, and she oriented him to the clinic policies and to the process he could expect receiving her services. José was surprised at how calm she was and how straightforward everything seemed. He wasn't sure what he expected, but it wasn't this. Her office had a desk and swiveling chair pointing toward her computer. There were pictures on the wall of photography from what could be Mexico, or maybe Cuba, or Puerto Rico. He couldn't tell. She had a bookshelf with a few pictures of children, probably her own, he thought. He sat on a comfortable but worn faux-leather chair while she sat across from him in a similar chair. It was all so ordinary. She asked him questions about what he was hoping to get out of therapy, whether he had been to therapy before, what he expected, and whether he was willing to complete home practices in between weekly clinic visits. She then began a series of questions about his mental health history and about the most recent panic attacks.

After José recounted his experiences of the past few weeks in minute and animated detail, Louisa asked him if he could recall ever having had similar attacks or sensations prior to these. Upon reflection, José realized that he had had these sensations before, during the trip to Miami. He recalled that the day after arriving in Florida he fell as he was walking down some steps toward the hotel pool. His injuries were not serious, but a cut on his arm was deep enough to require a couple of stitches. For the remainder of the vacation, José had momentary jolts of anxiety—including heart palpitations and mild dizziness—at the slightest indication of physical imbalance. He also realized now that since falling, he had been very tentative in his walking.

José tried to recall whether he had ever had similar attacks or sensations before the Florida incident. The only thing he recalled was an extremely upsetting experience from childhood. It was something that he had never discussed with anyone. It was a Sunday, and his father was home repairing a tractor in the field next to their house. José was 14 years old, and was helping his dad out, bringing tools to him from the garage. José was irritated that he had to help, but he knew this was always a good way to get to spend time with his father. He was in the garage searching for the tool for a long time. He was anxious that he would not be able to find what he was looking for, and that he would have to come back to his dad empty-handed. He decided to look behind a workbench, thinking maybe the wrench he needed had fallen behind and out of sight. When he moved the bench, he heard a shifting sound above his head, and before he could realize it a sledgehammer that had been hanging on the wall had become dislodged and fallen down, narrowly missing his head and neck as he bent over. It was a close call, and he knew it. His heart raced and his mind exploded with counterfactual thoughts about what *could have happened* if the sledgehammer had hit him. He stopped looking for the wrench, sitting down on the floor, crying uncontrollably. In that moment he felt the beating of his heart speeding rapidly. He felt his heart so palpably it was as if, like in the cartoons, his heart was literally extending his chest visibly, his tee-shirt pulsing heart-shaped protrusions. Louisa listened carefully, validated how difficult that most have been, and continued to ask additional questions.

After interviewing José and reviewing his medical reports, Louisa concluded that his condition met the DSM-5-TR criteria for a diagnosis of both panic disorder and agoraphobia. His panic attacks typically included several of the defining symptoms: breathlessness, heart palpitations, chest discomfort, tremulousness, sweating, and fear of losing control or going crazy. Moreover, he was almost constantly apprehensive about the possibility of further attacks. He was also diagnosed with agoraphobia, because he was beginning to avoid leaving the house except in Tita's company.

Louisa explained that the scientific literature on panic disorders suggested clearly that panic disorder and agoraphobia can best be explained by a combination of

According to research, people who are prone to panic attacks typically have a high degree of *anxiety sensitivity*. That is, they focus on their bodily sensations much of the time and interpret them as potentially harmful (Behenck et al., 2020). Research has shown that cognitive-behavioral therapy can decrease anxiety sensitivity, which helps lead to a decrease in symptoms of panic disorder (Craske, 2021; Morissette et al., 2020).

biological and cognitive factors. On the biological side, she outlined how panic attacks are similar to the so-called fight-or-flight response, the normal physiological arousal of humans and other animals in response to danger. The difference is that with a panic attack there is no true danger as a triggering event. From this standpoint, a panic attack can be considered a false alarm. The body produces its reaction to danger in the absence of any objectively dangerous event. People whose bodies repeatedly have such false alarms can develop panic disorder.

On the cognitive side, Louisa detailed what happens when people repeatedly *interpret* their panic attacks as something more than false alarms. They typically identify the physiological reactions as a real source of danger. They may conclude that they are suffocating or having a heart attack or stroke; or they may believe they are going crazy or out of control. Such interpretations produce still more alarm and further arousal of the sympathetic nervous system. As the nervous system becomes further aroused, the person's sense of alarm increases, and a vicious cycle unfolds in which anxious thoughts and the sympathetic nervous system feed on each other.

For many people with panic disorder, the panic experience is aggravated by hyperventilation. As part of their sympathetic nervous system arousal, they breathe more rapidly and deeply, ultimately causing a significant drop in their blood's level of carbon dioxide. This physiological change results in feelings of breathlessness, light-headedness, blurred vision, dizziness, or faintness—sensations that lead many people to conclude there is something physically or mentally wrong with them.

Even if people with panic disorder eventually come to recognize that their attacks are false alarms set off by their nervous system, they may live in a heightened state of anxiety over what their sympathetic nervous system might do. Many also develop anxieties about situations in which they feel a panic attack would be especially unwelcome (in crowds, closed spaces, airplanes, trains, or the like). Because of such anticipatory anxiety, their sympathetic nervous system becomes aroused whenever those situations are approached, and the likelihood of a panic attack in such situations is increased.

Given this integrated view of panic attacks, panic disorder, and agoraphobia, Louisa suggested a combination of cognitive and behavioral techniques, each chosen to help eliminate José's anxiety reaction to his sympathetic nervous system arousal. The cognitive techniques were designed to change his faulty interpretations of sympathetic arousal. The behavioral component of treatment involved repeated exposure to both internal (bodily sensations) and external triggers of the person's panic attacks.

Before they moved forward, Louisa asked José about alcohol use, noting that it is common for people with panic disorder and agoraphobia to use alcohol as a way to reduce physiological arousal, to cope with the anxiety or self-medicate. He told her sheepishly that he drank one to two drinks per day on average, and that

> The *fight-or-flight response* is so named because it prepares an organism to cope with a dangerous predicament either by fighting or fleeing. It primes the organism for a rapid use of energy by increasing heart rate, breathing rate, perspiration, blood flow to large muscles, and mental alertness.

> Panic disorder is similar to a phobia. However, rather than fearing an external object or situation, those with panic disorder come to distrust and fear the power and arousal of their own autonomic nervous system.

he drank more when he was worried about having a panic attack. She asked about his use over the past year. Looking at the photographs in her office, he responded by asking her to share more about herself. She acknowledged that it is important for him to trust her, and she would be happy to tell him more about her background. Louisa described her own family background and upbringing as a Latina in a predominantly white community. She told him about her favorite panaderia and the nearest place to get authentic food from her cultural background. She also talked about her intersecting identities as a cisgender, Latina woman from an immigrant family. It didn't take long, but learning this information about her helped him feel at ease. Believing he could trust Louisa, he recounted several times in the past year when he was so drunk that he blacked out, and a few other times when he drank more than he wanted to, had a hard time stopping drinking, and drank while driving. She went on to explain that alcohol is a central nervous system depressant, and that it has the effect of both calming and disinhibiting people, a natural recipe needed for those who are highly anxious and having panic attacks. Negative reinforcement, she further told him, is a process wherein the probability of a behavior, in this case drinking, will increase over time when the behavior functions to reduce an aversive state, like anxiety. And so in a way it made sense that he was drinking more and more as his anxiety and panic symptoms were increasing.

She diagnosed him with substance use disorder (alcohol), moderate, and told him they would incorporate this into their treatment plan. For starters, he would need to reduce his drinking to no more than one drink per day and would not be permitted to drink any alcohol when practicing the therapy home practice. They would monitor his alcohol use, and with his permission she would communicate back to his primary care doctor the need for ongoing monitoring of alcohol use and further consideration of higher level treatment, such as medications or more intensive outpatient therapy. As the evaluation visit with Louisa ended, she summarized the diagnostic impressions and outlined the basic steps for his treatment plan. José had received three psychiatric diagnoses and was oriented to the use of evidence-based cognitive-behavioral interventions for panic disorder and agoraphobia.

Session 1   To begin treatment, Louisa showed José a list of typical symptoms associated with panic attacks, including the mental symptoms "sense of unreality" and "fear of going crazy or losing control." She asked him which symptoms he had personally had. José was astonished to see his most feared symptoms actually listed on paper, and he seized the opportunity to discuss them openly at long last.

She explained to José that fears of going crazy were common among panic sufferers; indeed, many people found them to be the most disturbing aspect of the disorder. She emphasized, however, that the fear of losing one's mind on account of the panic disorder, although common, was completely unfounded. There was no

> Alcohol use disorder commonly co-occurs with anxiety disorders in general, and panic disorder specifically (Capasso et al., 2021; Smith & Randall, 2012).

> At least two-thirds of those who receive cognitive-behavioral treatment for their panic disorder fully overcome their disorder (Craske, 2021; Morissette et al., 2020).

chance of José going insane. Although visibly relieved to hear this, he wondered aloud why it seemed as if he were coming apart mentally.

The social worker gave him a quick sketch of the workings of the autonomic nervous system and the fight-or-flight response. She explained that José's symptoms could be due to extreme arousal of his central nervous system, a useful feature in an actual emergency but confusing when there is no concrete danger. This hyperarousal, she indicated, made it hard—but not impossible—for José to focus his thoughts, leading to the feeling of being out of control, disoriented, and fearful. As for his thoughts about rushing for the door of the airplane when he had the panic attack on the way home from Miami, Louisa emphasized that these were simply ideas: fleeting thoughts associated with the fight-or-flight response, but not actions that he was ever close to carrying out. Increasingly, José seemed ready to entertain the possibility that his condition was not as dire as he originally believed.

Louisa further detailed with some granularity the steps that would be taken to treat his panic disorder and the rationale behind them. There would be four basic components of treatment: (1) training in relaxation and breathing techniques, (2) changing his cognitive misinterpretations of panic sensations, (3) repeated exposure to sensations of panic under controlled conditions, and (4) repeated practice in situations that José was avoiding or apprehensive about. For the coming week though, he was instructed only to monitor his anxiety and panic attacks, as well as his alcohol use.

Session 2   At the next session, the social worker reviewed the records José had kept during the week. He reported drinking only one drink per day at most, and only on four days of the week. She validated his successful reduction of alcohol use. He explained his motivation to change was based on his desire to have a successful family and marriage, and to not lose everything he had always wanted in his life as an immigrant. She encouraged him to keep being aware of these goals and reasons to change when he considers pouring himself a drink. He agreed and felt proud. In addition, it turned out that he had not had any panic attacks during the day since the last appointment. However, he was still avoiding going out except with Tita, and he was waking up almost every night with breathlessness, palpitations, a feeling of unreality, and fear of losing control. Louisa asked José what he did when these symptoms occurred, and he explained that he simply lay in bed, fervently hoping that the symptoms would subside. To help him recognize some of his cognitive misinterpretations and to begin changing them, Louisa had the following exchange with José:

Louisa:	You said that when you got those attacks in the middle of night, you just lay in bed. Why is that?
José:	Well, it could be dangerous if I got up.
Louisa:	Why would it be dangerous?

Panic disorder can also be treated by medications that lower the arousal of a person's sympathetic nervous system. At least two-thirds of those who receive certain antidepressant drugs (i.e., selective serotonin reuptake inhibitors) or certain antianxiety drugs (i.e., benzodiazepines) experience considerable improvement (Baldwin & Huneke, 2020; Roy-Byrne, 2020). Selective serotonin reuptake inhibitors are now the first line of defense, and regular use of benzodiazepines is typically discouraged because of the risks associated with their chronic use (Kriegel & Azrak, 2020).

José: I might have a heart attack, or something else serious might happen.

Louisa: What did the cardiologist say about your heart?

José: He said it was fine; all the tests were normal. But my heart is pounding so hard, and it's so hard to breathe, I can't think of any other explanation.

Louisa: Let's review what we discussed last time about the physiology of panic attacks and why people get certain symptoms with these attacks.

Louisa described in greater detail the fight-or-flight response, the physiological changes it produces in various organ systems, and the role of hyperventilation. In addition, she gave José a written summary of this material for him to study at his leisure. She explained that the most important conclusion to be drawn from this material was that his panic attacks, although extremely unpleasant, were ultimately harmless to both his physical and his mental well-being. Then she resumed the discussion with José about his nightly panic attacks.

> Very close biological relatives of people with panic disorder (for example identical twins) are up to six times more likely than the general population to develop the disorder.

Louisa: In light of what we just discussed, how might you respond differently to the attacks you're getting at night?

José: Well, according to what you say, there would be no danger in my getting up. After all, the cardiologist did say my heart was fine. But I wonder if I might keel over just from the panic attack.

Louisa: What has happened on other occasions when you had panic attacks and were sitting or standing up?

José: I certainly never keeled over. In fact, when I had the big one out in the street, I even managed to walk several blocks to get back home.

Louisa: So it seems that your fear of keeling over might be unfounded. Do you think you would prefer to get up for a while when you wake up with an attack, rather than lie in bed?

José: I suppose it would make more sense. When I have trouble falling asleep under normal conditions I certainly don't just lie in bed doing nothing. I usually get up and putter around or do a little paperwork at my desk.

Louisa: From now on, why don't you try getting up when you awaken with a panic attack and do the things you would normally do. We'll discuss how this works out next time.

In the remainder of the session, Louisa had José carry out a standard progressive muscle relaxation exercise. Under her direction, he alternately tensed and relaxed various muscle groups, with the goal of achieving complete relaxation in all muscle groups by the end of a 20-minute training session. This widely used exercise teaches patients to recognize excess muscle tension and to relax the tension at will. Louisa felt that José could benefit from the relaxed feelings that the exercise produces and that the relaxation training might also lay the groundwork for an additional exercise in breathing control.

The breathing control exercise trains clients both to prevent hyperventilation and to cope effectively when hyperventilation occurs. For this exercise, patients practice breathing using the diaphragm as opposed to the chest. Use of the chest is discouraged because it fosters pressured breathing, promotes hyperventilation, and can produce chest pain or discomfort when employed regularly. With diaphragm breathing (the so-called natural way to breathe), the chest is almost immobile; only the abdomen moves, ballooning out as the person inhales and collapsing as the person exhales. Use of the diaphragm promotes slow, unpressured breathing of the sort necessary to prevent or counteract hyperventilation.

Louisa recommended an app that José could put on his phone or tablet that had progressive muscle relaxation and breathing control exercises. He was to practice his relaxation and breathing once a day and record his level of physical and mental stress before and after his practice session.

Session 3　José and Louisa again reviewed the records he kept during the preceding week. As advised, José had continued to reduce his alcohol use and also changed his response during the nightly panic attacks. Rather than lying in bed, he got up and did minor chores, reminding himself as he did so that the sensations he was experiencing were not dangerous. After following this practice every night, José noted that the nightly attacks were getting shorter; one attack subsided after only 5 minutes, as opposed to the 20 minutes or so that the attacks used to last.

Louisa took this result as an opportunity to point out the cognitive component of panic, specifically how overestimating the danger of panic sensations fuels the attacks, whereas assessing the sensations realistically allows the sensations to subside. José's more realistic mind-set about the nightly attacks this past week had resulted in shorter and less intense attacks by the end of the week.

Session 4　When José returned the following week, he reported that he still was waking every night with his panic symptoms; but as instructed, he was trying to appraise the sensations realistically and function normally, regardless. As a result, the symptoms seemed to be getting weaker and not lasting as long; in most cases now, it was only a matter of minutes before they subsided, aided, he felt, by his use of slow diaphragm breathing. Still, he was leery of venturing outside on his own.

Louisa gave José several instructions for the coming week. First, he was to continue with his current strategy for handling the nightly attacks and to continue practicing the diaphragm breathing exercise daily. In addition, he was to venture out of his safe, familiar house and work settings at least three times on his own, if only to walk to the end of the block and back. If he had any panic sensations, he was to handle them as he did the nightly sensations: breathe slowly and with his diaphragm, appraise the sensations rationally, and behave normally. In addition, he continued to report that his drinking was infrequent and, when it occurred, was not interfering with his cognitive-behavioral therapy home practices.

Panic disorder frequently precedes the onset of agoraphobia. That is, after experiencing multiple unpredictable panic attacks, persons become increasingly fearful of having new attacks while in public places. According to DSM-5-TR, agoraphobia is diagnosed separately.

Session 5 José reported that he had slept through the night three times this week, and on the nights when he was awakened, his symptoms had subsided within a few minutes. As instructed, he had gone out three times to the end of his block and back. In so doing, he had typical panic symptoms: heart palpitations, breathlessness, light-headedness, and unreality. The first time he did this exercise, José felt so fearful he almost returned home before completing it. However, he followed the psychologist's instruction to complete the assignment regardless of any symptoms. The second and third times, José also had symptoms but was better prepared for them and carried out the assignment without any thoughts of abandoning it.

Next, Louisa proceeded with the interoceptive exposure exercises—repeated exposures to panic sensations under controlled conditions. She explained that he would do several exercises designed to produce sensations similar to those arising from autonomic arousal and that therefore might trigger panic symptoms. The goal was to progressively extinguish his anxiety reactions to these sensations, to give him opportunities to practice more accurate cognitive appraisals of such sensations, and to help him develop behavioral coping skills. The specific exercises that were carried out are listed in Table 1-4.

After each exercise, José reported his specific physical symptoms and rated the symptoms with respect to (a) intensity, (b) resemblance to panic, and (c) level

> Procedures that are used by researchers or therapists to induce hyperventilation or other panic sensations are called *biological challenge tests.*

Table 1-4	Interoceptive Exposure Exercises and Individual Reactions*			
Activity	Duration (seconds)	Intensity of Symptoms	Resemblance to Panic	Anxiety Level
1. Whole body tension	60	3	0	0
2. Breathe through straw	120	1	0	0
3. Shake head from side to side	30	6	1	1
4. Place head between legs and then lift	30	3	2	2
5. Stare at spot on wall	90	2	2	0
6. Hold breath	30	5	5	3
7. Run in place	60	6	6	4
8. Hyperventilate	60	7	7	5

*José's ratings on a 0–10 scale. Exercises were derived from Craske, Wolitsky-Taylor, & Barlow, 2021; Craske & Barlow, 1993.

of anxiety provoked. Louisa instructed José to practice the mildest of the three panic-producing exercises—holding his breath for 30 seconds—three times a day in the coming week. In addition, he was asked to continue taking short trips on his own, this week to a nearby store at least three times.

Sessions 6 to 9   José continued to progress over the next few weeks. By now his alcohol use was no longer seeming to be a significant concern. He had moved the bourbon and rum to a different part of the house, and, at Louisa's suggestion, had placed a sticky note on the bottle of alcohol with a note to remind himself why he was not drinking as much as he used to—*"family, friends, work, live the dream!"* By session 9, he was carrying out on a daily basis three interoceptive exposure exercises—shaking his head from side to side for 30 seconds, staring at a spot on the wall for 90 seconds, and hyperventilating for 60 seconds—and getting minimal panic effects. In addition, his nightly awakenings were becoming infrequent, and he was traveling farther and farther from home without Tita. For session 9, he traveled to see Louisa alone without Tita for the first time. Although José arrived at that session with stronger panic sensations than he had had in weeks, he simply mentioned his symptoms to Louisa and proceeded to describe the other details of his week as if the symptoms themselves were a minor annoyance. Within a few minutes, they subsided.

José's instructions for the coming week were to continue practicing the interoceptive exposure exercises three times a day, and to travel freely, without allowing fear of a panic attack to restrict his behavior. The next session was scheduled for 2 weeks away.

Session 10   José reported that he had been panic-free for the entire 2 weeks. In addition, he was going wherever he needed to go on his own and without apprehension. He continued to perform the interoceptive exposure exercises, but at this stage they evoked no reaction; they mainly bored him.

Now he had a new concern. Tita was determined that they take a trip back to Miami in the next couple of months. They would have to fly, of course, and the idea revived painful memories of his experience on the plane from Florida, where his problem began. José had visions of reliving that terrible episode. Louisa outlined a program of progressive exposure over the next couple of weeks to images and situations involving airplanes. This would include multiple viewings of movies involving airplanes and trips to the airport twice each week.

Sessions 11 and 12   When José returned 2 weeks later for session 11, he had spent the intervening time immersing himself in airplane-related images and situations. As anticipated, initially he was anxious while watching the airplane movies, but by the second week he was watching them without emotional reaction; he and Tita had also made it out to the airport three times, and each time José felt more at ease. Two weeks later, José and Louisa met for the last time before the trip to Miami. At this meeting, he was panic free but still apprehensive about the trip. His parting words were, "I'll see you in a month—if I survive." On the way home from the appointment, he thought about the trip ahead and how he would be tested. He realized he had not eaten in a long time, and he started to feel dizzy. The traffic was stop-and-go, and José began feeling that familiar feeling in his chest. He had made so much progress, but what was happening? His breathing picked up, and his hands started to sweat. Then his mind leapt off the starting block and into a frenetic pace around and around. What if this wasn't a panic attack? This felt different, like maybe how heart attacks might feel. He decided to drive straight to the emergency room. As he waited to be checked in, he tried as hard he could to summon all of the knowledge about panic attacks he had learned from Louisa. He recalled in bits and pieces what she had taught him. He remembered the breathing exercises and the cognitive strategies she helped him learn to do. He closed his eyes to get focused, and practiced these cognitive and behavioral coping skills as best as he could—imperfectly, he knew, but as he sat there and worked to reduce his arousal, to restructure his thinking, and to remind himself about the probability that this was a heart attack he heard his name being called. Looking up, he saw the emergency room staff asking him to check in. He stared at her, kept his focus, then closed his eyes again, this time breathing in a bit more deeply. He was regaining composure, though slowly. He ignored the staff member when she called his name again. He knew in that moment he was not having a heart attack. He knew it was a panic attack, and he came to the conclusion that he was capable of coping with panic attacks, even when least expected. José finally stood up, looked around, and told himself he would never need to return to the emergency room again for panic attacks. He had the skills to manage them himself. He knew he had just been tested on all he had learned in therapy. "Yes, and I passed," he said as he walked to his car. When he came home, he told Tita everything. They cried together, holding each other, seeing how far he had come. And then they finished making plans for their trip to Miami.

Around 60% of people with panic disorder receive treatment for it (NIMH, 2017a; Wang et al., 2005).

Epilogue The Final Conquest

José returned triumphant from his trip to Miami. Though he did feel some anxiety, he had no significant problems on the plane or anywhere else. He felt his problem was behind him now. Louisa chatted with him for a while about the trip and said she was glad that things had turned out so well. She and José reviewed the treatment program, including strategies he would follow should he have any symptoms in the future. José was feeling better—enormously better than he had for many months. Most of all, he felt that he had regained control over his life again.

Assessment Questions

1. In the case of José, what event precipitated his panic attack?

2. How is José's development of panic disorder different from that of most cases?

3. What are the symptoms of most panic attacks?

4. Why do individuals first suspect a general medical condition?

5. Why was the social worker convinced that panic disorders are "best explained by a combination of biological and cognitive factors"?

6. Describe the four steps the social worker took to help José overcome his panic attacks. List each of the interoceptive exposure exercises that were part of José's treatment.

7. How did José's avoidance of going outside by himself contribute to his panic disorder?

8. How did his pattern of previous alcohol use complicate treatment for José?

CASE 2

Obsessive-Compulsive Disorder

Table 2-1

Dx Checklist

Obsessive-Compulsive Disorder

1. Occurrence of repeated obsessions, compulsions, or both.
2. The obsessions or compulsions take up considerable time.
3. Significant distress or impairment.

(Information from APA, 2022, 2013.)

Cherita, a 31-year-old Black cisgender accountant, nervously tapped her pen on a yellow legal notepad as she stood in the hallway preparing to leave her apartment for work. She had made a list of things to do, things to check, and things to make sure would be taken care of before she could leave. The top sheet of her notepad was clean, organized, and detailed, days of the week listed with tasks each day, check marks neatly spaced to the left of completed tasks. She had done everything she needed to this morning, but she wasn't quite satisfied. The back door had been locked and double checked to be sure. The oven was off. That, too, was double checked. The closets were full of supplies in case of any emergency. It was the same checklist as each day. And, as on other days, Cherita labored hard over what she may have forgotten. *Something* could have been missed. Something important. There could be grave consequences. This possibility, infinitesimal as she knew it to be, could not be ignored. "Even if it is unlikely," she muttered to herself, "I couldn't live with myself if I overlooked something." Her catastrophic obsessions were an unwelcomed and unstoppable doomsday prepper renting space in her head. These thoughts were distressing, exhausting, and kept Cherita from getting to work on time many days. So she stood for a few minutes longer, thinking harder, searching her mind for anything, anything at all she might need to add to the list and complete before leaving for the day.

Cherita and her younger brother grew up in a comfortable middle-class environment in an ethnically diverse suburb on the east coast. Her family and community were strong, important parts of her sense of identity. As a Black woman, she felt some pressure to perform well in school and work and to conduct herself in a manner that was beyond reproach, as though the slightest misstep might increase her vulnerability to prejudice. This was more true with words than with numbers. On occasion when she might misspell or incorrectly enunciate a word, she would reflexively hold her breath and clench her stomach, waiting to be corrected. Even worse were patronizing declarations about how "articulate" she was—for someone her age, the commenter might self-consciously clarify.

Cherita had been an excellent student and was considered a model for other children to follow. By junior high school, it was apparent that she excelled in mathematics, and even at that early age she had set her sights on a career in accountancy. Her seriousness as a student continued through high school, where she described her social life as conservative. In college, where she majored in mathematics and accounting, her commitment to academics continued. She was well on her way to success, and with how easily numbers came to her, she dreamed of being a highly paid certified public accountant one day, maybe even leading her own accounting firm.

Cherita Early Worries and Odd Behaviors

Cherita had been a worrier for as long as she could remember. For example, she always seemed more concerned about safety than other people did. She recalled that in college she sometimes would check the lock on her door three or four times before she could walk away from her dormitory room. And even then, she was often left with festering doubt, as though the door still hadn't been locked properly and someone would break in because of her negligence. She dreaded the losses her roommate might sustain if there was a theft. Curiously, her own losses didn't seem to matter so much; it was more the idea of being responsible for another person's misfortune that troubled her.

Similarly, other areas of anxiety had produced some difficulties for Cherita over the years. For example, paying her bills online often posed problems. Although she always carefully checked her bills and made sure she entered the correct amount online, when it came time to click submit, she doubted that everything had been done properly. Thus, she would stare at the computer, rereading the numbers three or four times and checking the due date as well, before actually submitting the payment. After receiving her confirmation number, she always felt a sense of unease, as though something irrevocable had just taken place. Occasionally Cherita's doubts were so strong that she would have to call the company to see if it had received the payment. She explained to her friends and family that she was simply being diligent, being careful. It's the kind of thing that accountants do.

Obsessive-compulsive disorder usually begins in adolescence or early adulthood and typically persists for years, although its symptoms may fluctuate over time (Rosenberg, 2021; ADAA, 2020).

Cherita Beyond Worrying

Around 7 years ago, soon after graduating from college, Cherita's worries and excessive behaviors began to worsen. This change first occurred after Cherita was the target of an attempted sexual assault. As she was about to enter her car after seeing a movie with some friends, she was accosted from behind by an acquaintance who tried to talk her into letting him into the vehicle with her. When Cherita refused, the man tried physically to force his way in, grabbing her arm and roughly stroking her face as she turned away from him. She struggled and screamed for him to stop, and the man backed off. They didn't know each very well, but they had met before through mutual friends. He apologized, saying he had too much to drink that night and was so sorry.

She wasn't sure if she had been sexually assaulted or not, but she was very angry about what happened. He had forcibly touched her and tried to get into the car with her. What was he trying to do? What if she had let him in? What if she had not told him to stop so assertively? What *could* have happened, she wondered? As time passed, Cherita began to have increasing feelings of insecurity in public. She compulsively looked behind her as she walked to her car, even in daylight. She started to check her door lock several times before going to bed at night. Gradually this practice extended to the checking of windows, then other objects, including the oven, faucets, appliances, and anything that she could control to increase her sense of safety.

Cherita's feelings of insecurity and her accompanying checking rituals continued to increase during the next several years, to the point that they were making it impossible for her to lead a fully normal life. Mornings were a particular problem: she was finding it more and more difficult to leave and get to work. Each morning, Cherita felt compelled to perform a large number of rituals to verify that everything in the apartment was being left in a safe condition. Her biggest fear was that her negligence would cause a terrible event, such as a fire or flood, that would damage both her apartment and—more important, it seemed—her neighbors' apartments.

Cherita's ritual included checking that the stove had been turned off, the faucets turned off, and the windows closed, and that various appliances were unplugged, including the hair dryer, the microwave, her laptop, and the television, among others. Just checking all the items once would have been a chore, but Cherita typically felt compelled to check each item several times. Often, after checking one item, she would feel compelled to go back and check everything all over again.

Sometimes she would go back to check an item even having checked it seconds before. It seemed she could never be reassured completely. Sometimes she would stand and stare at an item for a full 5 minutes, hoping that this would be enough to persuade her that the item had been properly checked. However, even this was often not enough, and within a few minutes, she would find herself checking the item all over again.

On a bad morning, it could take Cherita up to 2 hours to get out of the apartment. Occasionally, after completing all of her checking behaviors and getting out of her apartment building, she was suddenly seized with doubt about a particular item—had she really checked the stove satisfactorily, or did she just think she had?—and she would have to return to her apartment to end her suspense. A few times, she missed work altogether due to this checking. More often, she was able to break away after a certain point and would arrive at work late.

Studies reveal that many people with obsessive-compulsive disorder have unusually high standards of conduct and morality that are coupled with an inflated sense of responsibility (Taylor et al., 2020; Davey, 2019).

The 12-month prevalence of OCD in the United States is 1.2%, which is similar to prevalence rates in other countries (ADAA, 2020; NIMH, 2020b).

Fortunately, she had a flexible schedule, and it didn't matter when she showed up at the office, only that she got her work done. This she was able to accomplish by staying late. Indeed, she was highly valued for her abilities and had been promoted several times since beginning work at her firm 2 years before. However, her life in the morning had become, in her mind, a "living hell."

When Cherita returned home in the evening, the urge to check would be revived; she felt compelled to make sure that all was in order before going to bed. This nighttime checking was not as severe as the morning routine, however. She was somehow able to tell herself that everything had been checked earlier that day, and if she avoided using the stove or appliances before going to bed, a less thorough inspection would suffice. The next morning, however, the urge to carry out the complete checking routine would start anew.

Cherita also had another set of symptoms, which would manifest as she was driving to work. These other symptoms had begun a while before, after she drove past a minor accident one day. Soon after passing the accident, she ran over a bump of some kind. She looked in the rearview mirror to see what she might have hit but observed nothing. After driving for another 15 minutes, Cherita was suddenly seized by the thought that she had struck another car or person. In the throes of this anxiety, she got off the highway and doubled back to where she had felt the bump. She was trying to determine if there was any evidence of an accident there—a disabled car or a body in the road—to confirm or disconfirm her fears. She discovered nothing, however, so she went on to work, still in a state of anxiety that she might have been responsible for an accident.

The next morning, similar doubts arose on the way to work, and the problem continued thereafter. Now, almost every day while driving, she would wonder if she had accidentally hit a person or another car. Any irregularity in the feel of the car could set her off: a bump, a swerve, or even just the realization that she hadn't been concentrating very hard on her driving. To reassure herself, Cherita would scrutinize the road through the rearview mirror. Most of the time she could reassure herself enough to keep on driving. Occasionally, though, she would feel compelled to double back on her route to confirm that no accident had occurred.

Since these driving doubts had arisen, Cherita had also been experiencing other intrusive images of havoc and destruction. The slightest thing could provoke them. For example, if she saw a book of matches on a desk at work, she would get a mental image of setting fire to her office building. Sometimes, after walking away from the matches, she would half wonder if she actually had set fire to the building; she would then review in her mind the sequence of events to reassure herself that no such thing had occurred. Occasionally, she would go back to obtain visual proof that the matches were still resting safely on the desk. In another case, she might see a knife on a table in a restaurant and get an image of stabbing somebody. Again, as she walked away, she would half wonder if she actually had stabbed

Compulsive acts are often a response to obsessive concerns. People who repeatedly perform cleaning rituals may be reacting to obsessive fears of contamination. Similarly, individuals who repeatedly check to make sure doors are locked and that they have their cell phone may be reacting to obsessive fears that their life is unsafe.

someone; then, as with the matches, she would review the sequence of events in her mind or return to the scene to establish that the knife was still there and she had not in fact carried out the imagined act. At other times, she would imagine less catastrophic events, such as insulting someone or neglecting to leave her car keys with the parking lot attendant.

James Trying to Understand

Cherita and James met during their senior year at college. They were in an accounting class together, and as James would tell friends, "The numbers added up quickly." He was totally taken with Cherita. He found her to be beautiful, effervescent, and caring. She took herself seriously, in a good way he thought — always wanting to be of service to others and to do the right thing in the right way. And as a bonus, they had similar interests, particularly in the business world: She wanted to be an accountant, and he was determined to make it as a small business owner. He felt that she was perfect and that their relationship was perfect.

As it turned out, things were not perfect. In fact, perfection was part of the problem. As James and Cherita grew closer, he became aware that she had some very odd habits — behaviors that she would repeat again and again according to certain rules until she was certain that everything was okay. At first he found her behaviors — checking locks again and again, meticulously making lists, and the like — to be kind of funny, like a personality quirk. But over time they became less funny. He saw that Cherita was a prisoner of her rituals. They made her very unhappy, they made her late for everything, and they prevented her from living a spontaneous life — but she couldn't stop them. When James pushed her for explanations, Cherita was clearly embarrassed. She would say she just felt that she had to do these things and that she felt very anxious otherwise, but she didn't offer much more.

Concerned (and often annoyed) as he was, James believed that Cherita's behaviors were more or less tolerable — a price that he had to pay to have a relationship with an otherwise great woman. The two of them continued to grow close and eventually were engaged.

Unfortunately, his fiancée's strange habits had grown stranger still since the start of their engagement. The behaviors that he himself witnessed — constant checking, no longer just of locks, but of windows, faucets, appliances, and more — were certainly odd, but even more disturbing were the rituals that a desperate Cherita told him about one evening: the endless morning rituals in her apartment and the doubt-ridden drives to work. And then there were those mystery areas, the way she would go cold and freeze with apparent fear whenever she saw matches or came into contact with a knife. What was going through her head at these times?

Obsessive-compulsive disorder is equally common in men and women and among people of different races and ethnic groups (Taylor et al., 2020).

What was she worried about? She would not discuss these reactions with James at all, as close as they were and as much as she trusted him. She confided only that it was too dark to discuss and that if he loved her, he would let it go and let her be.

James did love her, and so, after much thought and heartfelt talks with a close friend, he decided to stay in the relationship with Cherita. Their wedding date was now 6 months away, and he decided to focus on all the positive things about Cherita and go full steam ahead with the marriage plans. He asked one thing of her, however—that she seek treatment for her problem, whatever it was. His request was not an ultimatum or condition of marriage, but rather, he explained, a plea from the man who loved her greatly and who worried that all of their wonderful plans could unravel if she continued as she was doing. Cherita more than understood the request. She knew, even better than James, how disturbed she was and how much worse she had been getting. And although James was not threatening to end the relationship, she knew that there was probably only so much that he could take. She loved him and didn't want to lose him. Even more, she was tired of living this way.

Within a few days, she called to make an appointment with Dr. Marlene Laslow, a psychiatrist whose name came up first in online searches for treatment and whose website looked welcoming. After calling Dr. Laslow, Cherita waited patiently for several weeks for a call back. After not hearing from her, she called Dr. Laslow again, leaving a slightly more assertive message asking to be called back as soon as possible. Weeks passed with no return message. Cherita was frustrated, and so was James, who reminded her that there are other people she could see for help. "But I had my mind *set* on Dr. Laslow," Cherita pleaded. James then told her to call Dr. Erin Norton, whose treatment of obsessive-compulsive disorders had received some attention in a recent news feed online. To her delight, Dr. Norton called Cherita back within several days, leaving a very welcoming and kind voicemail. After playing voice mail tag for another few days, they finally spoke. Dr. Norton calmly informed Cherita that she had a long wait list and it could be several more months, possibly longer, before she could begin to see her. Cherita was devastated. This time, she did not wait for James to give her another name to call. This time Cherita contacted her primary care doctor via the electronic medical record and asked for a name of someone who would be likely to be available and knew how to treat obsessive-compulsive disorder. Before the day ended, she learned about Ms. Joyce, a licensed professional counselor who often took referrals from her primary care doctor for anxiety or obsessive-compulsive-related disorders. Ms. Joyce worked in a local community clinic, accepted Cherita's insurance for payment, and was able to see her in the next week. They scheduled an appointment, and Cherita, for the first time in as long as she could remember, felt hopeful that she could free herself of her obsessions and compulsions.

Treatment for Cherita Eliminating Obsessions and Compulsions

Cherita recognized that her fears and rituals were in some sense absurd, but she also acknowledged finding them too compelling to resist. As she put it during her first visit with Ms. Joyce, "When I describe it to you here, I can practically laugh about it, because I know it's so dumb. But when I'm in the situation, I just can't stop myself, the feeling is so overpowering."

After hearing Cherita's description of her thoughts and rituals, Ms. Joyce concluded that she did indeed have obsessive-compulsive disorder. Like most people with this disorder, the client exhibited both obsessions and compulsions. Her obsessions consisted of thoughts that some disaster (fire, flood, burglary) might happen if she did not take special precautions; thoughts that she might have caused a serious road accident; and thoughts and images of setting fires, stabbing people, or carrying out other more minor antisocial or negligent acts. Cherita's compulsions included her morning and evening checking routines, her unusual driving habits, and her repeated mental reviews of events to reassure herself that she had not run anyone over, burned down the house, or harmed someone.

Cherita asked Ms. Joyce whether she should do talk therapy or take medicine. Ms. Joyce informed her that the research indicates that antidepressant drugs, particularly the selective serotonin reuptake inhibitors, significantly reduce the obsessions and compulsions of many people with this disorder. But the gold standard approach with the best evidence in support and, arguably, the longest lasting effects is treatment with cognitive-behavioral therapy, specifically exposure and response prevention. Ms. Joyce's usual practice was to try the cognitive-behavioral approach first, referring clients to a psychiatrist for medication only if they failed to improve with this approach. Cherita listened as Ms. Joyce continued to elaborate.

In exposure and response prevention, clients are repeatedly exposed to anxiety-provoking stimuli, typically stimuli that are the subjects of their obsessive fears and thoughts. Then they are prevented from performing the anxiety-reducing compulsions that they would usually feel compelled to follow. The repeated prevention of compulsive behaviors eventually shows clients that the compulsions serve no useful purpose. Ms. Joyce got animated, even seeming excited. "Cherita, we're gonna retrain your brain," she pronounced. She went on to explain that the rituals are not needed to prevent or undo the clients' obsessive concerns, nor are they needed to reduce anxiety. In short, clients learn that nothing bad will happen if they fail to perform compulsive behaviors. At the same time, this approach helps them increasingly learn that their obsessive concerns are groundless and harmless, and so their anxious reactions to the obsessions lessen.

In addition to exposure and response prevention, Ms. Joyce also described how she would use a cognitive intervention. The cognitive approach to treatment involved helping Cherita to recognize that intrusive thoughts are a very common occurrence in most people and that the problem was not the thoughts themselves but the way Cherita was interpreting them. She told Cherita she would help her to recognize that having an intrusive thought or image didn't mean that she was more likely to act on that thought. Instead, Ms. Joyce outlined how she would help Cherita realistically assess the amount of responsibility she held in a variety of situations in an effort to reduce Cherita's beliefs in her excessive responsibility for herself and others.

Session 1   In the first session, after Cherita described her symptoms and their background, Ms. Joyce spent some time discussing Cherita's views on the danger posed by the objects of her obsessions. Cherita knew that her morning efforts were excessive. She acknowledged that the danger from plugged-in appliances or dripping faucets was minuscule, but she felt compelled to take repeated measures "just in case, because if anything did go wrong, it would be horrible." Cherita was also aware that it was extremely unlikely that she could hit someone on the road, set a fire, or stab someone and not know it. "It just seems that I want to know for certain that it isn't true; if I review it in my mind or go back to check that the person is okay, I feel relieved."

Cherita was less confident about her violent thoughts and intrusive images. Occasionally, when talking to someone, she would get an image of a knife in the person's chest, or on seeing a book of matches, she might get the thought of setting fire to the building. Cherita was frightened by these images and thoughts because she assumed they indicated she was capable of committing such acts, even though all her life she had conscientiously obeyed every rule and regulation. She had never lit a fire even in a fireplace or campground. And she would never dream of harming someone on purpose!

Ms. Joyce explained that these images should be viewed in the same spirit as the dripping faucet or the plugged-in hair dryer: They provoked anxiety, but they posed no objective danger. The counselor pointed out that most people occasionally experience a bizarre image or a thought of doing something outlandish or destructive; however, they just dismiss these thoughts as meaningless or unimportant. Cherita, on the other hand, kept reading disproportionate significance into such images; thus, she kept monitoring them closely and becoming extremely anxious in their presence.

Cherita:	But isn't there a problem with these thoughts? I mean, if I am thinking such things, doesn't it mean I'm capable of doing such things or want to do such things?
Ms. Joyce:	Do you have any conscious desire to do these things?
Cherita:	Of course not. They are the last things I would ever want to do.

> Thought-action fusion (TAF) is a cognitive bias characteristic of individuals with obsessive-compulsive disorder. The construct of TAF has two components: (1) the belief that having the thought makes the event more likely to happen and (2) the belief that having the thought is as bad as engaging in the behavior (Taylor et al., 2020; Davey, 2019).

Ms. Joyce:	I think the reason the thoughts scare you so much is that you've been assuming that their very existence means that you are in danger of carrying them out. The fact that you think something doesn't mean you want to carry it out or would ever carry it out. In fact, in spite of having the thoughts hundreds of times, you've never once made even the smallest gesture implied by the thoughts.
Cherita:	True. But sometimes I feel so close, like I have to put away the knives if anyone comes over, or if I were to touch a knife in someone's presence I would lose control.
Ms. Joyce:	Again, these are just assumptions on your part. The problem is not the thoughts or images themselves; it's your incorrect assumptions about them and your excessively anxious reaction. During this treatment, you will learn through experience that these assumptions are not valid. When you are ready, we will do certain exercises in which you start coming into contact with knives more frequently, in fact more frequently than the average person. In doing this, you will learn that your fears are unfounded, and you will become less anxious when these thoughts and images arise. As you become less anxious, you will also become less preoccupied with the thoughts and images and will probably start having them less frequently.
Cherita:	Are there are other people with the same problem as me? With thoughts about stabbing people or setting fires?
Ms. Joyce:	Yes, lots. In fact, the thoughts and images you describe are very typical of people with obsessive-compulsive disorder.
Cherita:	That makes me feel better somehow. I guess I assumed I was the only person in the world with such bizarre and perverse thoughts.
Ms. Joyce:	No, not at all. In fact as I said, most so-called normal people will have a bizarre or perverse thought on occasion. The difference is that you become excessively preoccupied with these thoughts, whereas most people simply dismiss them.

> A common practice in the cognitive-behavioral treatment of obsessive-compulsive disorder is to cite research showing that over 90% of community and laboratory samples of people have at least some intrusive thoughts. Furthermore, many of the intrusive thoughts contain content similar to that of individuals with obsessive-compulsive disorder (Taylor et al., 2020; Salkovskis & Harrison, 1984).

For the remainder of the session, Ms. Joyce further explained the exposure and response prevention treatment, describing the principles behind it and indicating how it would be applied to Cherita. The client indicated that the treatment plan made sense to her and that she was ready to proceed.

Ms. Joyce recommended an app that Cherita could download to keep track of her obsessions and compulsions for the coming week. Then, at the end of the week, Cherita could easily print out her data and take it to her appointment with Ms. Joyce.

Session 2   Cherita dutifully completed her home practice between therapy appointments. She self-monitored her obsessions and compulsions, tracking and recording them with precision. Three separate categories of obsessive-compulsive anxieties were identified: (1) household anxieties, (2) driving anxieties, and (3) anxieties over destructive thoughts and imagery. Cherita and Ms. Joyce spent the session setting up exercises that would pertain to the household anxieties.

To begin, they made a complete list of all of Cherita's household checking compulsions. The items that Cherita felt compelled to keep unplugged included the hair dryer, the microwave, the toaster, the laptop, the television, and the air conditioner. Light switches and lamps merely had to be shut off, not unplugged, to Cherita's way of thinking. Other items that she felt compelled to check were the stove (to make sure the burners were off), the faucets (to make sure they were not dripping), and the door (to make sure it was locked).

For exposure and response prevention exercises, Ms. Joyce proposed focusing first on the items that Cherita felt had to be unplugged or turned off. The counselor suggested not only that Cherita plug these items in before leaving for work but also that she turn a few of them on (specifically, the television, the air conditioner, and some lights) and leave them running for the whole day.

Cherita said she couldn't see any way she could bring herself to do what Ms. Joyce was proposing. Accordingly, a less extreme procedure was devised. Cherita would not be required to leave any items on; instead, she would simply plug them in. Beginning the next morning, she was to plug in each of the feared appliances and leave them that way for the rest of the day. Cherita felt that this exercise was within her capability and agreed to carry it out. In addition, she was to allow herself only one check of the lights, faucets, stove, and lock each morning.

Ms. Joyce cautioned Cherita about not surrendering to any urges to do unauthorized checks, no matter how strong. She compared obsessive-compulsive disorder to a machine that needed fuel, explaining that every time Cherita yielded to a compulsion to check, she was adding fuel to that machine, whereas every time she resisted the urge, she was taking fuel away. Therefore, whatever benefit might be provided by the exposure exercises would be undone if Cherita gave in to the urge to check. She instructed Cherita to tell James about this plan, so that he would not inadvertently collude to relieve her anxiety.

Session 3 Cherita reported that she had carried out the instructions every day in the past week. By the end of the week, she found to her surprise that plugging in the appliances was producing no anxiety whatsoever. On the other hand, the urge to recheck the stove, lights, faucets, and lock was still present, although reduced. Nevertheless, as instructed, she had succeeded in limiting herself to one check for each item.

Cherita was pleased by her accomplishment and encouraged by the practical benefits of the new morning procedure. Instead of spending an hour or more with her checking routine, the current procedure could be accomplished in a few

Between 50% and 70% of clients with obsessive-compulsive disorder significantly improve when treated with cognitive-behavioral therapy (Rosenberg, 2021; Kulz et al., 2020).

minutes, essentially just the time it took to briefly unplug and then replug the various appliances. This was already having a significant impact on her quality of life. Ms. Joyce suggested that now was the time to start limiting the checking even further. After some discussion, it was decided that Cherita would stop checking all light switches, while still allowing herself one check of the stove, faucets, and lock.

The counselor also spent some time reviewing with Cherita her ultimate fears about household items. Cherita reiterated what she had stated in the first interview: Her greatest fear seemed to be a fire or a flood due to her negligence. She could envision the havoc and destruction and being blamed; the very thought of it made her visibly upset.

Ms. Joyce suggested that in order for Cherita to overcome her preoccupation with this thought, some of the emotionality associated with it would have to be reduced. She proposed that the treatment of Cherita's household anxieties include prolonged and repeated exposure to images of her building being destroyed.

> **Obsessions may take such forms as obsessive wishes (for example, repeated wishes that one's spouse would die), impulses (repeated urges to yell out obscenities at church), images (fleeting visions of forbidden sexual scenes), ideas (notions that germs are lurking everywhere), or doubts (concerns that one may make the wrong decision).**

Cherita:	You are saying it would be beneficial to eliminate or reduce the anxiety I feel when thinking of my building being destroyed. But isn't this anxiety appropriate? I mean, isn't it normal not to want the building destroyed?
Ms. Joyce:	Yes, that is normal. But there is a difference between not wanting the building destroyed and getting anxious at the very thought of it. The first is appropriate, but the second is causing you difficulties. Of course you don't want the building to be destroyed, but you also don't want the mere idea to cause you such extreme anxiety.

Ms. Joyce then explained the mechanics of exposure to anxiety-provoking thoughts or images. Cherita would have to develop a detailed description of the building being destroyed, perhaps by fire and flood simultaneously. The description would include the hideous aftermath, the people whose lives would be lost or ruined, their awareness that Cherita was to blame, and their everlasting loathing of her. Together the counselor and Cherita worked on a written scenario. Next week, the session would be devoted to recording a 50-minute description of the event. Cherita would then listen to it on her phone a number of times throughout the week.

Cherita's instruction for the coming week was simply to keep all appliances plugged in and not do any checking except once for the stove, faucets, and door lock. She was to follow the same procedure before going to bed. Like all the weeks before, Cherita complied, and despite feeling ambivalence and distress about this new way of managing her obsessions, she continued to trust Ms. Joyce that this was the best path forward.

Session 4 Cherita reported that she had been able to keep to the new morning and evening checking procedure 95% of the time during the past week. She continued to keep appliances plugged in all the time, saying it now felt totally normal to her. She mentioned, however, that she did make one or two unauthorized checks of the stove. These extra checks seemed to have been provoked by her use of the stove that morning or evening.

On hearing this, Ms. Joyce instructed Cherita on a new exposure and response prevention exercise. Specifically, Cherita was to use the stove at least once in the morning and once in the evening every day, even if only to turn it on and off. Then she was to walk away without checking it further.

The remainder of the session was devoted to recording her script of her building being destroyed. Cherita sat back with her eyes closed and imagined the scene as vividly as possible. She then began her verbal description: "I accidentally leave the water running as I leave the apartment. The overflowing water reaches an electric outlet, causing a short circuit. The walls ignite. Flames start shooting up to the apartment above me. The people are trapped . . ." Cherita continued for about 10 minutes, ending with the destruction of the building and her being blamed by the survivors. The counselor then provided a second description, Cherita a third, and so on until a 50-minute recording was produced.

In addition to the stove exercises discussed earlier in the session, Cherita was given an assignment to listen to her script daily, rating her anxiety prior to each visualization, at its peak during each visualization, and at the end of each visualization.

Session 5 Cherita reported she had been able to listen to the recording 5 times during the week, and she was indeed becoming less reactive to it. She also reported that her general feelings about causing a disaster seemed to be undergoing a shift of sorts as a consequence of listening to the script. She noted that in thinking about being blamed for a disaster, her reaction was becoming one of "healthy defiance." Specifically, she was thinking, "I suppose I could cause a disaster, but so could anybody; if I did do it, it wouldn't be on purpose, and to hate me for it would be ridiculous."

Cherita was enthusiastic about the positive effects the recording appeared to be having on her, and she even seemed to look forward to listening to it again this week, feeling it led to more positive attitudes with each listening. Each time she listened it seemed more and more unrealistic that any such catastrophe could occur. If it did, she began to think, it surely would not be her fault that is started, with all of the care she took to prevent such disasters.

Regarding her other exposure exercises, Cherita continued to keep all appliances plugged in. She also limited herself to one check of the stove, faucets, and lock in the morning and evening. As a new exercise, Ms. Joyce asked Cherita to leave several lights on every day while she was away at work and to stop checking faucets.

Next the counselor raised the idea of Cherita starting to limit some of her compulsions during the drive to work: the excessive inspection of the rearview

Certain antidepressant drugs (for example, *clomipramine*, *fluoxetine*, and *fluvoxamine*) may also bring improvement to 50% to 60% of those with obsessive-compulsive disorder (Rosenberg, 2021; Szechtman et al., 2020). Selective serotonin reuptake inhibitors (SSRIs) are usually the first-line medication treatment for the disorder.

Most people with compulsions recognize that their repeated acts are unreasonable, but they believe that something terrible will happen if they do not perform them.

mirror, driving too slowly, mentally reviewing events on the road to reassure herself, and keeping lane changes to a minimum. Ms. Joyce suggested that instead the client now start normalizing her driving habits, driving at least 50 miles per hour on the highway and making at least five unnecessary lane changes while driving both to and from work. She also instructed Cherita to check the rearview mirror only as required for monitoring traffic.

Sessions 6 and 7 At the sixth session, Cherita reported that she had been able to follow through with the new instructions about changing her driving habits. To all outward appearances, her driving habits probably now seemed normal. More important, these changes seemed to have reduced Cherita's obsessions about causing accidents.

It was decided that the next 2 weeks would be devoted to consolidating all of the changes that Cherita had made thus far. In addition, during the first of the 2 weeks, the client was to leave her laptop on all day while she was away at work, and during the second week, the television. In driving she was to continue with the current procedures.

Regarding the recording, by session 7 Cherita reported that she could listen to the disaster scenario with hardly any reaction at all; if anything, she was getting bored with it. Accordingly, Ms. Joyce said she could stop listening to the script.

In summary, by session 7, Cherita's household obsessions and compulsions had virtually been eliminated. When driving, she was checking the rearview mirror much less frequently and even felt free enough to listen to morning radio broadcasts rather than obsessing over the possibility of an accident. The next step was to work on her anxiety about committing deliberate destructive acts: stabbing people and setting fires. For the coming week, Cherita's task in this area was simply to use her app to keep track of the thoughts and her behavioral responses.

> Repeated cleaning and repeated checking are among the most common kinds of compulsions.

Session 8 Cherita reported that over the past week she had continued to maintain her gains in the household and driving areas. In fact, she sometimes amazed herself with how different she had become in household matters.

As instructed, she had kept records of any anxieties associated with destructive thoughts. She reported several typical incidents. Twice, while out to lunch at a restaurant, she was disturbed by the thought of stabbing her lunch companion. More frightening to Cherita, the same thought occurred when James came over for dinner at her apartment. Similarly, thoughts and images about setting fires still arose whenever Cherita saw matches.

She also tried to observe her behavioral responses to these images or to her obsessions about knives and matches in general. She noted that she took pains to keep all knives hidden in drawers while at home, particularly if she had company. She also made a point of never having any matches in the house.

Ms. Joyce proposed that they begin working on this problem with some in vivo exposures. First, as a response prevention measure, Cherita was to stop avoiding knives and matches. Indeed, she was to make special efforts to start exposing herself to these items. Specifically, at home she was to take all of the knives out of the drawers and leave them on the kitchen counters for the entire week. In addition, she was instructed to buy a box of matches and place several books of matches in plain view in each room of her apartment.

Session 9   Cherita reported that she had carried out the instructions concerning knives and matchbooks throughout the week. At first it had made her quite anxious to have these items out in plain view, but after a couple of days her anxiety subsided and she became accustomed to it. Still, she wondered how she would fare if anybody came to her house while the knives were accessible. She was concerned that the thoughts of stabbing someone might be overwhelming.

At this point, Ms. Joyce proposed some new exposure exercises for the coming week. Cherita was now to carry a Swiss Army knife in her purse at all times, to give her prolonged experience with having a knife accessible. In addition, the counselor suggested that Cherita have James over to dinner with all of the knives laid out on the kitchen counter. If practical, Cherita was actually to use a sharp knife in his presence; for example, she could have him come into the kitchen to chat while she cut vegetables.

In addition, Cherita was to increase the intensity of her exposure to matches. Specifically, she had to strike several matches every day, blow them out, and then discard them.

Finally, Ms. Joyce suggested that the next session be devoted to recording another imaginal exposure exercise, one involving the violent imagery associated with knives and matches. Cherita herself suggested that the scenario focus on her fiancé, since he was often the subject of her violent imagery, a factor that made the images particularly disturbing.

Sessions 10 to 13   In session 10, Cherita and Ms. Joyce recorded the new visualization exercise: a 50-minute description of Cherita stabbing James and then setting fire to his building. As with the first exercise, the client reported high anxiety while visualizing the scene, but the anxiety tapered off slightly by the end. For the next 2 weeks, Cherita listened to the recording daily, and as with the first visualization exercise, her anxiety lessened with each listening. It was almost comical, she realized, that she would even think she could possibly hurt James or anyone. During session 13, she informed Ms. Joyce that she was barely feeling any emotional reaction at all when listening to the recorded scenario.

During this 2-week period, Cherita also kept a Swiss Army knife with her constantly. At first, the knife made her anxious, fueling her image of herself as "some kind of secret killer." However, as time passed, the knife seemed no more remarkable than her keys or wallet. It was just another item in her purse. She even used it on several occasions to slice tomatoes for lunch at her desk.

Cherita also scheduled the fateful evening with her fiancé. James came for dinner, and she deliberately handled knives in his presence in the kitchen. In so doing, she experienced the usual violent image—she had an image of stabbing him—but she followed the instruction not to try to force the image out, as she had in the past. Instead, she just let the image occur and carried on normally with her conversation and dinner preparations; as she did so, her anxiety eventually subsided. Cherita also invited James over a second and third time during this period. On each occasion, she still saw the image, but she became less and less anxious and preoccupied with it.

In the other areas—household and driving—Cherita had been faithfully following the specified procedures, which were beginning to feel like second nature. Now, in the morning, she was free of any extraordinary urges to check and often did not bother with her one allotted check of the stove and lock. In driving to work, she felt like any other bored commuter. Occasionally, she said, she had a flashback to one of her former obsessions (about causing a car accident), but now it felt like just a vague memory of former times.

At session 13, it was decided that Cherita would stop carrying out any active therapeutic procedures, which by now consisted mainly of turning on items before leaving for work and listening to the recorded slash-and-burn scenario (as Cherita called it).

> Therapists will often explain to clients how "forcing the image out of their mind" is counterproductive. By trying to get rid of the image, the client focuses more attention on the thought itself, which increases anxiety. Also, holding the belief that one must force the image out reinforces the belief that the thoughts were bad and dangerous in the first place.

Session 14   Cherita reported on her first week of "normal life." She was not feeling anything more than an occasional urge to check, which she resisted. A plan was made to meet at 2-week intervals for the next two sessions and at 3-week intervals for the two sessions after that. The goal was simply to keep an eye on Cherita's status and advise her on adjustments to any new situations. As it happened, in 3 weeks' time, Cherita and her fiancé would be married and beginning their life together in a new apartment. Everything was working out as planned. The timing was perfect.

Sessions 15 to 18   These follow-up sessions were held over a period of 2½ months. Throughout this period, Cherita was free of obsessions and compulsions in the household and driving areas. Living with James, now her husband, turned out to present few unexpected challenges. As expected, however—and Ms. Joyce had advised the client about this—Cherita had initially experienced more frequent violent images. However, in keeping with all she had learned, she did not try to force the images out and did not treat them as a threat. After the first couple of weeks with her husband, the images lessened markedly.

Because everything continued to go well during this period, they decided not to schedule any more therapy sessions. Ms. Joyce asked only that Cherita return for one more visit in 6 months' time to report on her progress and consider whether she needed any additional follow-up appointments.

Epilogue

At her 6-month follow-up visit, Cherita reported that all was continuing to go well. Her only lingering symptom was an occasional violent image. What was amazing, she said, was that such images were causing hardly any anxiety. Generally, she was extremely pleased, and she expected that these images would continue to lessen with time. Overall, she reported feeling like a different person, certainly different from the woman who had entered therapy a year ago and also different from the person who had had less severe obsessions and compulsions for several years prior to that. Now able to focus on events and activities without the constant intrusion of frightening thoughts and images, and without the burden of complex compulsions, she found life much easier and more enjoyable than she had ever thought it could be.

Around 40% of people with obsessive-compulsive disorder seek treatment (NIMH, 2017b; Phillips, 2015).

Assessment Questions

1. When do obsessive-compulsive behaviors begin for most individuals?

2. What were Cherita's primary obsessions and compulsions?

3. Why did Cherita finally decide to seek treatment?

4. Which specific treatment did Ms. Joyce decide to try to help Cherita overcome her obsessive-compulsive disorder? Why was this a type of cognitive-behavioral therapy?

5. Ms. Joyce asked Cherita to keep track of her obsessions and compulsions. What did Cherita learn from entering this information, and how did Ms. Joyce use this information to assist in her treatment program?

6. What was the purpose of recording Cherita's visually imagined disaster scenes?

7. How many sessions did it take for Cherita to overcome her household obsessions and compulsions?

8. Obsessions may take different forms. List three forms cited in the text.

9. How many sessions were necessary for Cherita to overcome her obsessive-compulsive disorder?

CASE 3

Social Anxiety Disorder

Table 3-1

Dx Checklist

Social Anxiety Disorder

1. Pronounced, disproportionate, and repeated anxiety about social situation(s) in which the individual could be exposed to possible scrutiny by others; typically lasting 6 months or more.
2. Fear of being negatively evaluated by or offensive to others.
3. Exposure to the social situation almost always produces anxiety.
4. Avoidance of feared situations.
5. Significant distress or impairment.

(Information from APA, 2022, 2013.)

Xian was a 24-year-old, single, cisgender Chinese citizen from Beijing on a student visa living in the Los Angeles area. She was working on her doctoral degree in cognitive neuroscience at a large university and living alone, with few close friends. She spent most of her time on schoolwork: going to class and meetings, reading, running experiments, analyzing data, and writing. She loved her work, and hoped after receiving her Ph.D to return to China and work as a professor. She came from a very close family, and although she was an only child, Xian had grown up around her two cousins, both girls nearly her age and practically sisters to her. They were home in Beijing, along with her parents and their small white dog, Cassidy.

Xian had lived in the United States for several years and often missed her parents, both of whom had been loving and attentive to her needs throughout her life. She missed the way her mother would sit with her for long, quiet periods of time reading, or how her father would encourage her, even in her most stressful times, to "look inside yourself and find strength." She missed her cousins, two of the only people she could be around without feeling much stress or anxiety. There were so many things she wished she could do with them back at home: walking through Jingshan Park in April to witness the annual explosion of peonies and tulips, wandering the fragrant mazes of hutongs near Shichahai until sundown, or slowly sipping her favorite ba bao cha, a sweet eight-treasured tea. More than anything, she longed to walk with her cousins through the familiar malls and markets and endless family-owned restaurants back in the Haidian District, where she was born and raised.

Xian's parents were academics. Her mother was an English teacher at one of the large universities north of the city center and her father was a professor of psychology at a university in the growing outskirts of Liangxiang, near the sixth outer ring road of the city. Xian always wanted to become a professor or teacher—a laoshi—like her parents. She had carved her own professional path by focusing on science and anatomy. As a freshman at the most prestigious university in China, she had considered becoming a physician, but her ambitions changed after taking classes in experimental methods and abnormal psychology. She loved those classes, found them relatively easy, and got an A in both of them. Her professor told her she had a natural aptitude for scientific reasoning. This was something both her parents had told her too. She changed her mind, shifting away from a plan to attend medical school, deciding she wanted to become a scientist and study the brain. Years later, as an international student in her third year of graduate school, Xian was confident that she was succeeding as a young scientist and well on her way toward achieving her professional goals.

Unfortunately, despite everything Xian had going for her, she had an ongoing problem that was causing significant emotional distress and interfering with her life. It was something she had been dealing with as long as she could remember, and she felt ashamed about it. Putting it simply, Xian was terrified of social situations. During childhood, she was carefree and easy-going around her parents, cousins, and a few close friends. But she was shy, anxious, and somewhat aloof around almost everyone else. It was like she was always waiting for something bad to happen when she was around people she didn't know. It was a sense of worry and dread, trepidation that others would make fun of her, judge her, or humiliate her. The thing she feared the most was that someone would know how anxious she was and would embarrass her about it in one way or another. She carried these worries with her everywhere, unable to shake them even when her mind would try to convince her that a social situation was safe, that there were no threats to be found, and that others were not going to reject, ostracize, or poke fun at her.

Xian grew up on the 15th floor of an apartment building in a gated residential community. She knew her neighbors on the same floor and was always polite to them. They were a kind and quiet family with a son younger than her. Many days they would see each other in the elevator. She would smile and say hello, then hold her breath, clench her jaw, and stare at the floor. Sometimes she would pretend she was exhausted in the elevator, closing her eyes and slumping her shoulders, feigning fatigue and hoping her neighbors would leave her alone. They made her anxious. She didn't know what they thought about her. Even as a little girl, she worried they would talk to her and that she wouldn't know what to do or say. She thought it was stupid and foolish. After all, they had never done or said anything to her to give her reason to believe they would judge or criticize. And it wasn't just them. Most people made her nervous. Still, every time she saw her neighbors she felt desperate to avoid conversation.

> Shyness is a normal part of childhood and does not necessarily develop into social anxiety disorder.

Her elementary and secondary schools were both within walking distance of home. There were many girls her age in her building and the ones nearby. She was friendly with some of them, but she always found it hard to know what to talk about, so she mostly avoided them, even at school. Xian liked routines, and after school each day would wait for her cousin An Xin to get out, so they could walk back home together. An Xin was easy-going and comfortable talking to people. Her presence made Xian feel safe. With An Xin, she didn't have to worry about anything. If someone wanted to ask them a question, An Xin would answer. If they saw a friend or classmate together, An Xin knew what to say. Whatever Xian's anxieties might be, with An Xin in her presence they were lower. After school every day they would stroll over the canal bridge through the fitness park, across the busy third ring road intersection, and into their neighborhood, effortlessly dodging the cyclists and scooters until they got to the familiar iron gates of their apartments and the old guard with a missing tooth who smoked and always smiled when they arrived, welcoming them home.

Home was a safe place. Her parents were devoted to her development and supported Xian in every way they could think of. They had helped her learn several musical instruments, spoke Mandarin and English in the home so she would be bilingual, and had given her extensive resources to succeed academically outside of school, with tutors and evening classes after dinner most weeknights. Xian was grateful and felt loved by her parents. Besides her cousins An Xin and the younger Jingbo, there were rarely other children in the apartment. Unfortunately, because she limited most of her socializing to time with her cousins, Xian was not exposed to a sufficient number of different social situations to help her overcome her worries about interacting with others.

Xian Problems at School

Xian was a disciplined and intelligent child. Academic success came naturally to her, and she was always at the top of her class. Instead, her biggest challenges at school were always social. Whether it was working in small groups, giving class presentations, or introducing herself to classmates each year, it was all harder for Xian than it seemed to be for the other kids. Her parents hoped that she would learn to cope better with social situations as she got older. But when she was in her first year of high school, Xian's social anxiety emerged as a major problem. She had a project that required her to give a speech in front of the class. She wasn't friends with any of the other students and was terrified that they would judge her harshly. What if she stumbled over her words or forgot what she wanted to say? Or worse, what if they realized how anxious she was and made fun of her for it? Sure, it is normal for kids to worry about being judged by their peers. It was probably true that many of her classmates also worried about what others would

In the majority of cases, social anxiety disorder emerges during late childhood or adolescence and may continue into adulthood (ADAA, 2020).

think of them after their class speech. But Xian was more than worried, more than nervous. She was stricken with a debilitating fear, mentally paralyzed each time she thought about the presentation. As a result, when she should have been preparing she avoided the class project, usually by studying for other classes or doing some other genuinely important task. She was so scared that she never prepared a speech.

When it was the day to give her speech, Xian awoke after sleeping poorly to a wave of dread and a sense of impending doom. She didn't have anything planned to say. For the first time, she was not at all ready and would be at risk of failing the project. Xian felt completely nauseated at the prospect of facing her teacher and classmates unprepared. Her parents saw that she was behaving differently and asked her if she was feeling well. She impulsively lied and told them she was feeling sick. It was rare for her to be ill, and her parents took it seriously, telling her to stay home and contacting the school to inform them of her absence.

Xian was relieved that she didn't have to give the speech, but the feeling was quickly overwhelmed by a sense of guilt and helplessness. When her parents left for work, she cried, tears coming easily from a familiar fountain of shame. Her social anxiety had kept her from doing countless things in the past. She had skipped birthday parties, politely declined invitations to socialize, pretended to sleep on the bus, and stayed quiet in group gatherings. But this was the first time her social anxiety had prevented her from succeeding academically.

She cried until she was too exhausted to cry anymore, at which point she looked up and saw that her mother hadn't left for work after all; she was standing in the doorway, clearly aghast at her daughter's behavior. Xian completely broke down, sobbing in abject humiliation. Her level of shame and anxiety peaked at the highest level she had ever experienced. Xian's mother was compassionate, but when her daughter had calmed down, she reprimanded her for lying about being sick, and told her that they would go to the school together to speak to the teacher about her transgression. Xian begged for mercy, but to no avail.

This event led her parents to realize that Xian's social anxiety was worse than they thought. They knew she had always been slow to warm up to new people and quiet in social situations. Most of the time they interpreted her actions as being polite, demure, or conscientious. But after talking with her and hearing her explain why she didn't do the class project, this time it was clear — she was so worried about what others would think about her that she avoided preparing for her speech, missed school, and now she had to talk to the teacher about it all. Her anxiety was a problem that needed to be addressed.

Xian was sent by her parents to the psychological services clinic at her mother's university. They told the clinic that Xian was socially anxious and asked that she be evaluated for an anxiety disorder. Xian was mortified, feeling like she had confirmation about a core belief she had been thinking for some time: There was something fundamentally wrong with her. She feared that a core part of her was biologically broken, or maybe that she was born defective and incapable. On top of it all, she had failed herself and her parents, and now she had to talk about it with a stranger. This was about the worst thing she could imagine.

The counselor was a female graduate student in clinical psychology supervised by a faculty-level psychologist. They talked for about an hour. Xian sheepishly answered all of her questions and left as quickly as possible when the appointment ended. The counselor-in-training told her that she seemed to meet diagnostic criteria for social anxiety disorder. It was recommended that she return to the clinic for cognitive-behavioral therapy (CBT), an evidence-based approach known to work well for social anxiety disorder. Xian respectfully neither said no nor committed to treatment, saying she would talk with her parents about it. She later would convince her parents that she did not need treatment but would instead make major changes to how she dealt with her anxiety. It was the first time she had ever openly acknowledged her social anxiety like this to her parents, and they capitulated to her pleas that going to therapy could make her feel worse about herself. At the time, it felt like a low point in her life. But years later, as a graduate student herself, Xian would recall her experience with the student counselor as an important moment in her life. She had learned that she did have social anxiety, that it was something she could get help for, and it was something that explained why it was always so hard for her to be around people.

After this experience, Xian committed to never again letting her social anxiety interfere with her schoolwork. She went back to school with a renewed sense of dedication and determination, mostly out of fear. She simply would not allow herself to avoid schoolwork out of fear of what others might think of her. She had apologized to her teacher and family and promised her parents she would not avoid her schoolwork like that ever again. It all felt horrible. And this motivated her the next few years of high school to consistently do her homework, prepare for class projects, and study in advance for all quizzes and tests. During class, to ease her social anxiety, she avoided eye contact with other students, looking at her notes and at the teacher whenever possible. When not in class, she walked with her head down and put headphones in to avoid hearing anything that might increase her anxiety. This way she didn't have to worry about seeing people she didn't want to talk to. She could avoid their uninterpretable facial expressions and their laughter (were they laughing at *her*?). Instead, she stuck to her rituals: walking home with her cousin An Xin, talking and laughing, making her way home over the familiar canal bridge, through the usual park past nameless exercising retirees and parents with their children, all the way to the comforting smells and sounds of the Chengdu-style restaurant around the corner from home. When she saw the gate to her community, she knew she was about to see that same guard and his crooked cigarette-mouthed smile.

Around 7% of individuals in the United States and other Western countries experience social anxiety disorder in any given year (ADAA, 2020).

Like Xian, people with social anxiety disorder often perform "avoidance" behaviors that help prevent or reduce the chance of social interactions or anticipated social embarrassment (Kleberg et al., 2021; Ashbaugh et al., 2020).

Xian Adjusting to Life in the United States

After graduating with straight A's and an impressive track record doing undergraduate research, Xian was admitted to graduate school outside Los Angeles. She was thrilled to get into this doctoral program. It was highly ranked and difficult to get into. She was ready to get to work right away when she arrived in the United States. Her parents paid for her costs to travel and live. She rented an apartment within walking distance from the university and set it up in a spartan manner. Her living area was a one-bedroom studio with no TV or couch, only a foldable plastic table and chairs along with an outdoor wicker chaise lounge. She found a used bed online using WeChat and purchased it from a friendly Chinese neighbor, a graduate student in engineering. Her new neighbor suggested Xian get together with her and her friends sometime. They could go out, get a bite to eat, or check out the new movie theater, she said. Xian, as she done so many times before, graciously thanked her neighbor for the offer, then declined. It was the last time she would see her, as Xian from that point forward felt embarrassed and regretful that she did not befriend the neighbor. Instead of trying to change her emotions by getting to know the neighbor, Xian maintained distance, afraid that if she ever did see her again the neighbor would ignore her, or even say something mean to her. She would walk an extra block home to avoid her neighbor's apartment building, each time with her eyes fixed on the sidewalk or her phone.

Her graduate program was small, and her classmates were all Americans. Although Xian was fluent in English (her mother was an English teacher, after all), she had never lived in the United States. The customs of everyday behavior—everything that was expected of her by others—all seemed unfamiliar and sometimes puzzling. When class ended, for example, Xian would routinely raise her hand to ask the professor questions. She kept her focus on professors, locking eyes with them during their responses to avoid seeing others looking at her when talking, a tactic she had acquired during high school as a way to bravely speak up around strangers—and to make a favorable impression among her professors. She noticed that she was usually the one student asking questions at the end of class, and that 5, 10, even 15 minutes after the time class was supposed to end, she would still be fully engaged with the professor, astutely taking notes like it was still class time. Sometimes when she would finally look around the room, she noticed that few students remained. Most of the time students would leave at the end of class. But for Xian, when class ended, she considered it appropriate and respectful to ask questions. This was a normal thing she and others did growing up. But it was out of place in the United States. One day a classmate explained to Xian that students in the United States consider the end of the scheduled time for class to be the time to end class. "We all want to leave when class ends," she explained, "so don't be surprised if you are the only one left after class." Xian then realized, her

People with social anxiety disorder typically overestimate how poorly things have gone in social situations (Hofmann, 2021; Tonge et al., 2020).

face going white with humiliation, that she had been following customs common in China and had not noticed how her actions may have been perceived. She was so focused on the professor and so expert in avoiding eye contact with others that she didn't even see how the other students were reacting. Once again, Xian felt overwhelmed with social anxiety, but this time in a foreign country with unfamiliar cultural norms. Now that she was aware of this social gaffe, she wondered what else she had done. They must think I am so selfish, she surmised, ruminating and perseverating until she had determined that she must be disliked by all the other students.

Xian was doing well academically in graduate school. She kept to the stringent academic approach that had worked for her during high school and college. Home alone most of the time, she would write results from her studies up for publication, analyze data, and write grant applicants for her next studies. She was confident as a scientist and had the support and admiration of her advisor and graduate school colleagues. She was surely destined for success as an academic. But her advisor and classmates all had commented to her many times that they hoped she was "taking care of herself" and "living a balanced life." Xian hated it when people commented on her personal life. It made her wonder if they were all watching her, noticing her habits and patterns. Maybe they thought there was something wrong with her? "Yes," she told them each time, "I am feeling balanced and happy." But she wasn't living a very balanced life. She worked 12 hours or more every day. She spent her nights and early mornings before she started to work mostly looking at things online that reminded her of the comforts and safety of home.

She wasn't particularly happy, either. She couldn't get around the city very easily, like she could back home. She didn't have a vehicle, and her bicycle could only get her so far. Xian missed everything about home. She wished she could taste her favorite Beijing-style noodles or shop for clothes with her cousins. She missed her parents and her playful dog Cassidy. Because she spent most of her time alone, she was lonely. As anxious as it made her to be around others, Xian wished she had friends. She longed for time spent casually and recreationally. She had grown tired of her apartment. It made her sad being alone all the time, but it was extremely mentally exhausting for her to try to make friends. Ironically, despite her social anxiety, Xian was liked by her peers. She was collegial and friendly to her classmates and had developed one close friendship. Mara was a graduate student in the Social Psychology program. They met after a scientific presentation. Xian had asked the speaker questions after her talk, and Mara stuck around with Xian to listen, the three of them eventually walking out of the room together for an extended conversation about the latest trends in cognitive neuroscience. When the speaker abruptly said she had another meeting to go to, Xian was left alone with Mara. It went well. They talked about shared academic interests, their

> Approximately 60% of individuals with social anxiety disorder are female (ADAA, 2020).

respective labs and graduate programs, and, finally, about their backgrounds and families. Mara seemed somewhat safe for Xian. She was from Germany, also on a student visa, and though they came from very different cultural backgrounds, Xian felt a sense of shared experience with her. Over time, Xian would confide in Mara that she had social anxiety, at which Mara pretended to be surprised.

Xian Asking for Help

After Xian opened up to Mara about her anxiety, they had become closer friends. They both prioritized work over everything else, and on some weekends and the American holidays, the two of them would occasionally get together. Mara was more outgoing than Xian, and had a group of friends. She also had a boyfriend, Ander, a tall, outgoing Danish student in the Film Studies program who played ice hockey. Mara had been dating Ander on and off for about a year, and she wanted to introduce him to Xian. "We should all have dinner together," Mara suggested. "Um, OK," Xian responded. Mara knew her friend would be uneasy meeting Ander. "Xian," Mara said, "I know it could be stressful to meet him, but it would mean a lot to me. And I think you'll like him. He's a lot like me." Xian reflexively tightened her jaw and felt her face begin to flush. She looked away, down at her phone, acting as if she had just received an important text message. After a moment of awkward silence, she looked up and smiled at Mara. "Sure. I would like to meet him," she lied. Mara felt uncomfortable, but she was hopeful that Xian meant it. She looked at Xian and smiled back. They planned to get together in several weeks, for an American Thanksgiving dinner. As the holiday neared, Xian started to get increasingly anxious about the dinner and meeting Ander. What would they talk about? What would she do if Mara went to the bathroom and left Xian alone with him? What if he wanted to talk about film or theater, or worse, ice hockey? Xian knew almost nothing about these topics. She feared he would find her dull, or think she wasn't very smart. As much as she liked Mara, her worries about Ander's negative evaluations grew and grew, overwhelming and terrifying her. It felt like too much. Xian texted Mara. She apologized matter-of-factly, saying that she was feeling sick and would be staying home. Mara was irritated but texted back that she understood and hoped she felt better soon.

Xian was relieved but also thought she had made a huge mistake. She tried to get her anxiety down by thinking about other things, but it didn't work, and her emotional distress escalated. This time, she had avoided a social gathering with a friend who had told her how important it was that she meet her boyfriend. This time, she was in America and couldn't retreat to the comforts of her home. She didn't have An Xin or Jingbo to go to, and she felt too embarrassed to talk to them or her parents about what she had done. If she lost Mara as a friend, she would have to start all over again getting to know someone. And Mara had been

> Most people with social anxiety disorder believe that they are always in danger of behaving incompetently in social situations and that their inept behaviors will lead to terrible consequences (Kleberg et al., 2021; Mobach et al., 2020).

there for her, a true friend when she needed one. Xian wished she had the ability to act opposite to her fears by going to the dinner with Mara and Ander. She closed her eyes and imagined doing it, telling herself the encouraging things her father had told her when she was a child. She tried to summon the courage to go but finally concluded that she didn't have the capability to do so. She admitted to herself that her anxiety was too debilitating. It froze her behavior, keeping her from doing the thing that in her heart she valued doing for her friend Mara. It overcame her body, her heart racing and skin sweating as though, like being alone on an ice flow with a hungry polar bear, there was a true and imminent threat to her safety. It stormed her mind, seeking to hold her accountable to a conspiracy theory that because there was something inherently wrong with her, Ander, like all the others she had avoided before him, would discover it if she let herself socialize. The surge of fear was too much. Xian put her head on her pillow and wept. Unlike what had happened in high school when she avoided her class project, this time Xian knew it was time to do something about her problem. She remembered her time with the counselor-in-training who diagnosed her with social anxiety disorder. She made a promise to herself to get help.

Xian Treatment Using Process-Based CBT

In the weeks after she missed the Thanksgiving dinner, Xian occupied herself with her work. A grant application was due in two months, and she dedicated every spare moment to it. She and Mara exchanged a few text messages but didn't talk to or see each other. In the moments when she was not working on her grant or something else, Xian was thinking about how she would go about getting help for her social anxiety. She looked online, but the choices for treatment providers seemed endless. Besides, they all seemed to say the same thing: "I provide compassionate, evidence-based care that is personalized to meet your needs," or something like that. She didn't know how to choose, and she didn't want to randomly call therapists.

She looked to the university psychological services clinic, which was free, but decided she did not want to be treated by a therapist trainee with no experience. She was finally ready to get help for social anxiety after all these years and was hoping to find an expert. Turning to the academic medical center's website, she found a psychologist who was an assistant professor of psychiatry and who described himself as having expertise in the treatment of social anxiety. The psychologist, Dr. Robert Weir, was an academic who did research, taught psychiatry residents, and had a cognitive-behavioral therapy clinic specializing in anxiety disorders. Xian was excited, thinking this could be a good fit for her. She reached out to schedule an appointment, first with the clinic's intake coordinator for a standard psychosocial evaluation. In this meeting, she learned, she would be asked about

Around 40% of individuals with social anxiety disorder are currently in treatment (NIMH, 2017c).

a range of questions related to overall health, history, and current mental health symptoms. That appointment happened 2 weeks later, and at the conclusion of the evaluation, the intake coordinator told Xian she appeared to meet diagnostic criteria for social anxiety disorder. Like the counselor-in-training back in Beijing, the intake coordinator suggested Xian receive CBT, an evidence-based treatment for social anxiety. Unlike the last time she received this diagnosis, however, Xian now felt determined and resolute to come back for treatment. She eagerly asked if she could be seen by Dr. Weir and scheduled an appointment with him. Leaving the clinic, Xian felt excited and hopeful about her upcoming treatment with Dr. Weir. Finally, after all these years, she was seeking help.

Sessions 1 and 2   Xian met with Dr. Weir in his office at the medical center. He told her that he had reviewed the electronic medical record and the note from her initial evaluation. He then oriented her to the process of the session, telling her about limits to confidentiality (for example, if she had plans to harm herself or others, he would be bound ethically to address these plans with her even, if needed, at the expense of her confidentiality), his credentials as a licensed psychologist in California, and his training as a cognitive-behavioral therapist. He went on to explain that he would work with her to more carefully assess problems with social anxiety before beginning any specific treatment, but that if appropriate he would be able to use CBT for social anxiety. When Dr. Weir asked Xian what brought her to treatment, she hesitated, slowly taking in a deep breath, and replied, "For most of my life I have been afraid of what people will think of me. I am always afraid of being judged, being made fun of, or of people seeing how anxious I am and then thinking negatively about me. I have been dealing with this for a long time, and I am ready to do something about it." Dr. Weir listened, supportively acknowledged Xian's willingness to come to treatment after all these years, and asked her to share more about her history of social anxiety. Xian anxiously disclosed how she had long ago learned to avoid social contexts if possible, and when she couldn't she would find ways to inhibit her behavior to prevent getting into conversations or receiving attention from others. She told him stories about her limited social experiences as a child, the class project she avoided in high school, and her most recent problem avoiding Mara's boyfriend at Thanksgiving dinner.

Dr. Weir explained to her that social anxiety disorder can develop in people who were shy and inhibited when younger. He compassionately explained the nature of the human neurobiological defensive motivational system and associated freeze, flight, and fight responses to threatening stimuli. Xian courteously reminded Dr. Weir that she was studying to be a neuroscientist and had intricate knowledge about neural and peripheral nervous systems associated with perceptions of threat. Dr. Weir didn't miss a beat, stating that psychoeducation is a small part of treatment for social anxiety, and that he was glad she had such knowledge already. He noted the distinction between knowing about how the brain works and being able to skillfully change one's responses to perceived threat cues. "Knowledge is important, but it is not enough to change social anxiety," he proffered. Xian nodded, and he continued, "If we decide to do CBT for social anxiety, we will work together to identify and change patterns of responding to social cues that elicit anxiety responses and get in the way of your life." He asked her if they could talk about the things that trigger her social anxiety, and she hesitantly agreed.

Doing what he called a "functional analysis," Dr. Weir asked Xian to talk about the typical kinds of people, places, things, and experiences she had before, during, and immediately after she felt intense social anxiety. She asked if she could use a specific example from last week. "If it is representative of what typically happens, sure," he replied. Xian described the situation first. She was in a lab meeting with her peers and faculty advisor. An unfamiliar person was sitting at the conference room table with them, talking to her advisor quietly. When the meeting began, her advisor announced that they had a guest joining the lab meeting that day, a colleague and expert in computational decision making who was giving a lecture on campus later that day. Xian described how she immediately and automatically began to hold her breath and clench her muscles, feeling the pace of her heart rate increase. She recounted how she froze in her seat, made no eye contact with anyone, and started to think she would have to introduce herself and tell the speaker about her research interests. This thought led to her feeling her heart beat even faster, and she noticed her face felt hot and her hands started to sweat.

"What happened next?" Dr. Weir probed. Xian explained that they introduced themselves and their year in the program to the speaker, but no one was asked to talk about their research interests. "And," Dr. Weir said, "what did you immediately notice in your body or in your thoughts, or what did you do behaviorally?" Xian felt embarrassed but described how the speaker began to talk about their program of research, and Xian tried unsuccessfully to listen. The speaker talked for about 30 minutes, and Xian had hardly remembered a single word, instead obsessively thinking about her physiological symptoms of anxiety and whether anyone might notice.

The functional analysis of this situation took about 25 minutes to get through, and all along the way Dr. Weir was taking notes. When they finished, with several minutes left, he showed her his sheet of paper and what he had written. It was a grid with three columns entitled "before, during, and after" and rows labeled "thoughts, feelings, physiological sensations, and behavior." He had filled out the cells in the grid based on the information she shared with him. He held the sheet

Research suggests that social anxiety disorder is sometimes linked to a genetic predisposition, a hyperactive brain fear circuit, traumatic childhood experiences, and/or overprotective parent–child interactions, among other factors (Buzzell et al., 2021; Rose & Tadi, 2021; Schneier, 2021; Lai, 2020).

up for her to see and told her that he had some ideas about what might be eliciting and maintaining her anxious responses, that these were hypotheses, and that together they would explore these hypotheses to try to better understand the things that were causing her social anxiety.

At the end of the first session, Dr. Weir told Xian that he believed she met criteria for social anxiety disorder and that he was confident that he could help her using a CBT-based approach. He was careful not to guarantee that she would be completely symptom free after therapy, because he knew that, while CBT was an empirically supported treatment for social anxiety, it was not a cure. However, Dr. Weir believed that CBT could bring her significant emotional relief and improve her social functioning. Xian was excited and felt hopeful.

In the second session, Dr. Weir described the cognitive-behavioral model of social anxiety to Xian. He explained that her learning history of avoiding or escaping from social cues that could disconfirm her worries may be an environmental root cause of her social anxiety. She may have been biologically vulnerable to anxiety as a child, and her avoidance and escape responses to social situations prevented her from learning to be less anxious. He went on to say that there is a lot of evidence to suggest that social anxiety stems from a combination of problematic beliefs, avoidance, and escape behaviors. CBT would help target changing those same cognitive and behavioral patterns that had been learned. Xian felt confused and a bit blamed.

Xian:	Are you saying it is my fault?
Dr. Weir:	No, not at all. People who develop social anxiety tend to have a history of avoiding and escaping from situations that create intense worries about being rejected or negatively evaluated in some form or another.
Xian:	Yes, doctor, that describes me. But are you saying I did this to myself?
Dr. Weir:	No. We all learn as we grow up, and we continue to learn throughout our life. Learning is complicated, and there are many different learning processes. You didn't do this to yourself. But you did learn escape and avoidance behavior as a primary strategy to cope with your worries and feelings of anxiety in social situations. And your thought patterns were also learned. Unfortunately, the assumptions, interpretations, and automatic thoughts you have had related to social situations were not disconfirmed enough. If they were, you would be less likely to continue having these thoughts, and even if you did, you would be less distressed by them. What you and I need to do is create a process where you can gradually learn to identify and challenge these automatic thoughts, while learning to approach instead of avoid or escape from some of these social situations. If we do that, and work together to track your efforts to change, there is a good chance I can help you.

Cognitive-behavioral therapy brings improvement to around 55% of clients with social anxiety disorder (Stein, 2020b; Stein & Taylor, 2019).

Xian:	I want to get better, and I trust you. But it sounds difficult. How is this different from talk therapy?
Dr. Weir:	CBT is a kind of talk therapy, just one with structure and focus, with targets for change and measures of progress. We would be working together to solve everything, like we did in our first session when we did the functional analysis.
Xian:	How long will it take?
Dr. Weir:	Well, our department policy at the medical center allows us to have 10 weekly sessions for up to an hour, so we will start there. If you need additional weekly sessions after we end, our clinic is committed to helping you find the resources you need based on your insurance.
Xian:	Is 10 sessions enough?
Dr. Weir:	Good question. We are on session two, which gives us eight more to make change. We will not be following a single specific week-to-week manual. Instead, we will use what has been called a process-based CBT approach. We will flexibly use CBT interventions known to work for social anxiety in a way that meets your needs and our 10-session department policy. I am confident we can do it, but only if you are committed to working hard in between sessions to do home practice. This is where most of the change will happen. Kind of like if you have ever been to physical therapy, most of the change happens when you leave the physical therapist's office and practice stretches each day. The same is true in CBT for social anxiety. I'll give you home practice based on what you learn with me in each session, and when you complete the home practice you should begin to see improvements.
Xian:	I am giving my commitment. And even though I am nervous about it, I know it is what I need to do. What do we do next?
Dr. Weir:	One of the core processes of treatment we could use is something called cognitive reappraisal. This is an evidence-based way to help people monitor and label problematic learned ways of thinking about social situations, and then challenge the truth of such thoughts by looking for alternatives and facts that are incongruent with them. After you leave today, I will ask you to begin completing a daily self-monitoring form that will help you track and challenge your automatic thoughts about social situations. Is this something you might be willing to do?
Xian:	To be honest, I don't know. I have lots of evidence to support the truth of my thoughts. So many things have happened to make me think it is true that people will negatively evaluate me. I can't simply tell myself it won't happen, because it does.
Dr. Weir:	People will be negatively evaluated sometimes. That is true. But perhaps if we look closely it may not be as often or with as much negative

Research indicates that certain antianxiety drugs or antidepressant drugs may also help reduce social fears for around 55% of social anxiety disorder clients (Rappaport et al., 2021; Neufeld et al., 2020). People treated with cognitive-behavioral therapy are less likely to later experience a relapse (Stein, 2020b).

judgment as your brain tells you. There is another evidence-based process for social anxiety that takes a different approach to dealing with anxious thinking. Acceptance-based strategies also work, and they don't involve checking the facts about the truth of worries. Instead, using these techniques, you would learn how to change the context of how you think, rather than trying to change the content of what you think. Like learning to distance yourself and get perspective on your thoughts and internal experiences, letting go of needing to play tug of war with their truth.

Xian: That sounds like mindfulness. I am familiar with this concept.

Dr. Weir: I appreciate that feedback. If this is something that you are more open to, we can use this approach instead of cognitive reappraisal. Acceptance-based interventions in CBTs are used around the world to help people. And they do relate to the practice of mindfulness.

Xian: I think I would like to try that approach first.

Dr. Weir: OK, we will do that. The other core process I wanted to talk about us using is something that is called exposure therapy.

Xian: I was afraid you were going to say that. I have read about it. I read that exposure therapy means you would make me face my fears to get over them. But I don't think that will work. I have tried to face my fears. It didn't help.

Dr. Weir: I totally understand. You're right. It isn't easy. If it were, people would be able to do it on their own without the help of professionals. It's more complicated than the way you are describing it. Exposure therapies are a group of interventions that help people learn new associations, change expectations and assumptions, and be less emotionally distressed when encountering people, places, and things related to social anxiety. It's safe, structured, and systematic. It's not like what you may have heard. If I was trying to help you learn how to overcome fears of swimming, I would not throw you into the deep end of the ocean. We would go gradually, using a hierarchy of cues or situations that led to anxiety, starting with the least anxiety provoking and easiest, allowing you to safely learn to swim, or, in your case, to do the things you have been avoiding socially. The more you gradually and safely approach avoided cues and situations, and the more you do it in lots of different situations, the more exposure-based approaches should help your anxiety go down. Just as important, you should be able to stay in social situations more, fully participate in them, and prevent adverse consequences of escape and avoidance in school or any social situations.

Xian: I get it. But it makes me nervous.

> Exposure therapy has also been successfully applied in cases of phobia, panic disorder, obsessive-compulsive disorder, and PTSD, among other psychological disorders.

Dr. Weir: If it didn't make you nervous, it wouldn't be something that we need to do in therapy together. I'd like us to talk more about this next time we meet. Exposure will be a behavioral intervention that should change how you feel and also how you think about these feared social situations. The mindfulness and acceptance-based interventions we do will help you develop a new and more flexible way of having perspective on how you think and feel. Both the cognitive and behavioral interventions will equally focus on helping you live a life consistent with your values. That way, everything we do together will help you take steps toward living in a way that is true to your heart, true to the person you want to be, so that even if you have anxiety you still are able to do the things you care about the most and be as effective as possible in your school life, work life, and in relationships. Does that make sense?

Xian: Yes. I think so. But I am still nervous.

Dr. Weir: As long as you come to therapy and do the home practice, your anxiety and the way you make sense of your anxiety should change. And, even when you have anxiety, the work we do will help you take actions and make decisions that are the ones you care about the most, despite anxiety.

Session 3   Dr. Weir attempted to understand Xian's core values across different domains of her life (for example, romantic relationships, family, friends, career, physical well-being), how consistently she was living within her values across these different valued areas, and what was getting in the way of these values. They determined together that her social anxiety was preventing her from being authentic and honest with people who she wanted to befriend. Her worries about being negatively evaluated were triggering escape and avoidance behavior that kept her from exploring and experiencing new foods, local parks, and museums, all things that were consistent with her values of being curious, open-minded, and educated about culture and history. They acknowledged that her worrying thoughts regularly lead to her negatively judging herself and her ability to have a romantic partner, despite her value to be openly loving with someone. This last valued action was something Xian had thought about but never told anyone. It surprised her that she felt safe enough to tell Dr. Weir.

After clarifying values and how social anxiety interfered with her valued actions, Dr. Weir oriented her again to the role of mindfulness and acceptance, confirmed that this was what Xian wanted to learn, and told her they would do this work first then begin exposure-based procedures. Xian felt excited that she was trusting Dr. Weir, and they problem-solved how she could monitor her valued actions during the week, in order to look for any other areas of her life that social anxiety was interfering in.

Sessions 4 and 5 The next two sessions were devoted to teaching Xian some specific skills that would help her with what Dr. Weir called *psychological flexibility*. He taught her about mindfulness and cognitive defusion, which is the practice of separating one's sense of self from one's thoughts; then they practiced these concepts. Dr. Weir emphasized that talking about mindfulness and defusion is antithetical to doing mindfulness and defusion. He answered some of her questions but continually steered them back to various behavioral practices. Mindfulness techniques included an awareness exercise that led to Xian learning to silently, with her eyes closed, practice noticing different sensations in her body and thoughts, all as they occurred one at a time, like cars passing by on a busy highway. She noticed how to observe and then describe these sensations and thoughts without getting attached to the truth of the thoughts. She learned how to experience her thoughts with the perspective that her thoughts were not necessarily true, but were learned reactions to certain things that triggered them. Dr. Weir helped her put this into practice by observing her thoughts simply as experiences she had, rather than things that defined her. She learned to separate herself from her thoughts, undoing the learned fusion of her thoughts and sense of self. At the end of each session, Dr. Weir assigned Xian home practices, this time various daily mindfulness practices like the ones she was learning in the therapy sessions.

Sessions 6 to 9 During these sessions, Dr. Weir used exposure-based procedures. First, they constructed a fear hierarchy. Xian used a worksheet to write out a detailed hierarchy of people, places, things, and internal experiences (for example, thoughts about meeting people or having a boyfriend) that caused her to feel anxious and avoid social situations. They discussed the list together and added several items to make it quite long and thorough. Each item had a subjective units of distress (SUDs) rating from 1 (minimal) to 10 (most in her lifetime). After constructing the hierarchy, Xian was asked to gradually approach the lowest and least distressing items. Every day, Xian used a worksheet to approach items in her hierarchy. She rated her distress before, during, and after exposure to each item, and did this repeatedly. Because they had worked previously on using mindfulness and defusion skills, she also practiced mindfulness each day and rated her ability to observe the thoughts she had during exposures without accepting them as truths or as part of her identity.

During the session, they would practice exposure by having Xian imagine, rehearse, or role-play social scenarios on her fear hierarchy. Dr. Weir would assess her SUDs before, during, and after all of these exposure practices. She practiced

In addition to exposure-based treatment and other cognitive-behavioral procedures, some clients with social anxiety disorder may also benefit from social skills training groups to help them develop better social skills and perform effectively in social situations (Pina et al., 2020; Olivares-Olivares, Ortiz-Gonzalez, & Olivares, 2019).

looking directly in Dr. Weir's eyes as she role-played meeting a new friend, initiating conversation with an imaginary person on a date, and talking with a new friend about her fears and insecurities. Xian gradually learned through this process that the things she was most afraid of were unlikely to happen. She was feeling the beginning of newfound social confidence. And the mindfulness and defusion helped her deal with her worried thoughts about doing the exposures. They were only thoughts, not truths, and she was beginning to see the difference. True, each time she did exposures she felt anxious, but she was starting to see that even if she felt anxious, she could still approach and not avoid the things that were on her fear hierarchy.

By week 9, the top of the hierarchy was in sight, and in the last week of home practice she approached her most feared situation. She, Mara, and Ander had dinner together. And Xian, despite her biggest fear that she would be rejected and ostracized, shared with Ander how she felt unsure of her future, unsure of whether she would ever get married, and worried about whether she would ever be successful as a neuroscientist. To her surprise, Ander was compassionate and easily related these experiences to his own and to almost everyone he knew. He told her funny stories about his own insecurities. He told her how he had been in therapy for depression, and he joked about how everyone in Denmark is probably depressed but they don't know it because it is too cold most of the year and they are too busy trying to stay warm. He even suggested she come meet some of his friends, and told her about a friend of his who was single and who she might want to meet sometime to see if they hit it off. Xian's SUDs were as high as an 8 at one point, but by the end of the dinner she felt relieved that her SUDs had gone down to 4. She went home and tried to notice how her appraisals of the dinner were neither true nor untrue, but simply thoughts that she, as an observer of her mind, could notice as ephemeral experiences that would come and go without controlling her actions. She texted Mara and told her she wanted to get together again for dinner. And, to her delightful surprise, she impulsively asked to meet Ander's friend next time. Mara wrote back, texting hugs and heart emojis.

Session 10 Xian had completed a brief process-based CBT approach. She completed a self-report assessment of functioning and symptoms, and with Dr. Weir compared her results to her pre-treatment scores. She had improved. They reviewed her home practice data each week. There were ups and downs in her SUDs across weeks, but the trend was down in her peak SUDs over time. The exposures were not eliciting as much distress as they used to. They reviewed her mindfulness and defusion skills and how they helped her. And they talked about the expectations for possible relapse of social anxiety, and how she could come back to therapy for booster visits in the future.

Assessment Questions

1. What characteristics did Xian have as a child that are common in individuals who develop social anxiety disorder?

2. At what age do most cases of social anxiety disorder emerge?

3. What patterns of Xian's behavior were examples of negative reinforcement?

4. How did Xian's anxiety and related behavior affect her relationship with her friend Mara?

5. What kinds of biological and childhood factors have been linked in research to social anxiety disorder?

6. Describe the processes used in this cognitive-behavioral approach to treatment for social anxiety disorder.

7. According to research, how helpful is cognitive-behavioral therapy for people with social anxiety disorder?

8. List some of the beliefs Xian had about social situations that were at the core of her social anxiety disorder.

9. What principles of behavior change did Xian's therapist use to help her overcome social anxiety?

CASE 4

Posttraumatic Stress Disorder

Table 4-1

Dx Checklist

Posttraumatic Stress Disorder

1. Person is exposed to a traumatic event—death or threatened death, severe injury, or sexual violation.

2. Person experiences at least 1 of the following intrusive symptoms: • Repeated, uncontrolled, and distressing memories • Repeated and upsetting trauma-linked dreams • Dissociative experiences such as flashbacks • Significant upset when exposed to trauma-linked cues • Pronounced physical reactions when reminded of the event(s).

3. Person continually avoids trauma-linked stimuli.

4. Person experiences negative changes in trauma-linked cognitions and moods, such as being unable to remember key features of the event(s) or experiencing repeated negative emotions.

5. Person displays conspicuous changes in arousal and reactivity, such as excessive alertness, extreme startle responses, or sleep disturbances.

6. Person experiences significant distress or impairment, with symptoms lasting more than a month.

(Information from APA, 2022, 2013.)

At age 35, Julie, a new assistant professor of communication, had finally, after changing careers in her 20s and receiving her Ph.D, begun to live the life she had always envisioned. She was an energetic and outgoing woman, a social butterfly who enjoyed long talks with friends, traveling to the backcountry of exotic places on the cheap, and trying new foods. Having been raised in the exurbs outside Washington, DC, she considered herself somewhat of a city girl. She knew how to be in the city, how to be safe, to explore, to have fun, and then to return to the predictability and familiarity of home. But she didn't feel entirely safe in the city.

Her first job was in the suburbs of DC, on the Virginia side, working for a large consulting firm. She hated it. It was good money, sure, but for what? To help companies make decisions about how to maximize profits by "reallocating resources"? Firing people, she used to tell her friends over drinks in the corporate chain cookie cutter bars after work. I get paid to give CEOs spreadsheets and slide decks that they use to fire hard working employees. Nah. No thanks. After receiving her doctorate, Julie had moved to a small college town in North Carolina for her first job as a professor. Unlike her job as a consultant, teaching was very rewarding. She

Women are more likely than men to develop a stress disorder. About 20% of women who are exposed to a severe trauma develop such a disorder, compared to 8% of men (Carroll & Banks, 2020; Tortella-Feliu et al., 2019).

loved the feel of campus life and the rhythm and pulse each day. And she loved her students. Her favorite moments, the ones she would talk about endlessly with joy and optimism, happened when her students found themselves with a sense of purpose and meaning. She didn't care in which newfound direction they were headed, as long as she could see the spark ignite within them, something she herself had wished she could have felt as an undergraduate.

Julie A Bright Future

As a child, Julie had grown up free of any physical or mental health problems. Her parents, however, had not been so lucky. Julie's African American father, Roger, spent his childhood and adolescence in Alabama during the civil rights movement. During his senior year of high school, Roger began protesting in nonviolent marches and attending meetings with local leaders designed to plan solutions in the fight for social justice. As he would tell Julie many years later, during these years Roger had been in many, many situations where he feared for his life.

At age 14, Roger was the youngest of his friends to join the men from his neighborhood in protests outside the county courthouse. The first time he stood in the crowd, he knew he belonged. It was scary, but he felt like he had found purpose in standing for something bigger than himself. He would recount to Julie the pride he felt standing in awe listening to the reverend exhort the crowd of mostly young, Black men to stay strong, to believe in their cause, and to remain nonviolent. Every chance he could find, Roger attended events in support of the cause. It also put him at risk for being a victim of violence. By the time he was 15, he had been chased, grabbed, and shoved to the ground by the counterprotesting white men. When he was 16, he watched his friend's older brother get badly beaten and left to die by two men, their steel-toed boots breaking his ribs and brass-knuckled fists bloodying his face. Even as an older man, Roger wept as he recalled the details of this memory to Julie. He never forgot a moment of it. The smell of asphalt in the summer heat, the thick humid air, a driver honking their horn in delight after slowing to watch the gruesome scene. Roger had wanted to help, but he froze. He had stood behind a tree, alone, frantically turning his head every which way, looking for help, fearing he would be next. Sadly, this was only one of many violent incidents Roger had witnessed firsthand. By the time he moved north to Virginia and married Julie's mom Sandy, Roger had been exposed to no less than a dozen traumatic experiences. Roger had accumulated many emotional scars—stories he would share with Julie—that would impact him the rest of his life.

As Julie grew up, she heard her father's stories many times. Roger wanted her to know her family history, the struggles and sacrifice before her, who *he* was, so she too could bring focus and passion to the things that mattered most to her.

He had been significantly affected by what he witnessed. He felt survivor's guilt, wondering aloud why he was never the victim of violence. He witnessed horrific things happen, but he had never been physically injured directly. He told Julie these stories again and again. True to the nature of flashbulb memories, his stories had remarkable clarity and consistency. Details had been preserved in defiance of the distortions common to autobiographical memory.

Julie knew the parts he was most proud of, the ways he stood strong and firm, unwavering in his convictions during a tumultuous time of social and moral upheaval, and she felt inspired to do something meaningful with her own life. She also knew the parts of the stories that he was most sad about: all the loss, devastation, trauma, and imminent fear for his life. She felt these parts of his memories most profoundly. When he would talk about seeing his friend shot at, Julie could see it the way her dad would describe it and feel what he felt. Sometimes she would get so lost listening to his stories that she would forget where she was, practically feeling like she had traveled back in time to bear witness to the very same violence Roger had experienced. Sometimes she wished she could have been there with him. She loved her father so much it hurt to see him continue to be deeply affected by the events of his life so many years ago.

At the university, she threw herself wholeheartedly into her career, devoting her life to teaching, research, and writing. Her intense involvement in her work was obvious to those around her. Within her first few months, her colleagues were commenting about how much harder she worked than they did. They were playful about it, but it was clear to Julie that she was working long devoted hours as a new professor. It was a lot of fun, and she was beginning to make friends along the way. This was no surprise. Julie had always been sociable and made friends easily.

With her life taking shape as she had hoped, Julie was feeling excited about her future. She missed her family and friends back in DC, but she was making a new life for herself in North Carolina. She tried the local barbeque, Eastern-style with a balance of vinegar to offset sweetness. She frequented the farmer's market in the town center. She went out with friends to sample the local music scene, taking in unfamiliar singer-songwriters and acoustic sets with blissful lyrics that—along with a drink or two in her system—gave her a sense that she was on the right path. She was going to do what she had wanted since her miserable days as a new consultant. She was going to inspire others. Over time, her colleagues and students became like her family. Sensing her devotion, students packed her classes and requested her as an advisor. She won a teaching award in only her second year at the university, in near record time for a new professor. Everything was going so well for her. But one night, she was struck by a catastrophe that took her life and state of mind in a direction that she could never have anticipated or imagined.

Hispanic Americans, Black Americans, and American Indians are more likely than non-Hispanic white Americans to develop a stress disorder after confronting a severe trauma (Ellickson-Larew et al., 2020). The reason for this racial–ethnic difference is not clear.

People who have greater difficulty tolerating uncertainty in life and those who generally view life's negative events as beyond their control seem more prone to develop a stress disorder when confronted with a traumatic event (McGuire et al., 2021; Hancock & Bryant, 2020; Leonard, 2019). Nevertheless, even people like Julie, who have hardy attitudes and personalities, may develop a stress disorder.

Julie Disaster Strikes

Julie was walking back to her car after a night out with friends in a nearby town. She had parked a few blocks away from the bar where they had finished the night, but she thought she would be fine walking back on her own. After all, she had plenty of experience looking after herself in DC; she shouldn't have any trouble in this small city in North Carolina. She walked briskly toward her car, keeping a vigilant eye on her surroundings. It was darker than she expected, and eerily quiet, and she even noticed some signs of vandalism. She unconsciously picked up her pace as she got closer to where her car was parked. As she got into her car and quickly locked the door behind her, she breathed deeply and felt a surge of adrenaline. She was more scared than she had realized but was starting to relax now that she was on her way home.

As she drove to the first red light, she saw two men in what seemed to be a heated argument enter the crosswalk. To her alarm, they stopped right in the middle of the road, yelling and gesticulating wildly, pointing and angrily posturing toward each other. Julie froze. They didn't seem to even notice her, but she instinctively feared for her life. She wanted to honk but feared this would turn their aggression toward her. Time seemed to slow down dramatically as she saw two other men rapidly approaching from behind her car. Seconds later, she heard gunshots, five bangs that seemed impossibly loud. As the light turned green, the two men in front of her ran off into the night, and the others ran past her car, their shouts and cursing reaching her through the sound of her music. It was total chaos. The light turned red again, and she hadn't even moved. Without thinking, she hit the accelerator and sped away. She went a few miles out of town and onto the highway, then started to weep.

She was horrified. What if she had been shot? What if she was bleeding to death and no one could reach her? What if they had carjacked her? Held her hostage? She was so overwhelmed with fear that she did not even stop to assess whether she had in fact been hit by the gunfire. She didn't feel anything, but she also knew that if she had been shot, she might not immediately feel it. She knew she was alive, and she felt lucky.

When she got home, she called the police, and they arrived to take her statement and begin an investigation. While waiting, she checked her car and saw that it had been hit by gunfire. A bullet had passed through the rear quarter panel, missing the gas tank but going through her back seat. She felt numb. She could have been killed if the shooter had moved his arm just a little bit in a different direction. Her hands started to tremble, and she felt like she couldn't breathe. Everything she had worked for, all of it, could have been lost in a blink. She sat on the curb waiting for the police and sobbed. She tried to call her parents, but they didn't answer. She texted her friend from work. No response. It was chilly, and she started to shiver. When the police arrived, they could tell she was very upset.

Generally, the more severe or prolonged the trauma and the more direct one's exposure to it, the greater the likelihood of developing a stress disorder (Hyland et al., 2020, 2017).

They took their time with her, and Julie told them everything in as much detail as she could.

After about 15 minutes of gentle questioning, she realized they were starting to ask her questions that made her feel a bit uncomfortable. "What were you doing in that part of town, ma'am?" She was out with friends. "Why were you alone then, at that time of night, in that part of town?" She told them she had walked to where her car was parked, and that this was the closest parking available when she went to meet her friends earlier in the night. "Ma'am," they kept calling her in a way that felt dehumanizing, "if you don't mind, we'd like to take you in to ask you some more questions." It turned out that there was a major problem with drug trafficking in that part of town, and the police wanted to know if Julie was involved. She was shocked and angry. "I was out with friends," she reiterated, "I was just driving home. You think I had something to do with drug trafficking and the shootings?" She was now becoming agitated. "With all due respect, would you ask the same questions of someone who didn't have brown skin like me?" The police began to escalate in return, telling her to calm down. "Ma'am, we are asking standard questions we would ask anyone to understand the nature of the events that transpired." She repeated everything she knew and had already told them. "OK, ma'am," they said, "thank you for your time and we are so sorry for what happened to you." She was very upset; she had almost died, and instead of the compassionate help she had expected, she felt like she was being blamed or accused.

Before the police left, they told her they might come back the next day to ask some more questions. She spent the next 3 hours in a highly anxious state compounded by confusion and anger about the way the police had questioned her. She ruminated about calling a lawyer or going to the local news media. She couldn't sleep that night, and in the morning, she finally talked to her parents and a friend about what happened. They were emotionally supportive and were equally aghast at her description of the police questioning her.

Julie was relieved to be talking to people about what happened. She felt loved and understood by her family and friends. Still, she felt overwhelmed and exhausted. She couldn't imagine how she could ever get over the experience. Could she ever go out at night again? Could she trust that the police were on her side? What if the drug traffickers found out who she was and came after her? These thoughts spawned others, and her mind raced anxiously, tears uncontrollably streaming in between bursts of anger.

> Persons treated with dignity and respect by the criminal justice system after they experience a severe trauma such as robbery, shooting, or rape tend to have more successful psychological recoveries from their ordeals (Palmer, Scott, & Ting, 2020).

Julie Aftermath of the Trauma

In the weeks after the traumatic event, Julie had difficulties with sleeping, intrusive memories and nightmares interfering with her ability to get a good night's rest.

She was jumpy and hyperattentive to her environment whenever she left her home. Driving was difficult, even after her car was repaired and she no longer had to look at the bullet hole in her car. She took a week off from work to help her adjust at her friend and colleague's recommendation. During that week, she hardly thought at all about work, obsessively reading the local news and searching for information about the drug trafficking problems in the nearby city.

Her friends were sympathetic, and as time went on they kept asking her if she needed anything. But oddly, Julie found it difficult to answer their questions. What *did* she need, she wondered? She wished for it all to have never happened. She wished to never have to think about it again. She told her friends she wanted to talk about other things. She hated the blend of feelings she felt whenever she was reminded about her traumatic event. Her experience was becoming jumbled in her mind, and explaining it again and again required considerable effort. It was tiring just to talk for a few minutes about it. She talked to her father almost every day. He listened and shared his own stories of being treated unfairly by the police when he was younger. But after a month had passed and she still was struggling to return to her normal functioning, her dad told her she needed to get help from a professional. Julie felt relieved to hear that from him and decided to take his advice.

Julie Drifts Away A Friend's Perspective

During the weeks immediately following the event, Julie regularly talked on the phone to her friend Veronica, whom she affectionately called "Vee," sharing her experience. Vee was supportive at first, but over time came to dread her daily text messages and phone calls from Julie. In a later conversation with her sister, Vee tried to explain such a reaction and to describe the course that her relationship with Julie had gone in the time following the event.

"At first I hung on every word, trying to grasp the horror that had befallen her. I worried about her terribly, wanted to help her through this, wanted to be there for her. But after a few weeks our conversations all sounded the same. No matter what we talked about, Julie found a way of turning the discussion back to her situation and her emotions. If I told her about a funny YouTube channel I found, she would keep talking about the police or the problem with drugs in the area. Then she'd tell me for the 50th time how dangerous it can be to drive alone at night, how many crimes are committed in this part of the state, or some other tale of fear and crime. Eventually I felt unimportant to her, just an excuse to describe the danger she now saw everywhere. Sometimes, it didn't even seem as if she was even talking to me—just reciting her fears and anger out loud. It didn't matter that I was her friend—anyone would have done fine. Like I was an object to her. An ear to talk at and not a person who had her own things to talk about. It got

If a person's stress symptoms begin within 4 weeks of the traumatic event and last for less than a month, a diagnosis of *acute stress disorder* is appropriate. If the symptoms continue longer than a month, a diagnosis of *posttraumatic stress disorder* is appropriate. Many cases of acute stress disorder develop into posttraumatic stress disorder.

annoying real quick. Once I realized what was happening, I would try to divert her attention from these topics. I would offer gossip about someone at the university, bring up items from the news, or recall a funny or interesting event from past times. Nothing. Julie showed no interest in anything except her newfound fears.

"I would try to make plans to see her in person, rather than just talk on the phone. Julie would not consider going out to a restaurant or movie; however, she would 'let' me come over to visit her. Of course, during these visits we would just wind up talking about her fears again. Over time, the visits became shorter and shorter. Finally, I began to feel like a delivery person. Julie would 'allow' me to take groceries to her or to pick up some laundry from the cleaners. Our whole relationship became empty and superficial. I tried letting her talk about her fears; I tried not letting her talk about her fears. But nothing seemed to help. In time, it became a moot point, because Julie pushed me out of her life.

"By 3 months after the shooting, she had stopped calling me and would only occasionally answer my calls. Our communications were brief and very superficial, as if Julie couldn't wait for them to end. She seemed very fearful over what had happened to her and, worse, over what might happen to her in the future. Loving her, I truly felt for her. But she also seemed to become increasingly angry, nasty, and cynical, not at all the friendly and warm woman I have known. She acted as if she blamed me—I'm not sure for what—perhaps for not having gone through the same ordeal or maybe for not seeming to care enough or to do enough now. All I know is that after a while conversations or interactions with me seemed to further agitate Julie. If I suggested that she see her doctor again or gave her advice, she would act like I was bothering her and sticking my nose where it didn't belong. So I pretty much stopped. I stopped making suggestions or trying to coax her back into the world. It seemed easier for Julie that way; it was certainly easier for me.

"You know, in an odd way, I feel like I was a victim too. For the most part, I have lost my friend. I have been forced to stand by and watch her drift away. This warm, energetic, and fun woman who added so much love to my life has been replaced by a stranger—an obsessive, self-centered, angry woman—who seems to resent me and wants little to do with me. I am just so frustrated and sad and a little angry as well, I guess. For now, Julie and I have an implicit understanding to keep some distance between us."

Julie in Treatment Challenging her Fears

Over the next few months, Julie's life became more isolated. Her fearfulness did not improve, and her outdoor activities remained restricted to what she considered safe situations, although nothing felt completely safe. At her annual physical exam, she completed a set of standard screening questionnaires before meeting with her doctor. They included questions about her physical and mental health.

> Research indicates that people whose social and family support systems are weak are more likely than people with stronger support systems (caring, empathic, loving) to develop PTSD after a traumatic event (Sareen, 2021; Cowan et al., 2020).

Several of the questions asked if she had experienced an event in the past year that was traumatic, or where she worried that her life was in danger. When the doctor met with her, she asked Julie about these questionnaire items. Julie told her what happened. As she did, her countenance vacillated from angry to scared, and she voiced thoughts about her future that sounded hopeless. She told the doctor that she had been feeling numb and less interested in work or spending time with friends since the event. She told her about her difficulties with nightmares and her avoidance of people, places, and things associated with the event. She also shared her lingering anger toward the police. Even though they never did come back for more questions, she felt mistreated and blamed. Soon realizing that her patient was in need of psychological help outside the doctor's expertise, the physician suggested that Julie make an appointment with John Barlow, a licensed professional counselor affiliated with her medical practice who was an expert in posttraumatic stress disorder, just to discuss her situation and see if the counselor had any helpful suggestions about what to do. He was very experienced, she learned, and easy to talk to. The doctor described him as someone who has a special way with words. Julie trusted her physician. The next morning, after yet another fitful night's sleep, she decided to call Mr. Barlow.

At the counselor's office, Julie recounted her "nightmare experience" and how her life had unraveled overnight. She told Mr. Barlow that on the one hand, she felt that her current state was an understandable result for anyone undergoing such a horrifying experience. But on the other hand, given her previous level of functioning, she would not have expected to be so completely undone by what she knew objectively to be a fairly random event. Her whole identity had been consumed by this event and its aftermath. She felt like a different person.

After listening to Julie's story, Mr. Barlow concluded that her condition met the DSM-5-TR criteria for posttraumatic stress disorder (PTSD). First, she had been exposed to a traumatic event that posed a threat of death or serious injury; moreover, her response to the event entailed intense fear. Second, the traumatic event was followed by months of intrusive symptoms — in Julie's case, in the form of intrusive recollections and intense psychological distress in response to cues that resembled the original trauma (neighborhoods, stoplights, traffic, and strangers on the street). Third, Julie persistently avoided stimuli associated with the trauma and experienced numbing (in the form of diminished interest or participation in activities and the sense of a foreshortened future). Fourth, she exhibited persistent negative emotions and a significant change in her own thoughts about herself and the dangers of the world. Finally, Julie also exhibited increased arousal, including sleep difficulties, hypervigilance, and exaggerated startle response. This had been going on for many months now, and her functioning had been greatly impaired as a result. Mr. Barlow believed that Julie had developed an acute stress disorder in the immediate aftermath of the traumatic

At least half of all people with a stress disorder seek treatment, but relatively few do so initially (Korte et al., 2020).

About 3.5% to 6% of people in North America have acute or posttraumatic stress disorder in any given year; 7% to 12% have one of these disorders during their lifetimes (Sareen, 2021; ADAA, 2020).

event but that as her early symptoms continued and even intensified after the first month, she now had PTSD.

A specialist in stress disorders, Mr. Barlow knew that there were two kinds of cognitive-behavioral therapy (CBT) with a strong evidence base to treat PTSD. Although both were in the same CBT category, one was more behavioral and the other more focused on cognitive change. The behavioral approach, called pro-longed exposure, involves exposing the person—using *in vivo* exposure (that is, actual exposure) and *imaginal* exposure—to anxiety-provoking but safe stimuli. The cognitive approach, called cognitive processing therapy, guides the individual to identify ways that the trauma has impacted different areas of her life and to identify and change ways of thinking that are disrupting daily functioning. Both treatments could work well, and Mr. Barlow offered them both as options to Julie.

In vivo exposure is used to help clients react less fearfully to stimuli and events around them. The in vivo exposure procedure for the client with PTSD is similar to that used with other anxiety disorders, such as phobias. A hierarchy of anxiety-provoking situations, ranging from the least to most threatening, is constructed by the client and therapist. The individual is then given assignments to enter these situations and to remain there for a time, usually until the person has a significant drop in anxiety or a sufficient amount of time has passed. The therapist generally has the individual repeat the exposures on several occasions until a tolerable level of anxiety is achieved during the exposure. Such exposure assignments proceed up the hierarchy until the most threatening item is mastered.

Imaginal exposure is used to help clients with PTSD react less fearfully when recalling the original trauma. The individual repeatedly visualizes the entire sequence of events involved in the trauma for a long period. In visualization exer-cises, the client usually produces and then listens to a lengthy recorded descrip-tion of the trauma. The purpose of the exposure is to desensitize the client to the memory of the trauma in the same manner that someone would be desensitized to any phobic object through repeated exposure. In essence, the meaning of the traumatic memory as a danger signal is changed by the exposure, and it eventually stops producing a sense of threat. Ultimately, the traumatic memory can be readily integrated like any other long-term memory.

Cognitive processing therapy, which more directly challenges the accuracy of the individual's negative cognitions, brings about changes in the reactions of persons with PTSD in a different way. A client might be guided to write down an *impact statement*—a detailed description of the various ways the traumatic event has affected their life— and then over time to discover how broad, trauma-related themes may be pervading their daily experiences. The themes may focus on power, self-esteem, trust, safety, and intimacy, for example. "In your case," Mr. Barlow told Julie, "you have been having a lot of thoughts and reactions to everyday cues as though they are unsafe. In cognitive processing therapy, you

Some studies indicate that exposure may be the single most helpful intervention for people with PTSD (Peterson et al., 2020; Stein, 2020a).

might learn to practice less catastrophic, less self-damaging interpretations of daily events." Julie asked questions and then told Mr. Barlow that she wanted the best of both treatments. She wanted to work on the exposures but also wanted help with changing her ways of thinking. Mr. Barlow was trained in each approach and agreed that they could do a CBT-based treatment that included both exposure and cognitive processing. Under his care, Julie embarked on a treatment program that extended over 19 sessions.

Session 1   In the first session, Julie described the anxiety she had been feeling over the past months. She also described the traumatic event and its aftermath. She explained that the feelings resulting from that experience — mainly the fear of injury or attack — seemed to have colored her entire approach to life. "I just can't seem to get past this horrible experience. This is not me. It's like I've become somebody else. I've got to get my old self back."

Mr. Barlow said he was optimistic that Julie would be able to get back to her former self. He explained that she had PTSD, a constellation of symptoms that arises following an intensely frightening experience where one's life is immediately jeopardized. He also explained that after such an event most people go through a stressful period in which they feel especially vulnerable.

The counselor then outlined the basic treatment strategy. He said one component of the treatment would be to survey all of the different ways in which Julie's life had been changed by her current fears and anxieties, paying particular attention to curtailed activities. Then the two of them would arrange the activities along a scale ranging from the least to the most threatening. Together, they would construct weekly exercises in which Julie would enter — expose herself to — the situations she was avoiding, according to carefully specified procedures. Mr. Barlow explained that Julie's anxiety should ultimately improve after she repeatedly entered situations for specified durations and frequencies each week.

The second component of treatment, the counselor explained, also involved exposure, but in this case, exposure to the traumatic memory itself. He noted that the memory of the trauma was provoking a strong emotional reaction in Julie, and as long as this was the case, it would intrude on both her waking and her sleeping life. He indicated that the emotional reaction provoked by the traumatic memory could be reduced by prolonged exposure to the memory itself.

Julie was puzzled by the logic of this approach. She remarked that she already was repeatedly exposed to the traumatic memory; indeed, it seemed to intrude numerous times each day, but her emotional reaction remained as strong as ever. Mr. Barlow noted that with these naturally occurring intrusions, the exposure often lasts only a few minutes; in addition, people are inclined to block out some of the more disturbing elements of the intrusion. The counselor explained that in general, improvement occurred with prolonged exposure, perhaps as long as 45

Increasingly, a number of cognitive-behavioral therapists are including *mindfulness* interventions to further help clients with PTSD become more accepting and less judgmental of their recurring thoughts, feelings, and memories (Desormeau et al., 2020).

Research suggests that for clients who can stay with the intense memory exercises of prolonged exposure treatment (many cannot), that intervention is typically more helpful than gradual exposure interventions (Riggs et al., 2020; Sherrill et al., 2020).

to 60 minutes at a time, and only when all the elements, including the most disturbing ones, were faced.

For the coming week, he asked Julie to start monitoring her feelings and behavior. She was to note particularly any instances of fear and anxiety, including the circumstances that provoked the anxious reaction and any associated thoughts. In addition, the counselor asked Julie to start taking note of the various activities she was avoiding, so that he and she could begin constructing a series of in vivo behavioral exposure exercises.

Session 2   Julie began the next session by reporting that she had not kept any of the requested records. She explained that she was focused on work and getting back to her normal routines again. She went on to tell the counselor how she had too little time in the day to do the therapy homework. Mr. Barlow suggested that avoidance is a common problem in any therapy for PTSD, and that her mind would come up with reasons to avoid doing the exposures because they were eliciting fear, even though there was nothing dangerous that was being suggested in the exposures.

Julie understood and expressed concern that her avoidance behavior might prevent her from proceeding at a reasonable pace with in vivo exercises (that is, doing things she had been avoiding). Maybe she should do therapy another time, she mused. Mr. Barlow stayed firm. It was decided that for the time being, greater emphasis should be given to the imaginal exposure and that the next session would be devoted to discussing the traumatic event in more detail. Still, Julie would try a couple of brief shopping trips in the coming week if she felt physically capable.

They also began to explore how her traumatic experience had affected her life. She was asked to write an impact statement describing how the experience had changed the ways in which she thought about herself, others, and her future. First, she was asked to consider how the event had been influencing her day-to-day functioning. Then they uncovered the broad themes tied to these daily reactions, including how she thinks about issues of safety, trust, self-esteem and control. Julie acknowledged that she felt chronically unsafe, less trusting of people in authority, and less confident and hopeful about her life, and she sensed that she now had less control in her life more generally. They discussed how these themes would be explored and she would come to challenge thoughts that might be related to themes and interfering with her life, things he called "stuck points." Identifying and challenging trauma-related stuck points would, over time, become a central component of the CBT approach they used to treat her PTSD.

Session 3   Mr. Barlow asked Julie to relate the details of her traumatic episode, including the event and its aftermath with the police. Mr. Barlow made a recording of Julie as she began describing the episode matter-of-factly. She soon closed

---

Many clients with a stress disorder are also given antidepressant drugs (Duek et al., 2021; Stein, 2021, 2020a). Typically these drugs are relatively helpful for the symptoms of increased arousal and negative emotions and less helpful for recurrent negative memories and avoidance behaviors.

her eyes in a trancelike fashion, as if trying to focus her efforts on an intensely painful task. She then described the whole episode in a detailed monologue lasting approximately 45 minutes. She included rich sensory details and used first-person tense.

When she had finished, Julie appeared fatigued. Mr. Barlow praised her for her tremendous effort in recounting those experiences. He then asked her to estimate her level of anxiety at its peak during the monologue and at the end of it, using a 0-to-10 scale. Julie assigned ratings of 8 and 5, respectively, indicating that some reduction of anxiety had occurred by the end of the monologue.

Session 4   Julie and the counselor listened to the recording together. While listening, Julie closed her eyes and, as instructed, tried to imagine the events as vividly as possible. This time, she said she seemed to have had some new insights. First, she said she now realized that one of the most troubling elements of the whole experience was the sense of loss of control—in this case, being at the mercy of the stoplight while the men were shooting and not being able to fend for herself. She drew a direct connection to her childhood experience hearing her dad talk about his own litany of traumatic experiences, which she had believed could happen to her one day. She also realized that the event itself followed by the experience with the police had challenged her sense of normalcy and safety in her new hometown, a place that she had believed was safe. She felt sadness, loss, and anger about everything that she was losing.

Mr. Barlow tried to offer Julie a means of viewing the experience in a less negative fashion, suggesting that occasional episodes of loss of control are a normal part of life and that people are not necessarily diminished or demeaned by their occurrence. On hearing this, Julie seemed tentatively prepared to accept the idea. She said she could now see how it might be possible to view the recent shooting event in a similar light.

Sessions 5 to 8   During the next 4 weeks, Julie was instructed to listen to the recording almost every day. She recorded her peak anxiety level for about half of these imaginal exposures. Julie's anxiety level declined progressively, and by the end of the fourth week, her anxiety reaction to the recording was virtually extinguished. Decided shifts in Julie's thinking accompanied these reductions in anxiety. After about 2 weeks, when her peak anxiety had lessened considerably, Julie told Mr. Barlow that listening to the recording was making her feel that many of her fears had been overblown. By the third week, when Julie's anxiety had decreased still further, she said that the reduction in anxiety seemed to be carrying over to other parts of her life. She had resumed taking drives through places that she had been avoiding, at first with friends and then alone; moreover, she said she felt much closer with her friends, who had remarked on and rejoiced over the improvement

Studies indicate that, even prior to confronting a severe trauma, people who later develop PTSD have overly reactive brain-body stress routes (the *sympathetic nervous system* and the *hypothalamic-pituitary-adrenal axis*). Then, after confrontations with a severe trauma, their brain-body stress routes become even more overly reactive (Lopez-Duran et al., 2020; Zakreski & Pruessner, 2020; Speer et al., 2019).

Some people with a stress disorder also benefit from group therapy, where they can discuss with other trauma survivors their lingering fears and other symptoms, their feelings of guilt or anger, and the impact that the trauma has had on their personal and social life.

in her spirits. Julie also observed that repeated listening to the recording had made her feel that the episode was "now part of my experience." The memory was no longer constantly "in the back of my mind"; nor did she feel compelled any longer to shut it out when she did think of it. In other words, its intrusive properties had been eliminated. By the eighth therapy session, Julie reported that she had actually fallen asleep during a couple of listenings, so relaxing had the recording become.

During these same 4 weeks, Julie also spontaneously began to take trips to the area near where the event happened, as well as to places that she hadn't visited since it occurred (again, first with friends and later on her own). At about the same time, her fear of people on the street also declined.

The counselor felt Julie no longer needed to listen to the recording at this point, suggesting that the most benefit would come from Julie increasing the range of her behavioral activities through in vivo exposure. The therapist and client designed a plan for Julie to approach trauma-related cues that she was still avoiding at least once per day.

Sessions 9 to 13   During these sessions, held over a 4-week period, the emphasis remained on the in vivo behavioral exercises. Julie continued to become more comfortable driving closer and closer to the exact place where the shooting had occurred. She was, however, still having problems trusting the police and kept asking what could be done in treatment about this ongoing distrust.

Although she still wished she had been treated more compassionately after the incident, Julie felt intellectually that the police were on her side. Still, she could easily become angered when she saw a police officer, and she wanted to change this reaction. Thus, Mr. Barlow suggested that perhaps this anxiety could be reduced through some exposure to police-related cues. They created a hierarchy and used in vivo exposure to gradually help her. The first step would be to drive to the police station and look at police cars and police-related cues for 45 minutes.

Sessions 14 and 15   Julie carried out the assignment and reported on the changes. It turned out that she was less anxious or angry than she expected. She felt some anxiety initially, but it went away after several times sitting outside the police station in the parking lot. She even got bored. They probed the kinds of thoughts she had about the police during the exposures, and used cognitive restructuring techniques to change these thoughts together.

Sessions 16 to 19   During these sessions, Julie and the counselor spent all of the time exploring how her thoughts about the trauma-related themes of safety, power, and trust were occurring in response to daily situations. They used worksheets to check the facts about these thoughts, and she learned how to reframe her assumptions and interpretations in a more flexible manner. In the final session, they reviewed her progress, made a plan for relapse prevention, and talked about her journey in treatment. She noted how much the home practice had helped her. She had grown comfortable talking to Mr. Barlow, sure, but it was the days between therapy sessions where the majority of her growth had occurred. Doing the exposure therapy first helped her know, through experience, that the automatic thoughts she had been having in reaction to the event-related cues and situations were not necessarily accurate. She had tools now to challenge these thoughts and not let them control her emotions. Her PTSD symptoms now were significantly reduced. Julie had benefitted from CBT.

Epilogue

After treatment ended, Mr. Barlow contacted Julie via electronic medical record 3 months later and learned she had continued to be free of PTSD symptoms. They scheduled a follow-up for one year to check in, and he offered her an appointment anytime in the interim.

> Interest in stress disorders intensified during the Vietnam War, when clinicians observed that increasing numbers of returning veterans were having flashbacks (intense recollections of combat traumas) and were generally alienated from everyday life.

Assessment Questions

1. What event precipitated Julie's posttraumatic stress disorder?

2. How do the brain-body stress routes of people with PTSD generally react to stress, both prior to and after their traumatic event?

3. Why do friends and relatives eventually distance themselves from a person who has had a traumatic incident?

4. Why did Julie finally decide to seek treatment?

5. Why was Julie diagnosed with posttraumatic stress disorder rather than acute stress disorder?

6. What modes of therapy did Mr. Barlow select to assist Julie with her disorder? Give an example of each type of therapy.

7. Early in treatment, Mr. Barlow outlined the various components of Julie's upcoming therapy. Describe those components.

8. What was the purpose of producing a recorded description of the traumatizing incident?

9. Why did Julie initially fail to take notes of her feared activities as part of her treatment plan? How did Mr. Barlow handle this problem in his session with Julie?

10. What other incident in Julie's early life may have contributed to her posttraumatic stress disorder?

11. What percentage of people with PTSD seek treatment?

CASE 5

Major Depressive Disorder

Table 5-1

Dx Checklist

Major Depressive Episode

1. For a 2-week period, person displays an increase in depressed mood for the majority of each day and/or a decrease in enjoyment or interest across most activities for the majority of each day.

2. For the same 2 weeks, person also experiences at least 3 or 4 of the following symptoms: • Considerable weight change or appetite change • Daily insomnia or hypersomnia • Daily agitation or decrease in motor activity • Daily fatigue or lethargy • Daily feelings of worthlessness or excessive guilt • Daily reduction in concentration or decisiveness • Repeated focus on death or suicide, a suicide plan, or a suicide attempt.

3. Significant distress or impairment.

Major Depressive Disorder

1. Presence of a major depressive episode.

2. No pattern of mania or hypomania.

(Information from APA, 2022, 2013.)

Phillip was born in 1973 in Chicago, Illinois, and grew up on the infamous South Side. His parents were both from Chicago and their parents, his maternal and paternal grandparents, had immigrated to the area from Ireland in the early twentieth century. Trained as a masonry worker, Phillip's father had worked from company to company in the industrial areas of the South and Southwest neighborhoods outside the city. When Phillip (who was always called Phil or Philly by his parents) was in middle school, his father got a job as a supervisor in a manufacturing facility on the West Side. It paid a salary, which was better than the other jobs, which had been hourly. His father worked hard to succeed as a supervisor in order to maintain the steady income and consistent schedule. For Phil and his three younger siblings, everything was better after their dad started this job. Before being a supervisor, the rent or bills might not get paid on time, the power could be turned off, and some days they went without enough food for family meals. Worse, Phil's parents would scream and yell, fighting about how there wasn't enough money to meet the family needs. It was a hard childhood, and one that Phil would later describe as "scarring."

Most people who are clinically depressed have *unipolar depression*; that is, they have no history of mania and return to a normal or nearly normal mood when their depression lifts. *Bipolar disorder*, in which people alternate between depression and mania, is the subject of Case 6.

Phillip A Mason's Child

Phil worked during high school under his dad's tutelage as a mason's apprentice, learning many of the fundamentals of the trade. As he learned he became proud of his skills, and enjoyed the time spent with his dad. Phil had come from a working-class neighborhood. Most of the kids he knew would not go on to college. Many of them didn't finish high school. Some of them would end up in prison or in and out of jail for various crimes born out of poor education, poverty, and lack of opportunity. Phil had been in fist fights, narrowly avoided dangerous crossfire from gangs, and witnessed people being beaten or robbed dozens of times by the time he was 16. After high school graduation, Phil began working in the masonry business full time, landing an entry level job at his dad's company. He helped move pallets of raw materials in the warehouse, cleaned machinery, and made sure all the tools were safely secured for his more senior coworkers to use successfully. It was a decades-old family company that sold supplies to builders, hardscapers, and contractors in the tri-state area. Phil's family assumed that he would make a career for himself in the masonry supply business. Only an average student in school, he couldn't imagine what would have become of him if he had had to make it on his own. He was proud to carry his load in the business and had aspirations to make a salary and one day have a family of his own.

At age 23, Phil married Scarlet, whose family was also from the same South Side neighborhood. She was fun-loving, had a soulful singing voice, and was into the blues. They hooked up from time to time in high school but didn't get serious with each other until about a year before they were married. Phil came to realize after graduation that he was attracted to her and hoped to marry her one day. He courted her playfully at first. "You're not like other girls," he'd say. "There will come a time for us … You'll see … And you're gonna say you might as well … I think you know it. Lord, you can see that it's true." Scarlet was a South Side girl and she knew how to hold her own. She bantered with him and told him she wasn't ready to be serious. But the attraction was mutual, and eventually she came to see how much this man loved her. She felt respected and loved, and even though they both were fairly young in her mind, she said yes when he proposed. They were married in a large church wedding. They set up a relatively traditional household around the corner from the house she grew up in. Phil worked at the masonry company, and Scarlet worked part-time as a waitress as a local coffee shop in the gentrifying neighborhood nearby. Unlike Phil, she was taking college courses online and had plans to get a degree in graphic design. Within a year of marriage, she gave birth to a daughter; another daughter followed 5 years later, then a son, and then another son.

Phillip Everything Changes

At age 41, Phillip, having spent many years rising through the ranks of his masonry business, was now a supervisor and manager of operations. He had eclipsed his father's success in the company early in his 30s and had established himself as a respected leader among his peers and supervisors. Since his father's retirement, Phil had found an even higher gear of success, feeling confident in his knowledge and skills as both a masonry expert and as a leader. Scarlet enjoyed success as a graphic designer. She had become quite talented and worked full-time for a company that allowed her to work from home. Phil loved her very much and respected how hard she had worked while the kids were little and he was away every day at his job. He also appreciated how much money she was bringing in to support their family. They owned a home in one of the middle-class suburbs southwest of the city, along with two cars and an old class B camper van they called Bertha parked next to the house. The kids were all in school, healthy, and had friends. It was a normal life, as he would reflect to Scarlet in their quiet moments. Indeed, things were going well for Phil and the family. And then everything changed.

His brother, who was 3 years younger than Phil, died suddenly in what was initially thought to be a heart attack. He died in his sleep without any warning symptoms of any kind. Phil's entire extended family was shocked and deeply saddened. It made no sense. They had no history of heart disease in their family, and no one that they knew of had ever had a heart attack. Still, what else could have explained how he died at such a young age in his sleep? This was Phil's closest sibling in age, and he had spent much of his childhood with him. Phil was overwhelmed with grief. He took several weeks off from work and was beginning to have a hard time getting out of bed in the mornings. His mood was flattening, and he felt numb most of the day. The things that he normally enjoyed were less rewarding and enjoyable. Scarlet told him he looked depressed, but Phil had never been depressed before, and he chalked his changes up to grief and sadness. In the first month after his brother's passing, this interpretation made some sense. As the months went on, Phil continued to feel a melancholic mix of sadness, hopelessness, and worry. The simplest interpretation of grief was making less and less sense as time went on.

Four months after the funeral services Phil learned that his brother had been a regular user of prescription pills for years and most likely died from respiratory or heart failure caused by the combination of alcohol and legally prescribed but misused opioid medications. Phil was shocked. He had no idea his brother was addicted to painkillers, but as he thought about it he recalled many times when his brother would seem agitated and ask for money. His brother had been in an accident at the factory where he worked some years ago and had surgery on his

Significant grief reactions after the loss of a loved one are common and typically normal. According to DSM-5-TR, however, some bereaved people qualify for a diagnosis of "major depressive disorder", and others qualify for a diagnosis of "prolonged grief disorder" if their grief symptoms continue to appear daily for more than a year and cause marked distress or impairment.

back. He could have started to use the pain medications when he was recovering from surgery. Or maybe it started when he had the motorcycle accident last year and went to the emergency room? Phil remembered that his brother had told him they gave him some oxycodone, and it made all the pain better. Whenever it started, Phil wouldn't know for sure. But he did know that he couldn't stop thinking about his brother. He couldn't stop thinking about how he wished he could have known and helped him. He wondered if maybe he missed out on seeing the warning signs. It made him feel terrible that his brother was gone. Even worse, Phil felt guilty that he wasn't there to help.

Phil didn't use drugs and had never taken any painkillers other than the kind you can buy over the counter at the drug store. And Phil had no history of cardiac problems. But as time went on after his brother's death, he kept wondering about his own health and the health of his wife and children. He had a primary care doctor that he was supposed to see every year, but he hadn't been in several years. Scarlet regularly went to see her doctor, and they were diligent with the kids, going every year to the pediatrician. Phil always said he would schedule an appointment but never got around to it. Another year would pass, and Scarlet would remind him. He wasn't against going to the doctor. He just didn't ever seem to prioritize doing so. Now, almost a year after his brother's death, Phil scheduled an appointment.

He went to the clinic near his home in the suburbs. When he checked in, the person at the desk took his copay and then handed him a tablet to complete questionnaires in a kiosk adjacent to the wait area. Phil was surprised. A lot had changed in the clinic in the years since he saw his doctor last. He used the tablet to answer questions about his health history and any current concerns or medical problems. He clicked on the bottom of the screen. The next page asked him to answer questions about mental health. Phil started to feel uneasy. The questions asked about his mood, anxiety, alcohol and substance use, a history of trauma, and how he was coping with stress. As he answered them, Phil knew he wasn't telling the entire truth. He had admitted to feeling sad and anxious sometimes, but he downplayed his overall level of stress and the amount of alcohol he was drinking per week. He handed the tablet back to the man at the front desk, then waited for the doctor.

Instead of a doctor, Phil was greeted by a young woman who said she was the doctor's clinical assistant. They walked back, and she took Phil's vitals, then brought him to a clinic room. When his primary care physician arrived, they exchanged pleasantries, and the doctor completed a basic review of his systems. She explained that his routine blood tests taken before the appointment had come back normal. She asked Phil whether there were any concerns about his health. Phil told her he needed to exercise more and wondered if his eyes needed checking for glasses. "I'll make a referral to the ophthalmologist in the clinic," she said. They talked about his lack of exercise. She then asked him about the screening questions he had answered earlier. She related his lack of exercise to his reportedly lowered mood. Phil shrugged his shoulders. "Do you think your mood has been much worse than normal for at least the last two weeks or more?" she asked. Phil nodded affirmatively. She continued to ask questions about Phil's sleep, appetite, and weight. Phil acknowledged that he was sleeping much more than normal, nearly 10 hours per night. His appetite was lower than usual for him, and he had unintentionally lost roughly 10–15 pounds in the last 6 months. She continued, "Phil, in the last two weeks or more have you had less interest or pleasure in the things that normally would give you enjoyment?" Phil explained that this was definitely true, and that he didn't understand why or what was wrong. His doctor leaned toward Phil from her desk. She told him that he seems to meet criteria for major depressive disorder, and that she would like for him to consider one of several treatment options.

Phil couldn't help but agree with her that he may be depressed. After all, what had started as grief was now a long list of symptoms. His mood was down. He wasn't feeling enjoyment anymore. He wasn't sleeping or eating well, and he had lost weight. Phil was not thinking about suicide, but he did feel hopeless about his future and was spending a lot of time thinking about his own death. At work, he was moving more slowly and having a hard time concentrating. All of these things were bothering him, and his boss and wife had both noticed a change in him. Both had been frustrated with his lack of energy and the uncharacteristic number of times he seemed to forget his responsibilities. Phil knew when his doctor said the word *depression* that she was right. He was depressed.

She described his treatment options. He could begin on an antidepressant medication that she would prescribe, likely a low dosage of a selective serotonin reuptake inhibitor—possibly *bupropion*, to help boost his energy, she speculated. After she described the possible side effects (for example, headaches, constipation, insomnia), Phil asked about his other option. He told her he had always been someone that disliked taking medications and was feeling even stronger about this since his brother's death. She told him that the other option was a kind of talk therapy called cognitive-behavioral therapy, or CBT. Just like there are different types of antidepressants, there are different types of CBT he could do for depression.

She told him she wasn't the expert on CBT but that she could provide a referral in their electronic medical record to a colleague in an affiliated clinic. Phil demurred, "Talk therapy? Like seeing a shrink? How is that going to help me? Nah. I'm good doc." She told him that CBT is a type of talk therapy that is structured, brief, and has been shown to work scientifically. Phil said he would think about it. She validated how doing therapy could be uncomfortable at first, but that there were no side effects like there could be if he took medications. Noticing Phil's ambivalence about treatment, she asked if she could make the referral despite

Approximately 8% of adults in the United States have a severe unipolar pattern of depression in any given year, while another 5% have mild forms (Krishnan, 2021a, 2021b, 2021c, 2020; DBSA, 2020). About 20% of adults have an episode of severe unipolar depression at some point in their lives.

As many as 60% of people who take antidepressant drugs for unipolar depression are helped by them (Simon, 2019). To help prevent a relapse by such individuals, most medicators keep the clients on these drugs for at least 5 months after the elimination of the depressive symptoms (DeRubeis et al., 2020).

his uncertainty and he could decide later if he was willing to give CBT a try. He agreed. Before he left, she asked him if her colleague, a social worker in the clinic, could talk with him for a few minutes to answer any questions he had about depression and CBT. He nodded silently, feeling embarrassed.

The social worker knocked and entered the clinic room a few minutes later. She was a middle-aged woman named Peggy Olson with golden yellow hair and an elegant silver dove brooch pinned to her lanyard. They talked for about 15 minutes. Peggy mostly asked him about his depression symptoms and whether he wanted to change them. As he answered, she reflected and paraphrased back to him in a way that communicated she understood what he was saying. She asked him why he wanted to decrease his depression symptoms and in what ways his life would be different if he made changes to decrease his depression. Phil found himself feeling more motivated to change, more resolute and deter-mined that he needed to make changes, and more open to trying. Peggy smiled and graciously told him that they could talk again in the future, but that he could meet with a CBT therapist to begin having regular weekly therapy appointments to help him make the changes he had identified as important to him. Phil still felt ambivalent about talk therapy, but after his positive experience with Peggy, he agreed to try CBT.

Scarlet's View What Is Happening to My Husband?

Phil was not the only person affected by his emerging depression. His wife, Scarlet, and their children—the people who lived with him and cared about him—were hurt by it as well. And like Phil, they were confused by the dramatic changes that they had seen in him. As Scarlet explained to her sister:

> For years I lived with this strong man who was a good father and caring husband and who worked hard every day to provide a good life for all of us. Then over the course of weeks, I watched him change into a sad, frightened, hopeless person who could think of nothing but himself—his fears, his future, his unhappiness.
>
> It seemed innocent enough when it first started. When his brother died, we were all upset, and it was natural to think about how young he was and how something like that could happen to any of us. But while the rest of us—his siblings, his cousins, and I myself—got over it and got back to our lives, it seemed to trigger something in Phil that wouldn't let go of him.
>
> First it was his relentless need to talk about his worries that he could die suddenly like his brother. Then he became obsessed with me or our children dying. Then worry-ing about every little thing, overprotecting himself, seeing doom everywhere. I would walk into the family room and find him sobbing. Over what? He was healthy, he was successful, he had a beautiful family, yet he was sobbing.

Studies reveal that depressed people who have weak social supports, are isolated, and lack intimacy tend to remain depressed longer than those who have a supportive partner or warm friendships (Pastor, 2020).

Time and again, I tried to point out the brighter side of things, to snap him back to his old self, but nothing helped. I talked my guts out, but it was always, "Yes, but this" or "Yes, but that." He felt doomed and hopeless about everything; nothing made a difference.

It was horrible to see him so upset, but worse was the way he stopped doing anything. At home he stopped being a father and husband. The kids would need help with their homework or have to be driven somewhere. The sink or car would need fixing. Or I would need to talk about finances with him. He could do none of it. He would just sit there, usually staring into space, sighing, or crying. He became like a fifth child. Actually, it was worse than that. At least I could reason with the children, get them to do things, have fun with them.

At work it was the same. His boss called one day, wondering where Phil was, because he had not showed up to work for two days. He was forgetting things at home and work. He hardly was doing anything to help around the house as time went on. We all were walking on pins and needles worried we might upset him. The kids would ask me what was wrong with dad all the time. I kept asking him "What is happening to my husband?" He wouldn't admit to being depressed. Instead, he came up with excuses and reasons for all of these changes. But I knew better. It was like I was losing him.

I was relieved when he finally went to see the doctor. When he came home and told me what happened I was furious at him for not taking the prescription for medicine. It seemed like the easier solution. I don't really know if he will take therapy seriously. But I don't know what to do. Nothing I have done has made much of a difference. What if he decided to do something to himself? He certainly was headed in that direction. It's all so scary. I just want my husband back.

Between 6% and 15% of people with severe unipolar depression die by suicide (Schreiber & Culpepper, 2021; Halverson, 2019).

Phil in Treatment Behavioral Activation

Weeks after meeting with his doctor and the social worker, Phil scheduled an appointment with a CBT therapist named Rosemary for their first therapy session. The clinician was a master's level therapist who had devoted herself to years of training in CBTs since completing her master's in clinical psychology. He looked her up online before meeting her. She was an older woman who looked to be in her late 60s and who shared on her website profile that she had been trained in lots of different therapies in her career, including things Phil had never heard of before like Rogerian therapy, gestalt therapy, logotherapy, and something she called eye movement desensitization and reprocessing (EMDR). Phil's eyes scanned intently as he continued to read about her professional training and therapeutic style. He had been diagnosed by his doctor with major depressive disorder, and he was relieved when he saw that Rosemary described herself as someone who had expertise in the treatment of depression. For depression, she wrote, she commonly used something called cognitive-behavioral therapy, or CBT for short. This was the same type of treatment his primary care doctor had told him about. He still didn't think he knew what it was, but knowing Rosemary would use the same approach that his doctor suggested made him feel less nervous about seeing her.

As he scheduled the appointment, Phil wasn't sure what to think. On the one hand, she had lots of experience and looked like she knew what she was doing. On the other, this would be Phil's first time ever going to a therapist, a "shrink" as he called her, to get help. Before clicking "confirm" on the appointment request, Phil sat back and reflected. Growing up, he never heard of anyone seeing a therapist in his low-income, working-class community. People were just trying to make ends meet. A roof over their head, a decent job, food on the table—these were the things he remembered people he knew worry about. But he also recognized that there was a stigma he learned around mental health: the kid in sixth grade who everyone called "spaz" who was unmedicated and had behavioral outbursts in class all the time; the depressed neighbor his friends called "crazy Charlie" who, when Phil was 10, died by suicide after he lost his job and wife left him; the homeless man who sheltered under an elevated train platform, whom Phil and his friends used to make fun of by imitating his confused speech. Phil teared up thinking about all of the people he had come into contact with in his life that may have had depression or other mental health problems. He had so little compassion or empathy for them, and now he was one of them. He clicked "confirm" and saw on his phone an immediate confirmation e-mail that said he would be contacted by Rosemary or her staff to schedule an appointment.

Session 1   Phil waited nervously in Rosemary's waiting room. He kept his head down but managed a forced courteous smile when Rosemary introduced herself. Her hair was long and silver and she walked slowly and with purpose. When she smiled as she extended her hand to meet him, Phil saw that her face seemed welcoming and kind. She had a scent of vanilla and cardamom and well-defined crow's feet. They walked back to her office. It was cozy. There were two comfortable-looking reclining chairs seated facing each other and flanked by bookcases that were adorned with an abundance of succulents, gemstones, and books. She invited Phil to sit and welcomed him, then gave a well-rehearsed orientation about the limits of confidentiality and clinic policies. She asked him if he wanted any hot tea and got up to pour herself some. "There," she said as she handed him a mug of probiotic peppermint, "now we are ready to begin."

Most of the first session of psychotherapy was devoted to a discussion of Phil's current condition and the events leading up to it. In spite of his obvious distress, Phil related the events of the past year in a coherent and organized fashion. At the same time, the desperation on his face was almost painful to observe, and his voice trembled with distress. She assessed him for symptoms of major depression, just as his primary care doctor had recently. His answers were no different. He was still depressed, and Rosemary noted that he met criteria for more than five symptoms of major depressive disorder. She told him that she was going to be diagnosing this and including it in her notes and the insurance billing. Phil nodded and said that made sense.

Rosemary then began describing CBT as a general approach for depression that she suggested. She began by talking about the "C" in CBT for depression. Her style was irreverent and engaging, and even though Phil was very nervous—and still unsure about doing treatment altogether—he found Rosemary someone he thought he could trust. Rosemary explained that "the 'C' stands for the term 'cognitive,' which is nothing more than a fancy word for thinking." She chuckled. Phil noticed as she talked that he felt less anxious. Using cognitive interventions, she could treat depression largely by focusing on a person's style of thinking. Although a disturbance in mood is the most obvious symptom of this disorder, she highlighted that research suggests that disturbances in cognition have an important—some think primary—role in the disorder. People with depression have a severe negative bias in their perceptions and interpretations of events, a bias that leads them to experience themselves, events in their lives, and their futures in very negative—depressing—terms. The goal of cognitive interventions is to change this negative bias and style of interpretation, and in so doing, remove the source of depression.

Phil was listening and tracking this. It seemed clear: Ways of thinking are at the core of depression, so they could change the ways of thinking to reduce depression. Before Phil could say anything, Rosemary segued into a description of the "B" in CBT for depression. Decades of research had shown that *behavioral activation*, "BA" as she called it, was an evidence-based way to reduce depression. Using BA interventions, she could help him reduce depression symptoms by increasing the amount of activities Phil did every day that were consistent with his values, pleasurable, regulating, and gave him a sense of mastery. Rosemary explained that they could use either a mostly "C" or "B" approach, and both could work equally well. And no matter what they chose together, the process of using CBT strategies for depression would include psychoeducation, self-monitoring, willingness to trust and try new things on his part, and an openness to identifying and changing his problematic patterns.

He listened carefully but responded by saying he just wanted to know one thing: whether Rosemary believed that he could ever be cured. He stated that he was becoming a burden to his family, was struggling to keep up at work, and was at a loss for how to get better. He said he just wanted the straight truth: "Am I ever going to get back to normal?"

Studies have found that depressed individuals have a variety of biases in attention, interpretation, and memory for negative events. They recall unpleasant experiences more readily than positive ones, denigrate their performance on various tasks, and expect to fail in various situations (Krishnan, 2021a, 2021b, 2021c, 2020; APA, 2020a).

Like most mental health professionals who encounter a seriously depressed patient, Rosemary found herself wondering for a moment whether Phil would improve with treatment. The psychologist told him that nothing was guaranteed but that she had agreed to treat Phil because she had every expectation of bringing about a full recovery. Phil pressed the matter further, wanting to know specifically when he could expect to be restored to normal. "How many months?" he asked. "How long will it take?"

Rosemary felt no antagonism in Phil's close questioning about the timetable. Rather, she knew the questioning reflected his sense of desperation and fear that he might be a hopeless case. He was obviously hanging on to her every word, looking for some glint of reassurance.

The psychologist felt she had to walk a fine line. On the one hand, she wanted Phil to have confidence in getting better. On the other, given Phil's ambivalence about beginning treatment and his persisting questions about a timetable, Rosemary wanted to avoid setting up expectations for improvement by specific dates, foreseeing that if expectations were not met, it could fuel Phil's negative view of the future, worsening his depressive symptoms.

Rosemary: I know you're anxious to get better, and I don't blame you. It's natural to wonder when this is all going to end. As I said before, I'm seeing you because, as I told your primary care doctor, I expect I can help you recover from depression. The approach we are going to use can take as short as a month or two, but also could take longer than that. But you know Phil, I have been doing this for a long time, and I have learned that I can't predict exactly how long treatment will last for people. So I don't think we have to put an exact timetable on it, simply because it has been my experience that the rate of improvement varies from person to person. I could, of course, make a guess as to when you'll be better, but I'm concerned that if you don't have a complete recovery by that date, you might think it means more than it really does.

Phil: Good points. OK, so what then? I don't want to be in treatment forever. No offense. It's hard enough for me to get here. Now you are saying it could be a long time until I am better.

Rosemary: I think it is best that we leave the timetable open for now. We'll keep our eyes on how you are doing, and every so often I will ask you to complete a questionnaire that will help us use a consistent way to check in on our progress. I don't know if you can tell this about me yet, but I am a pretty straight shooter. I'll tell you things as I see them. And if I think we're not getting anywhere, I'll let you know honestly and we'll consider our options.

Phil: OK. I like that. I'm a straight shooter too. So, what next?

Rosemary spent the remaining 15 minutes of the session continuing her overview of the cognitive and behavioral models of depression and the related treatments rooted in these theoretical frameworks. She used Phil's sensitivity to the timetable of recovery as an example of how certain negative perceptions or interpretations can have powerful effects on the way one feels. In particular, the psychologist noted that a different point of view, one that placed less importance on the exact timetable of recovery, could result in a less catastrophic response to the absence of a full recovery by a certain date.

The psychologist went on to explain that a major part of therapy would be discovering those aspects of Phillip's thinking and behavior that were undermining his capacity to feel well and then helping him develop alternative ways of thinking and behaving that would ultimately reduce his depression. She explained that Phillip would be asked to monitor his emotional reactions throughout the next week, recording all thoughts or events that produced distress (sadness, anger, anxiety, or whatever) and rating their intensity. She asked him to use a daily tracking form to write down his activities each day, so that she could see hour by hour what he did with his day. They would use this information, she told him, to identify where and when he could begin to add in other activities that would help him be less depressed. In the next session, Rosemary explained they would discuss these tracking sheets and would begin to identify specific patterns of thinking and behaving that could be problematic. They would then work together, she assured Phil, to implement new and more effective ways of thinking.

At the end of the session, she asked him whether he had any feelings about using a more cognitive big "C" or a more behavioral big "B" CBT approach. Phil thanked her for asking, disclosing that he thought the behavioral approach, BA, seemed well-suited for him. "It just seems to be more simple," he told her. Phil took in a breath and exclaimed with some determination, "I've always been more of an action kind of guy, and it seems like BA is more action-focused. I'll let you get into my head with that cognitive stuff too, don't get me wrong. But can we try the BA thing first. Yeah let's do that. I think I will do better with that one." Rosemary smiled, handed him several worksheets to use for his first week of self-monitoring, and invited him to contact her via electronic medical record during the week if he had any questions about how to do the self-monitoring.

Session 2 Rosemary reviewed Phil's records of both his moods and his activities, and these provided the focus of discussion. Phil wrote down on most days that he slept 10 hours, went to work during the day, and at home mostly spent time in the living room watching TV and sifting through websites related to camping and traveling. He listed very few activities other than these, which included watching TV with the kids and with Scarlet. There were no social activities, no hobbies, no

When nondepressed research participants are manipulated into reading negative statements about themselves, they become increasingly depressed (Bates et al., 1999).

time spent doing anything spiritual or religious, and nothing that looked like it was recreationally fun on his list of daily activities. His mood was generally low all week, and went up somewhat in the hour when he returned home from work and when spending time with his family. Phil looked despondent as she reviewed his self-monitoring forms. "I'm such a mess, Rosemary. How did I get like this? I don't do anything except work, sleep, eat, and watch TV." Rosemary validated how distressing it is to look closely at one's patterns when depressed. She reassured him that this is what it usually looks like when she begins treating people with depression. She then shifted to the focus of the session. They were going to spend some time identifying what is important to him—values clarification, she called it.

Rosemary: Let's talk about how we can begin to make changes to your daily activities. We are going to do some things to help you activate, behaviorally, in order to have more experiences of pleasure, reward, and mastery.

Phil: Okay.

Rosemary: Remember last time I told you how the behavioral model of depression suggests that you are stuck in a negative feedback cycle?

Phil: Remind me.

Rosemary: Your mood is low which makes you more likely to avoid doing the things that give you joy and pleasure, or a sense of mastery, or the things that matter to you the most. But, by not doing these things, your mood stays low, and makes you continue to avoid doing those kinds of things even more, creating a negative cycle.

Phil: Yeah. That's true. I don't do anything anymore. Ever since my brother died, it's like my feet are caked in concrete, or like I am moving in quicksand. I feel stuck, slow, and unmotivated to do anything.

Rosemary: What would life be like if you did things that made you feel good, or that you were good at doing and wanted to be done? Or even things that didn't feel good or that you were good at doing, but things that you care about and value?

Phil: What do you mean?

Rosemary: I'd like to ask you to make a couple of lists for your therapy homework this week. One list will be all of the things you used to enjoy doing, the other will have things that you need or want to get done but have been avoiding, and things you are skilled at and capable of doing. A third list will be something we will work on in a few minutes. It will be a list of valued actions, meaning the way in which you care about living and being the most in different parts of your life. Let's start with the first list.

Phil: Well, I don't do anything fun anymore, but I used to love to camp with the family We'd go anywhere really. It didn't have to be far away. It was fun to just be away from the house and in the woods. I also loved working on the camper and learning how to do things with gadgets I have for camping. And I love traveling too, not just camping. Even thinking about traveling. Or planning trips. I used to do those things and talk about possible trips with my family all the time.

Rosemary: This is us getting on the right track. Let's list out as many things as possible that, like camping and traveling, used to give you a feeling of enjoyment.

With continued discussion, the psychologist helped Phil draft out a long list of avoided activities. Then they moved on to do the same exercise with a list of activities that give him a sense of mastery and accomplishment, as well as those that he had been avoiding that he wanted or needed to get done. Phil reported that he had been avoiding dealing with a broken sink and looking into a strange smell that came from his oldest son's bedroom. He had been wondering if it might be something electrical but hadn't gotten around to opening up the outlet covers to investigate. It was worrying him that perhaps there was a slow burning electrical outlet that he was neglecting. The whole house could burn down. They could lose everything. Still, Phil emphatically pointed out how depressed he was that he couldn't even get around to looking into the problem.

The two of them made a long list of avoided activities that he had the ability to do and either wanted or needed to complete in order to feel a sense of mastery and competence. Phil acknowledged sheepishly that he had thought about doing all of these things but couldn't bring himself to do them. "That's why you are here, Phil," Rosemary quipped. "We are going to do this together. If it was easy, you would already have done everything without my help." The session ended without having time to talk about the third list of valued actions. She assigned him therapy homework. He agreed to continue monitoring his daily activities and mood. In addition, he would also finalize his lists and hierarchically organize them by activities that were easiest to most difficult for him to complete.

Session 3 Phil appeared somewhat proud when he came in for the third session. He had completed his therapy homework and also had tried several times to begin adding pleasant activities into his day. He pointed her to those parts of his self-monitoring forms and showed her how his mood went up when he did enjoyable activities. "That's terrific," she responded, "we can build on this, Phil." They reviewed his week and identified other times and days when he could in the future add enjoyable activities. Then they talked about and problem-solved when and how he could begin taking on the easiest of the avoided activities that could build a sense of mastery. Rosemary explained that this should help give him a sense that he was no longer procrastinating but instead making progress dealing with things in his life that had been on the back burner for a long time. He agreed to look into the odor in his son's bedroom immediately. Then they clarified and iterated the list a bit more, adding new things he wanted to do that he had been

Studies have demonstrated that exercise compares favorably to either psychotherapy or antidepressant medications in mild to moderate cases of depression, especially when it is integrated with psychotherapy or medication (Dishman et al., 2021; Firth et al., 2020; Miller et al., 2020).

avoiding at work. When he told her he had been avoiding exercise but wanted to get back into shape again, they included exercising 3–5 times per week as a way to improve his mood. The session was now halfway done, and Rosemary transitioned into a discussion about values.

Rosemary: When we talk about values, we are really referring to the ways in which you care the most about being in all the different parts of your life. You have values, ways that, in your heart, you care about being across work, family, friends, your marriage, physical well-being, religious or spiritual well-being, your sense of community, and other areas of your life. To help identify them, we can use adjectives. For example, I value being authentic when I do therapy, so I try to be that way with you. When I interact with the staff here, I try to be respectful and non-judgmental, because I value being those ways with coworkers. Does that make sense? We all have values but don't always know what they are or let them guide us. When things are going well for us, values are like our moral compass, telling us what to do as we navigate life each day. When we are not living aligned with our values, we tend to be distressed. And we can look to each of the different parts of our life and clarify our values to then determine whether we are living consistently with them. Where we are out of step with our values, those are really helpful places to make behavioral changes in an effort to reduce depression and live a life that is valued.

Phil: You just said a lot Rosemary, but I think I get it.

Rosemary: I will give you a worksheet to fill out as homework this week. It will have different areas of your life and ask you to write out your values for each of those areas. I'll give you a list of common values to help you, but you should write down whatever your own values are for each part of your life. Then, the next step of this worksheet will ask you to rate how closely you are living within your values recently. Take your time to complete this. It will help guide us next week to figure out which valued activities to add into your daily routine and when.

They spent the remaining time problem-solving together how to do this homework, as well as how to add pleasurable and mastery-inducing events into specific times in the upcoming week. Phil left the clinic feeling like he was beginning to finally understand what CBT for depression would be like. He was still unsure how long it would take. And he continued to feel hopeless and sad. Still, he knew he could come home and be proud to tell Scarlet that he was making progress.

Session 4   Rosemary asked Phil first about the behavioral assignments. The client reported that he had checked his son's room and learned that the outlets in fact did have evidence of burning. He told her how relieved he felt to have fixed them. He also had cleared some brush behind his house over the weekend and organized his desk at work, both things on his list of avoided activities. Doing these things also improved his mood a bit. Turning to the values clarification homework, he handed it to her, and they reviewed what he had written. He valued being dependable, loving, and helpful as a husband. As a father, he valued most being physically present and available for his kids, something he had been doing hardly at all since his brother died. The list went on across each domain of Phil's life. He noted how he was not living within his values in any area of his life, but that he didn't really prioritize some areas as much as others. Family relationships were the most important set of values, and Phil cried as he told Rosemary how he had been failing as a husband and father. Rather than challenge the truth in his thoughts about his failure to live up to his values, Rosemary highlighted how they had more work to do in changing his behavioral patterns. She was reassuring in how she said everything, and with the tea and the vanilla–cardamom smell in her office, Phil felt soothed by Rosemary.

A large portion of this session was devoted to working out in detail the days and times that he would act in alignment with his values as a husband and father. They spent time problem-solving the barriers and did some role-playing and rehearsing together to help Phil practice. It was decided that he would follow a set routine upon returning home from work: (1) talk to his wife about her day; (2) eat dinner with the family, setting aside his own concerns and attending as closely as possible to the conversation, including asking the children some questions about their day; (3) assist the children with their homework; (4) go on a walk for exercise with Scarlet; (5) check in on and spend time with the kids before bed; and (6) spend the rest of the evening with Scarlet, being sure to ask her about her most recent work projects or things she was finding interest in. They would go to bed at the same time and in the morning he would help her get the kids off to school.

The main assignments for the coming week were outlined on paper. He would continue to record his daily activities and mood, and would take steps each day to do activities on each of his three lists.

Research indicates that individuals with marital problems are 25 times more likely to have a depressive disorder than people in untroubled marriages (Keitner, 2021). In some cases the individual's depression may cause the marital discord, but often the interpersonal conflicts and low social support of troubled relationships seem to lead to depression (Balderrama-Durbin et al., 2020; Williams & Nieuwsma, 2020).

Session 5   Phil reported that he had been able to follow the prescribed routine at home. He found that keeping his attention focused on the concrete tasks before him had a way of reducing his depressive feelings and thoughts. He told Rosemary he was pleased with his ability to do these things, and he was starting to enjoy more activities. In fact, he spontaneously decided to go outside a couple of times to play basketball with his kids and had a fun time.

The next discussion turned to Phillip's routine at work. He reported that he was spending about 6 hours a day at work (9:00 A.M. to 3:00 P.M.), but he found

People who consistently *ruminate*—that is, repeatedly dwell on their moods without acting to change them—are more likely to become clinically depressed than people who do not generally ruminate (Watkins & Roberts, 2020; McLaughlin & Nolen-Hoeksema, 2011).

himself frequently feeling depressed there. Apparently he had severely cut down his activities at work under the assumption that stress could exacerbate his condition. As a result, he had a lot of dead time on his hands, which he would spend sitting at his desk, staring at his computer and brooding over the extent of his disability and his rate of progress. Rosemary pointed out that he could increase his valued actions, pleasant events, or avoided tasks at work.

Rosemary:	You are making good progress at home. Can we do the same thing at work?
Phil:	Do things that are fun? It's work.
Rosemary:	Yeah, I know. But maybe there are things you can do here and there during the day that, even for just a minute or two, could boost your mood? And can we talk about the ways you value being a supervisor and coworker, because the last time we talked about this you wanted to be a responsive boss and helpful coworker to your peers. But you said you were neither of those things since your brother died. And is there anything at work you are avoiding that could be approached to help improve your mood?
Phil:	All of that is true. But I don't know. I am much more motivated to change at home, like we talked about.
Rosemary:	You have made really big positive changes at home. And you are seeing how your mood is improving at home. Our plan included also making changes at work, since that was your number two area of priority after family. Are you still willing to do this?
Phil:	I am willing. I just don't... This is hard, Rosemary. You gotta know how hard it is to make all these changes.
Rosemary:	I do. From my seat, I can't experience it the same as you, but I can tell you that I have helped many others with depression go through this same process. I get it...

Phil agreed to gradually start building up his activities at work. Specifically, he would (1) leave the office at 5:00 P.M. rather than 3:00 P.M.; (2) schedule previously avoided weekly meetings with his subordinates; and (3) resume attending daily managements meeting with his peers in leadership at the company. They would, as they had in previous sessions, problem-solve and troubleshoot how to not avoid doing all of the things he was scheduling to do in the upcoming week. Phil knew if he did each of these activities, he would feel better. The list was growing and long, but it included various pleasurable events alongside things that he valued that were not very fun (but he cared about doing). Once again, he left feeling hopeful about the changes he would make in the week and proud to tell Scarlet about his next steps in treatment.

Session 6 This session focused on Phil's adjustment to the fuller day at work. The client's overall impression was that it was going well. He noted particularly that when he was actively engaged in practical activities—talking on the phone to coworkers, attending meetings, speaking to his team about company concerns—he tended not to be as sad or depressed. In contrast, when he avoided them all and sat idly at his desk, he became caught up in depressive thoughts and feelings.

Rosemary suggested that Phil use this observation to his advantage and do what he could to minimize his brooding. The psychologist recommended that he keep reminders of his values about work in front of him while at his desk. She encouraged him to read his values each morning as a reminder, and to commit to Scarlet that he would continue to follow his treatment by not avoiding what he committed to doing at work.

Phil liked the idea of having concrete reminders about his values. But why couldn't he just sit and do nothing without getting depressed? Rosemary explained that avoidance or inhibition of doing what is important—valued actions—can lead anyone to feel stressed or down. She disclosed that she felt annoyed with herself when she had days at work that were incongruent with her values. Phil thanked her for sharing this. It helped to know she wasn't perfect, that she was a regular human who sometimes didn't do things well. She shared more about herself, telling him about her forays into treatments that were not based at all on any scientific evidence. She regretted it, she told him, but as evidence-based ways of helping people became more common, she realized that she needed to adapt to the times and learn them. Phil felt connected with and understood by Rosemary. And she continued to persist in her application of BA. Homework was assigned and problem-solved, and Phil left the office with a sense of increasing momentum. It had only been a few months since they started, less time than he thought it would take, but he was already feeling less depressed.

Sessions 7 to 9 Over the course of the next 3 weeks, Phil and Rosemary continued to increase his frequency and diversity of activities. They worked to generalize values across contexts, so that he felt confident that he was changing in as many relevant situations as possible. His life was being led more consistently with his values, he was procrastinating less at home and work, and he was spending time every day, multiple times, doing things that were enjoyable. He was feeling pleasure again, noticing how good it felt to sit with his wife and be with her, to play with his kids, and to plan their next camping adventure. As a result, he was feeling like he used to most of the time. He was participating fully in the family routine, and at work he was meeting the responsibilities he had set for himself. As he functioned better, it strengthened his conviction that he was not headed for a permanent mental collapse.

Almost two-thirds of people with severe unipolar depression or persistent mild depression are receiving treatment currently (NIMH, 2021a; Krishnan, 2020; Wang et al., 2005).

Most people with symptoms of unipolar depression improve to at least some degree within 6 months, some without treatment. More than half of people who recover from severe depression have at least one other episode of depression later in their lives (NIMH, 2021; Coryell, 2020; Kessing, 2020).

Sessions 10 to 12   In the 3 weeks comprising sessions 10 to 12, Phil had returned to full functioning and was in good spirits most of the time. His family had even gone camping together for the first time in over a year. They went north to the Wisconsin Dells, and Phil felt the joy of being in the outdoors with his family again. Accordingly, the therapy sessions themselves were now devoted to relapse prevention. The goal was to help Phil plan for ways to maintain and further generalize his gains over time. They spent time in their final session reminiscing about their time together, putting a fine point of emphasis on the specific behavioral strategies that Phil had learned. Phil completed a self-reported measure of depression. Rosemary told him he was below the cut-off for being considered minimally clinically depressed. They agreed that if he started to feel depressed again, he would call her and schedule an appointment.

Epilogue

At the one year anniversary of his brother's death, Phil began to feel depressed again. He called Rosemary, and she reminded him to stick with their relapse prevention plan. They had planned for this anniversary reaction, and she calmly reassured him that she knew he had the ability to follow his plan. He felt reassured, and they scheduled a therapy session. By the day of the appointment a week later, Phil was feeling better. He had implemented the relapse prevention plan by doing the things that had helped him when he was depressed. He made sure to spend extra time with Scarlet and the kids, and they planned a trip together. This time they would travel and camp out west, to a place Phil had always wanted to see called Bryce Canyon, in Utah. The planning for this trip alone was so much fun that it gave Phil great joy and raised his spirit. He thought about his brother often and wasn't afraid to do so. But when he did he made sure to stay active with his home and work valued actions, and, of course, to plan for their camping trip in Bryce Canyon.

Assessment Questions

1. What are the first signs that a person might be depressed?

2. Why did Phil initially see his primary care doctor?

3. What symptoms did Phil present that prompted his primary care doctor to suggest a psychologist?

4. What was the purpose of the social worker who talked to Phil after the primary care doctor?

5. Why did Phil choose cognitive-behavioral therapy over medications?

6. What helped Phil feel comforted by and trusting of Rosemary?

7. What concerns did Scarlet, Phil's wife, have about her husband's depression?

8. What type of psychotherapy did Rosemary use with Phil?

9. What were the criteria for Phil's diagnosis of major depressive disorder?

10. What are some of the methods that were used as part of behavioral activation?

11. Phil wanted to know how long it would be before he felt normal again. Why did Rosemary not want to give him a definite timetable?

12. What was the first assignment Phil was given for the first week of therapy?

13. Why did Rosemary want Phil to clarify his values near the beginning of therapy?

14. What was the homework assignment given in session 2? What was the purpose of this assignment?

15. Why was it important to get Phil to set up an evening routine of activity?

16. What were the three main components of BA that Rosemary used?

17. At approximately what point in treatment did Phil return to full function?

CASE **6**

Bipolar Disorder

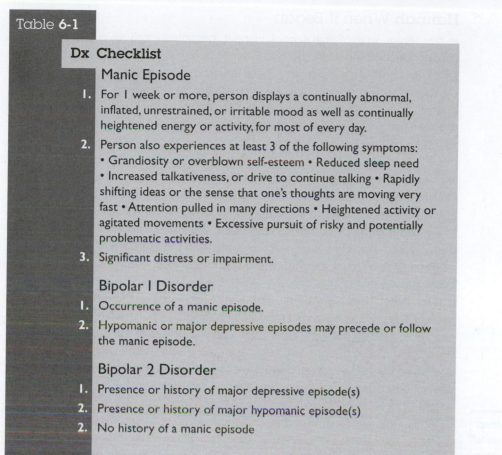

Table 6-1

Dx Checklist

Manic Episode

1. For 1 week or more, person displays a continually abnormal, inflated, unrestrained, or irritable mood as well as continually heightened energy or activity, for most of every day.

2. Person also experiences at least 3 of the following symptoms: • Grandiosity or overblown self-esteem • Reduced sleep need • Increased talkativeness, or drive to continue talking • Rapidly shifting ideas or the sense that one's thoughts are moving very fast • Attention pulled in many directions • Heightened activity or agitated movements • Excessive pursuit of risky and potentially problematic activities.

3. Significant distress or impairment.

Bipolar I Disorder

1. Occurrence of a manic episode.

2. Hypomanic or major depressive episodes may precede or follow the manic episode.

Bipolar 2 Disorder

1. Presence or history of major depressive episode(s)

2. Presence or history of major hypomanic episode(s)

2. No history of a manic episode

(Information from APA, 2022, 2013.)

Hannah, one of two sisters, was raised in an upper-middle-class family in the suburbs. Her father was a physician, and much of his work entailed the hosting of fundraising events to support charitable projects. Through these events, Hannah's family acquired a wide array of prominent people as family friends and acquaintances.

Hannah attended a highly competitive public school, where she excelled academically yet couldn't crack the top quartile in her graduating class. Growing up, she was a lot like most of the other girls. She did not seem to have any unusual psychological problems during childhood and early adolescence. An outgoing and popular girl who got along well with others, she had many friends. When she was 17, something happened that would change the trajectory of her life.

The onset of bipolar disorder usually occurs between the ages of 15 and 44 years (Kessing, 2020; Stovall, 2020). Bipolar disorders are about equally common in women and men.

Hannah When It Began

In her senior year of high school, Hannah became deeply involved in a school play production in which she had a minor acting role. As the production progressed, she became more and more absorbed in the work. Her presentation on stage during rehearsals became increasingly theatrical, and she became more involved in her costuming and makeup. The other students initially were in awe of the teenager's increased level of creativity and comfort on stage. However, with time, her behavior became bizarre. Once, for example, in the diner where students would gather after rehearsals, Hannah became so giddy and talkative that she approached strangers for rambling conversations, telling some that she was a famous actress. Once, she actually burst out in song, reveling in the attention she got, which was actually not admiring.

As these kinds of outbursts continued, the other cast members distanced themselves from Hannah. Over time, Hannah's impulsively joyful spectacles stopped happening. In their place, she became unsure of herself, worried excessively about what others thought of her, even paranoid. She became convinced that the other students were plotting against her, trying to undermine her road to fame and glory. She became increasingly guarded and ultimately withdrew from everyone, isolating herself socially. Over a period of weeks she became depressed, crying throughout the day and refusing to go to school; she believed that everyone hated her, and she wished she were dead. She wasn't sleeping well and rarely left her bedroom. Unable to cope with this dramatic turn of events, her parents sought professional help, and Hannah was soon admitted to a psychiatric hospital.

Antidepressant drugs can trigger a manic episode for some people who have a bipolar disorder (Baldessarini, Vasquez, & Tondo, 2020; Carvalho, Firth, & Vieta, 2020). Thus, clinicians must carefully monitor the impact of these drugs when prescribing them for people with the disorder.

While hospitalized, she improved with low doses of an antipsychotic (*olanzapine*, or Zyprexa) and antidepressant (*fluoxetine*, or Prozac) medication and was released after several weeks, feeling more or less like her old self. She received her high school diploma after making up missed work over the summer, and she began college as planned in the fall. Things progressed well during her first two years in college; Hannah found moderate academic success and began to develop a romantic relationship with a young woman she met in one of her classes, but in her junior year she had another depressive episode, which led to her doctor increasing her antidepressant medication. Coupled with a breakup with her girlfriend and a semester with very difficult classes, the increased dose of antidepressant may have contributed to her second manic episode and subsequent hospitalization.

Hannah Ups and Downs Worsen

During her junior year in college, Hannah became increasingly absorbed in her course work in business, often neglecting her other courses. She would spend large amounts of time at the library, reading and talking to anyone who might listen about her plan to create a global business empire within the next year. Her energy seemed to have no bounds. Nights were particularly problematic. While others were sleeping, Hannah couldn't quiet her mind. It raced frenetically, spinning and speeding around various topics related to her newfound destiny. She spent multiple consecutive days in her room almost without sleeping, plotting ways to disrupt this or that industry with paradigm shifts that would bring her instant fame and magnificent fortune.

Her apartment roommates eventually became aware that Hannah had stopped attending classes and was up at all hours of the night. When one of them asked her about her activities, Hannah offered an excited discourse on her marketing strategy and how it would eclipse those of Apple, Nike, and all of the most successful approaches. Realizing something was amiss, her roommate urged Hannah to visit the student health center, telling her that she looked exhausted. In response, Hannah got annoyed and stormed off. Her roommate finally decided that Hannah's behavior might be a health emergency and contacted her parents. They immediately drove to her off-campus apartment and realized that their daughter was in a state similar to the one that had preceded her depression in high school. Within days, her parents took Hannah to the psychiatric hospital for what was now becoming a pattern in her young life.

While she was hospitalized, Hannah's mania received psychopharmacological attention. She was given the antipsychotic drug *paliperidone* (Invega), which produced dramatic relief within a few days, restoring her to a normal condition. She was discharged from the hospital with a prescription for extended-release Invega, with the hope of stabilizing her mood for a longer time.

This medicine appeared to work well for her, and it became the mainstay of her treatment for the next several years. Later, the antipsychotic medication began to produce problematic motor control and coordination symptoms, side effects called *extrapyramidal effects*, so her doctor decided to change her to *lithium carbonate* (lithium) in combination with *eszopiclone* (Lunesta) for sleep. The problem was that Hannah felt incapable of taking medications consistently. Although recognizing the benefits, she often felt "straitjacketed" by the drugs she was taking. When medicated, she was free of manic episodes, but at the same time she felt she had lost her spark; her emotions felt dulled, and she sometimes longed for a few mild highs in her emotional life, a feeling of excitement or of "just being alive," as she put it. When the longing became intense, Hannah would stop taking the medications, often without immediate negative consequences and with a return of her desired emotional highs. Unfortunately, she also became more vulnerable to manic episodes and the depression that often followed.

The result, over these years, was a life greatly hampered by periodic bipolar episodes. Because of several further hospitalizations during the next few years and other disruptions caused by more depressive and hypomanic (that is, mildly manic) episodes, Hannah was unable to complete her bachelor's degree on time. She moved back into her parents' apartment and lived there for several years while taking a reduced course load at a community college. Ultimately she earned

Lithium is a silvery white metallic element that occurs in nature as a mineral salt.

a bachelor's degree and found work, ironically as a sales representative for a pharmaceutical company.

Unfortunately, Hannah continued to ride an emotional roller coaster after obtaining employment. Her manic episodes were more frequent than her depressive episodes and in her opinion more of an obstacle to her professional and social goals.

At the outset of any manic episode, there was no obvious indication that something was wrong. Rather, the first sign was usually a feeling of happiness that gradually grew to a glorious outlook on life. At this early stage, Hannah felt immensely pleased, considering herself the smartest, sexiest, most talented woman alive. These feelings were in sharp (and initially welcome) contrast to the feelings she would have when depressed, when she would consider herself the most miserable failure who ever existed. Even when not depressed, Hannah often would hold herself in somewhat low regard, unhappy with her work, her love life, and her appearance.

The feelings that preceded a manic episode were pleasurable and a welcomed respite from her general dysphoria. Hannah might go shopping for new clothes or electronics, often spending large amounts of money that she did not have. Her parents, wealthy enough and used to her spending sprees, provided her with a financial backstop whenever she overspent. Additionally, Hannah would become unbearably extraverted and gregarious, chatting with strangers on the bus or subway and calling up friends both new and old in search of stimulating conversation late at night.

As the euphoric feelings progressed, her behavior frequently crossed socially acceptable boundaries. She would ask people about highly personal matters or, conversely, disclose secrets about her own life to people she hardly knew. Most of the time this led to people shying away from her. But some people, in some contexts, were drawn to her manic behavior. This was particularly true with men and women who were sexually attracted to Hannah. When manic, she would often dress with more revealing clothes and talk to people in sexually provocative ways, drawing attention from men and women who took interest in her. Because of her family's social connections, Hannah often attended charity balls and other gala social events. When she was manic or hypomanic, these parties became settings for her to feel the rush of being looked at and, as she assumed, wanted by others. She would tease and flirt with the most attractive people in the room. After the second or third event, she found herself outside under a gazebo having sex with a man she had met minutes before. This was the beginning of a long pattern where she would channel her manic symptoms into heavy flirting and sex in the same evening with strangers. There was one extremely short red dress that she favored for such events. Her typical strategy was to put on that dress and then apply lavish makeup. When finished, she thought she could have been a Hollywood actress.

Unlike Hannah, most people with a bipolar disorder typically have depressive episodes more often than manic episodes (Baldessarini et al., 2020; Kessing, 2020). Moreover, the depressive episodes tend to last longer than the manic ones.

Bipolar disorders occur in people of all socioeconomic classes and ethnic groups. However, the disorders appear to be more prevalent in lower socioeconomic groups (Bressert, 2018; Sareen et al., 2011).

At most parties and social events, she would make a grand entrance in an effort to become the focus of attention. Hannah loved the surge of adrenaline she had when she noticed others giving her attention, and her sense of euphoria and self-satisfaction increased with each passing hour. As the typical event might progress, someone inevitably would suggest to Hannah that they leave the party together, and Hannah would automatically go. It felt great to be desired, and she felt a sense of control and dominance in these situations. Plus, it was such a different way to express her sexuality than her mother had when she was younger, marrying her father at 22 and having a child the next year. With these ways of making sense of her sexual behavior, Hannah had sex with over 50 people in similar circumstances over the course of several years.

Her work activities also offered opportunities for picking up men or women when she was in a manic state. One of her functions as sales representative at the pharmaceutical company was to coordinate conferences and meetings among doctors to promote sales. During her manic states, Hannah would arrive at meetings wearing the provocative red dress or a similar outfit. Her language would become flowery and fast-paced. Although she was often noticed at the meeting, it was after the conference, at the customary social hour, that she made her presence truly felt. As at parties, she found people to flirt with and inevitably wound up hooking up with one of them.

This behavior had its negative consequences. Aside from medical problems—she contracted a sexually transmitted disease—she acquired a reputation. Thus, even when no longer manic, she might be approached by people who assumed they could take liberties with her, given her behavior on prior encounters. On one occasion, word got back to her employer when the director of a medical department requested that Hannah's company send someone "a little more low-key" to organize the conference for the following year. Another time, a woman she had slept with accused Hannah of being sexually inappropriate with a different colleague. It led to an internal review by the company's human resources department followed by ongoing training, a change in job duties, and changes in how she was treated by her coworkers.

As her mania progressed, her contact with reality would increasingly slip away, and she was capable of developing many grandiose ideas. For example, she once became convinced that she had discovered a new and natural talent for interior design and was going to surprise her parents, who were on vacation, by redecorating their entire 5,000-square-foot house for them. Completely taken with this idea, Hannah got in her car and spent several days buying paint, wallpaper, curtains, and various furnishings.

Hannah ultimately purchased several thousand dollars' worth of supplies and furniture and spent the next few days stripping wallpaper, mixing paint, and pulling up carpet, a process she carried out on only a couple of hours of sleep per night. One week later, Hannah received a phone call from her mother on her way home

Like depressive episodes, some manic episodes include psychotic symptoms. Some persons with mania, for example, may hold delusions of grandeur. They believe that they have special powers or that they are especially important beings, even deities.

from the airport. When she heard her daughter talking about a "huge surprise" she had for them at their house and that she had been working on it for a week straight, she knew that Hannah was once again manic. Racing back to her house, her mother found her in their living room, looking like a creature from another planet—white as a ghost, covered from head to toe with various colors of paint and what looked like plaster. The living room and kitchen were painted with multicolored polka-dots; one wall had the wallpaper half removed; and there were many odd pieces of furniture and decorations that she didn't recognize.

Hannah excitedly told her mother that she planned to open her own interior design business and that their home would be featured in her portfolio. Her mother, who found it difficult to concentrate because of her anger, tried explaining that her idea was unrealistic and that she didn't have any experience with interior design, but Hannah became irritated with her mother's failure to support her. When her mother begged Hannah to call her psychiatrist, she refused, saying she had finally discovered her own special talent and all her mother could think about was putting her away. Eventually Hannah's mother called the psychiatrist herself and was advised to call an ambulance.

When the paramedics arrived, they tried persuading Hannah to come with them to a hospital where she had been taken once before. Only when they promised that she would be released right away if an examination by her psychiatrist proved that everything was all right did she agree to go.

Hannah was confined at the hospital on the basis of a *physician emergency certificate,* which allowed the hospital to hold her for 3 days without a court order. She was again given medications, and she lost her desire to return to her redecorating project, which she eventually saw as absurd. Hannah felt intensely guilty for what she had done to her parents' house. Her mother tried to pacify her by saying she had wanted to redecorate anyway, but Hannah knew her mother was just trying to reduce any stress in her life.

When she was depressed, Hannah's feelings were almost the mirror image of what she felt when manic. She lost all interest in normal activities, called in sick at work, and slept 16 hours each day. Even when awake she could barely leave her bed. Instead, she spent most of her conscious hours mindlessly surfing the Internet, sobbing, and thinking she was a miserable failure at every aspect of life. Occasionally she might put on some old clothes and go to the store to buy a few basic things, barely looking at anyone she might encounter. At such times, she had no concern for her appearance and ate only enough to keep going.

In between her mood episodes, Hannah was intelligent, responsible, serious about her work, and considered a capable sales representative by her employer. However, even then she was not completely free of difficulties. She suffered from chronic low self-esteem, shame, and hopelessness. Although perfectly capable in her work, for example, she often doubted herself, feeling ashamed and guilty for

Many states have established procedures by which physicians can temporarily commit patients to a psychiatric hospital in an emergency. The procedure is usually called a *physician emergency certificate.* Today, certification by nonphysician mental health professionals is allowed in many states.

things that she had not done as well as she wanted, or for not doing certain things at all. After organizing successful meetings, she would spend considerable amounts of time and energy ruminating about her perceived flaws or faults. Similarly, any hint of criticism had a way of overshadowing the praise that she generally received in her work. This sensitivity led to great anxiety and suffering. In her love life, Hannah's lowered self-esteem would interfere with her ability to find a suitable partner. In turn, her relations with men and women were mostly confined to sexual escapades while manic, even though she longed for a more long-term relationship.

> Identical twins of persons with a bipolar disorder have a 40% to 70% likelihood of developing the same disorder, while fraternal twins, siblings, and other close relatives have a 5% to 10% likelihood (Kessing, 2020; Mondimore, 2020).

A Friend's View This Is Difficult to Watch

It was a challenge, to say the least, to be friends with Hannah. Actually, it was easy—even fun—to become her friend, especially if a person met her during the early stages of a manic episode. Her wit, charming social presence, and upbeat disposition would win people over. But it was very hard to stay friends with Hannah. As she became increasingly manic, friends would find themselves confused, appalled, and ultimately frightened. When she was depressed, they might feel pulled down by the weight of her self-doubt, hopelessness, or endless preoccupation with her faults and inherent defects. After witnessing one of her manic or depressive episodes, some friends would decide to end the relationship. Others might understand that she had a severe disorder and would try to pick up the relationship where it had left off. But in many cases, such efforts were unsatisfactory. A line had been crossed; the friend's trust or confidence in Hannah and in her stability had been broken, and so things were not quite the same. A line had also been crossed for Hannah. Embarrassed and humiliated by how she might have acted, especially during a manic episode, she later found it hard to feel comfortable, or even respectable, in the presence of those who had witnessed her bizarre behaviors.

Izzy, another sales representative at work, was one such individual. Her relationship with Hannah started as a source of great joy, but it progressed, along with Hannah's manic behaviors, into a troubling, painful, and desperate experience that Izzy had trouble putting behind her. As Izzy would eventually say, it was hard to watch Hannah go through these cycles. She later described the relationship to Katina, one of the newer representatives in the pharmaceutical company:

> I didn't think too much about Hannah at first, because she generally kept to herself. The first year that I worked with her, we never talked too much, even when we were at sales meetings together. In fact, she kind of had a reputation for mostly keeping to herself. She didn't have a lot of people who seemed close to her. She was a really good salesperson, and she dressed well, but that was about all I knew

> The cause of bipolar disorders in not clear, although biological variables are pointed to most often, including genetic factors, abnormal brain structures and brain circuitry, problematic ion activity within cells, and abnormal neurotransmitter activity (Nurnberger, 2021; Quide et al., 2021; Sato, 2021; Churchull et al., 2020; Phillips & Drevets, 2020).

about her. Everyone seemed to have their own theory about her, and I heard some talk about her being bipolar or having manic depression, but I figured it was just a rumor. People like to talk about others, and I figured I'd get to know her myself before I'd believe any of those rumors.

So I was really surprised at a conference in Chicago when Hannah suddenly approached me and started talking to me. It was intense, you know, like she had big eyes and was up close in my business. It wasn't aggressive or anything. Just kind of out of the blue and took me off guard. She told me that she'd always wanted to ask me if my name was short for Isabel, Isabella, or from something more fun like Frizzy, since I have thick curly brown hair. I told her it had nothing to do with my hair, but that I was called Frizzy Izzy in elementary school. We laughed. And we sort of hit it off right then. It turned out that we enjoyed the same kind of music and we both enjoyed going out to clubs dancing. We also talked about movies and favorite TV shows. Looking back, it wasn't really what we talked about, I guess, but the way the talk happened. She seemed really excited to be getting to know me, and I was happy that I was making friends with someone at work. Soon we arranged to sit next to each other at marketing meetings, and we would start to have little private jokes that we'd share. She was cool.

I was having a lot of fun with Hannah. I guess the first time I noticed that something might be a bit off was half a year or so after we started really being friends. One night she called me up at 4:00 A.M., which was very unusual, and I immediately assumed there'd been some sort of emergency. She seemed extremely excited, and when I could get her to calm down and tell me what was going on, she said, "You know that guy Dave who reps for us in Seattle. Well, you'll never guess. I totally hooked up with him! I went home with him and we had an amazing time!" I tried to find a way to get off the phone, but she just kept talking a mile a minute, telling me every detail I didn't want to know.

I was pretty shocked that she was having sex with someone from work who she hardly knew. Then she told me that she'd hooked up with a whole lot of people who worked for the company. A few months later, Dave was transferred to our office. By the end of his first week there, Hannah was telling me that she was deeply in love. After a couple of weeks of hearing about her perfect relationship, I must admit I was getting pretty tired of it, but I had to be polite. Then, by the end of just a month, she was talking to me about marriage. I would say, "Listen Hannah, don't you think this is a little fast? I mean, you guys aren't ready to be talking about marriage."

She wasn't even fazed. "Oh, Dave and I are going to do this; it's gonna be like that." She even asked me my opinions on flower arrangements for the wedding.

Finally, I said to her, "Listen, I think this is too soon. As your friend, I have to say I just don't think you're ready to get married, and it doesn't sound like Dave is either. I mean, you guys haven't even told anyone at work besides me that you're seeing each other, and you won't even let me tell him that I know."

Genetic studies have linked bipolar disorders to possible gene abnormalities on at least 13 different chromosomes (Nurnberger, 2021; Stovall, 2020).

She screamed at me, "I love him so much! He's the one! You're the best friend I've ever had and you're going to be my maid of honor. Why would you say we're not ready to get married?" This really scared me. We were good friends, but I didn't realize she considered me to be her best friend.

I decided I had to do something. She was starting to make me nervous; she was so jumpy all the time. There seemed to be a real desperation to the way she felt about this relationship, and so I decided to talk to Dave about it.

First thing he said was, "How did you find out about that?"

I just said, "Look, Dave, I know, okay? She told me. And because she's my friend, I want you to know I am not sure if she's ready for marriage." And he just stared at me like I was from Mars. He told me he'd seen her a couple of times but it was no big deal.

Now I was really scared, so I told her what happened. She got so mad at me, screeching over the phone, "You ruined everything. We were taking it slow, but I know he wanted to marry me, and you ruined it!" She hung up on me and wouldn't talk to me for months. At work, her behavior kept getting stranger and stranger, more and more outrageous. Needless to say, Dave wanted nothing more to do with her, and quite truthfully, after a while, I began to feel the same way. I mean she was so bizarre and frightening. By then, of course, I realized that she was terribly troubled. Yet for a long while I couldn't shake the thought that I had done something terribly wrong. Now that I know about her problem it makes more sense. We're still friends, kind of, but not nearly like before. I went on one of those rides with her for several months, and I'll never forget it. On the other hand, what must it be like for her to live through them again and again?

Hannah In Treatment Again

As Hannah approached age 32, she decided to seek treatment with a new psychiatrist. Her emotions were stable at the time, due largely to a combination of the medications lithium and eszopiclone. Nevertheless, she knew from experience that this stability would eventually change unpredictably, because of either changes in her reactions to the medications or a change of heart about taking them. She had grown weary of the roller-coaster ride, weary of making and losing friends, weary of all the unpredictability and pain, and she hoped that perhaps a new psychiatrist could help her gain better control over her symptoms.

She contacted Dr. Ainsley Stanley. She had heard of Dr. Stanley from an online friend, a man whom Hannah had first met a few years before in a Facebook support group for people with mood disorders. The friend himself had been treated by Dr. Stanley. He said that the psychiatrist had been able to help him settle down and stabilize his life. He couldn't have been more positive, and so Hannah, feeling that she was running out of time to live a normal life, decided to see Dr. Stanley.

More than 60% of patients with bipolar manic episodes improve while taking lithium or another mood stabilizer (Carvalho et al., 2020; Kessing, 2020). Such drugs are less successful at alleviating bipolar depressive episodes (Stovall, 2021; Vieta et al., 2020).

It was certainly worth a try. Thus began a doctor–patient relationship that was to continue for 17 years.

A Psychiatrist Prepares for Treatment A Delicate Balance

Experience taught Dr. Stanley that medicating mood disorders, especially bipolar disorder, is complex and can involve a certain amount of trial and error. The stereotype of the bipolar patient who simply takes lithium, a mood stabilizer, to be free of symptoms was, unfortunately, more the exception than the rule. Most such patients require other medications at different phases of their disorder. Many need a combination of antidepressants and antipsychotic drugs (usually second-generation antipsychotic drugs) for both their major tranquilizing and their antipsychotic effects.

Dr. Stanley knew that when prescribing lithium it is necessary to achieve a balance between the drug's therapeutic efficacy and its unpleasant side effects — side effects that often would lead patients to just stop using it. In addition, a special problem in the case of bipolar disorder was the pleasure that patients often would get from their manic symptoms. Even with minimal side effects from lithium, the patients might be tempted to discontinue the drug to get the high.

> Some antiseizure drugs—lamotrigine (Lamictal), carbamazepine (Tegretol), and valproate (Depakote) — are also used in the treatment of bipolar disorder. They are each about as effective as lithium and often have fewer side effects. In many cases, certain antipsychotic drugs are combined with these mood stabilizers (Mondimore, 2020).

Added to this was the issue of helping patients with bipolar disorder to accept the reality that they have a lifelong disorder and that they probably will have to be on medications for most of their life. Dr. Stanley knew well that the psychological management of patients was an important adjunct to medication management. Routine and regulating daily structure, like balanced eating, sleeping, exercise, and social interactions collectively have an important role in preventing manic episodes and managing depressive symptoms. These behavioral changes could be difficult to implement and maintain. Additionally, a psychiatrist had to be sensitive both to the patient's concerns about medication side effects and to the changes in emotional life brought about by the medication. On top of this, treatment often had to include behavioral strategies to help patients and their family members learn how to recognize and seek help for their manic episodes before the episodes fully blossomed.

The First Session After gathering a description of Hannah's symptoms and history, Dr. Stanley was certain that the patient's condition met the DSM-5-TR diagnostic criteria for bipolar I disorder. Hannah had had both manic and depressive episodes. Her manic episodes were characterized by inflated self-esteem (sometimes called grandiosity), decreased need for sleep, increased talkativeness, increase in goal-directed activity, and excessive involvement in activities with a high potential for painful consequences (especially risky sexual behavior and buying sprees). Conversely, her depressive episodes were marked by severely depressed mood, loss of interest in nearly all activities, excessive sleep, fatigue, feelings of worthlessness, and loss of appetite. Moreover, the episodes brought significant distress and impairment.

The psychiatrist explained to Hannah her basic plan for treating bipolar disorder. She noted first that Hannah was encountering a common problem for people with bipolar disorder, namely difficulty in adhering to the medication regimen. In discussing this problem, Dr. Stanley felt it was important not to convey this observation in a critical fashion. Given Hannah's somewhat girlish self-presentation and her involvement with her parents even at this stage of her life, the psychiatrist wondered if there might have been an adolescent-type rebellion in Hannah's problems with medication compliance in addition to the usual reasons patients fail to take their medications.

Since Dr. Stanley would now be assuming the role of an authority figure, she worried that Hannah might decide to resist her recommendations as another way of demonstrating rebellion. Thus, Dr. Stanley's first tactic was to empathize with Hannah's spotty record of medication compliance. She remarked that the medications used to control manic episodes often had the effect of reducing even a normal sense of high spirits, and as a result, many patients were tempted to omit their medications occasionally.

Hannah readily agreed, and she began to open up about the dilemma posed by medications. The feelings that resulted from omitting the medication were indeed pleasurable; moreover, once her feelings progressed to a manic phase, she was no longer capable of rationally considering the advisability of taking medication or of getting medical help. Hannah wondered out loud how she could ever be helped out of this dilemma; it seemed she had to choose between a chemical straitjacket and destructive bipolar episodes.

The psychiatrist explained that the first step was to see what could be done to maximize the antimanic benefit of medication while permitting a greater range of emotional feeling. She remarked that there had been some inconsistency in Hannah's care to date, as her hospitalizations had led to involvement with a variety of mental health professionals, none of whom had been able to follow her for any length of time. The psychiatrist said she would like to set matters on a different course and asked for Hannah's commitment to remain in treatment with her for the next year. Hannah agreed, and the first stage of treatment was devoted to finding a medication regimen with which Hannah could comply.

The First Year of Treatment

Dr. Stanley's goal during the first months of treatment was to determine the lowest therapeutic dose of lithium for Hannah—specifically, a dose that would keep the patient's moods stabilized but that was not so powerful as to flatten Hannah's mood completely or produce intolerable side effects.

Hannah typically had *full* manic episodes. In contrast, a *hypomanic* episode is an abnormally elevated mood state that is less severe than a full a manic episode. It produces much less impairment. In bipolar I disorder, full manic episodes alternate or intermix with major depressive episodes. In bipolar II disorder, hypomanic episodes alternate or intermix with major depressive episodes.

Between 1.0% and 2.8% of adults around the world have a bipolar disorder at any given time (Carvalho et al., 2020; Stovall, 2020).

Possible side effects of excessive lithium doses include gastrointestinal irritation, vomiting, diarrhea, tremors, metallic taste, cognitive dulling, weight gain, excessive thirst, muscular weakness, seizures, heart irregularities, and/or kidney dysfunction (Fernandes et al., 2020).

Routine and regulating patterns of behavior, such as healthy sleep and balanced eating, are helpful in managing bipolar disorder.

When Hannah first consulted the psychiatrist, she was taking 900 mg of lithium daily and 2 mg of eszopiclone for sleep. Blood tests ordered by the psychiatrist at first seemed to indicate that this dose of lithium was operating at a therapeutic level. However, after listening carefully to Hannah, the psychiatrist suspected that the patient's medication compliance problems in the past year might have been due not so much to her search for emotional highs as to impaired judgment brought on by her repeated manic episodes. That is, as Hannah declared again and again that she had really been trying in the past year to take the medication properly, the psychiatrist came to believe that the main problem might be that her dose of lithium was too low.

Dr. Stanley discussed this impression with Hannah and suggested that as long as she was taking medication, she might as well be taking enough to get some of the intended benefits. The psychiatrist proposed increasing Hannah's dose gradually, with the goal of raising the patient's blood level to the higher end of the therapeutic range. Hannah agreed to this proposal, and over the course of the next couple of weeks, the daily dose was gradually raised.

Months 2 and 3   Unfortunately, even this higher dose did not bring about the desired results over the next few months. The first sign was Hannah's arrival at a treatment session dressed more strikingly than Dr. Stanley had yet seen her. There was nothing outlandish in her appearance; she was simply wearing more jewelry and makeup than usual. Hannah said she had decided to start dressing up a little to present a more professional image. She added that colleagues seemed to treat her more professionally when she attended more to her appearance. In fact, she thought she might be considered for a promotion soon and wanted to look the part in case there was any chance of her influencing things favorably.

Dr. Stanley asked Hannah if she was continuing to take the lithium at the prescribed dose, and she replied that she was. In fact, she said she was very satisfied with the medicine. She took it regularly and felt that it was controlling her moods and helping her get back on the road to recovery. To be on the safe side, the psychiatrist asked Hannah to visit the lab for another test of her lithium blood level.

A few days later the lab report came back indicating that Hannah's blood level was the same as before—the lithium blood level had not increased despite the increase in medication. In the meantime, it soon became clear that something was indeed amiss behaviorally, as Hannah failed to appear for the next scheduled session with the psychiatrist. It turned out that she was in the midst of a 10-day manic episode, marked by increasing euphoria and flirtatiousness, which culminated in a one-night stand with a participant at one of her medical conferences. When Hannah's sexual partner informed her the next morning that she was headed home to her partner, Hannah grew furious and began hurling hotel furnishings around the room, smashing lamps and the TV. When the hotel manager was called

Hannah was ejected, along with her companion, who was grateful to have someone intervene on her behalf.

Hannah descended on her parents' house, where she encountered her mother. Recognizing a manic episode, Hannah's mother asked her daughter when she had last seen her psychiatrist and insisted that Hannah get in touch with Dr. Stanley right away. Hannah said she was fine and didn't want to bother. Her mother insisted and then made the call herself, which made Hannah furious. She was a grown woman, and her mother was calling the doctor for her. It made her feel angry. As her mother spoke on the phone, Dr. Stanley could hear Hannah shrieking in the background. Eventually, Hannah came to the phone and sheepishly agreed to come to the psychiatrist's office that evening.

Hannah arrived in the company of both parents, who wanted to ensure that their daughter kept the appointment. During the session she was irritable and pouty. She berated her parents for treating her like a child but at the same time was very much acting the part of a child. On their side, Hannah's parents—her father in particular—made snide references to Hannah's "need to grow up and take life more seriously" and her general failure to live up to their expectations. Throughout it all, Hannah was extremely agitated; she spoke rapidly in a shrill voice and periodically rose from her seat and gestured wildly to emphasize a point. She was exasperated and petulant, trying to make her case to Dr. Stanley as though she was arguing a case in a courtroom.

After listening to everyone, Dr. Stanley asked to speak with Hannah alone. After making sure that her patient was still taking her medication, the psychiatrist concluded that the dose was inadequate. Hannah at first resented this pronouncement, complaining that "everything good that I do is called an illness." Dr. Stanley was wary of confronting Hannah with the facts of the past 10 days. She elected instead to validate and support Hannah. She calmly focused on Hannah's current state, asking her how she felt and whether she was up to going to work. Hannah acknowledged that she probably needed help to return to work. The psychiatrist therefore advised her to increase her dose of lithium yet more; at the same time, she gave her the powerful antipsychotic drug chlorpromazine to calm her right away.

The next evening, Hannah called the psychiatrist, now in a much calmer state because of the chlorpromazine. She had gone back to her own apartment and had made arrangements to resume her work appointments on the Monday of the following week. She would take time that week to get regular sleep, physical activity, and balanced eating.

Early that week, Dr. Stanley met with Hannah once again and determined that her mood had indeed stabilized. The psychiatrist ordered blood tests, and this time her lithium blood level came back at the high end of the therapeutic range. The plan was to taper off the chlorpromazine with the hope that the higher dose of lithium, if taken properly, would prevent further bipolar episodes.

Around half of all people with bipolar I or bipolar II disorder receive treatment each year (Stovall, 2021; ADAA, 2020; Carvalho et al., 2020; Kessing, 2020; NIMH, 2020d, 2017d; Wang et al., 2005).

Lithium and other mood-stabilizing drugs also help prevent bipolar episodes, particularly manic episodes (Vieta et al., 2020). Thus, clinicians usually continue to prescribe these drugs even after a mood episode subsides.

Months 4 to 8 The new medication regimen appeared to control Hannah's mood swings. In fact, she was calm for the next 4 months, meeting all of her work demands and leading a quiet and stable personal life. During this period she practically went out of her way to avoid social gatherings in the evening.

After about 4 months of this existence, Hannah began to grow increasingly more cynical about her "boring" life. She started wishing she could have more fun, meet more people, and feel more stimulation. Finally, she decided to stop taking her lithium. She called Dr. Stanley and told her that she just couldn't see herself living this way indefinitely. She had grown up with enough "domination" from her parents, and now she said she was being dominated chemically; she felt she was being deprived of her freedom. Furthermore, the new level of lithium seemed to produce enormous thirst, which led her to gulp water constantly, leading in turn to constant trips to the bathroom. She stated she just couldn't take it anymore. The psychiatrist strongly advised Hannah to keep to the medication, reminding her of her last manic episode. But all that Dr. Stanley could really do at this point was urge the patient to keep her informed about how she was doing and to call her at the earliest sign of either a manic or depressive episode.

Months 9 to 12 For the next couple of months Hannah felt fine. She was happy to be off the lithium and feeling more like her "normal" self. As the weeks progressed, however, her feelings of contentment progressed to euphoria and then mania, which led to one of the most traumatic experiences of her life.

It began at a society fundraising function where Hannah, now in her manic state, began flirting with a philanthropist from Toronto. As the evening progressed, the man suggested that Hannah fly back on his private plane to his country that night. Hannah, in high spirits and needing little encouragement to do almost anything, readily agreed, and the two headed for the airport directly from the party. On the plane, Hannah was in a boisterous mood, feeling she was on top of the world. Her companion was so taken with her vivacity that, upon arriving at their destination, he had a stretch limousine take them to a hotel in opulent style.

At the hotel, Hannah and her companion settled in for a high time of fine dining, alcohol, and sex. After 3 full days of an extravagant, reckless existence, Hannah's companion raised the idea of Hannah's "entertaining" a couple of his friends. Hannah was shocked by the suggestion but ultimately agreed, and there followed what she later described as "the most degrading week of my life." It all came to an abrupt end when her companion, tiring of the arrangement, checked out of the hotel, leaving Hannah on the curb with nothing but cab fare back to the airport. Alone in an unfamiliar city and with only a few dollars, Hannah called her parents and explained her predicament. Her father immediately made plans to retrieve his daughter. Hannah spent the next 24 hours awaiting her father's arrival, sitting on a lonely seat in the airport fuming to herself and kicking at any objects within reach.

If people with a bipolar disorder have four or more mood episodes within a year, their disorder is further classified as *rapid cycling*.

Once home, Hannah spent 2 weeks in her parents' house, now overcome with depression. She felt she was a complete misfit who would never succeed in life or love, and all she wanted to do was die. In view of her condition, her parents begged her to get back in touch with Dr. Stanley. Hannah agreed to schedule a visit, and she tearfully related the episode to the psychiatrist.

Dr. Stanley prescribed the anticonvulsant drug *lamotrigine* (Lamictal) to treat Hannah's acute depression and reinstated the previous high level of lithium. Hannah's depression lifted somewhat several weeks later. After a couple of months, the psychiatrist gradually tapered the anticonvulsant in the hope that Hannah's mood could be stabilized once again with just the lithium.

Hannah had thus come full circle. She was once more taking the lithium that she so detested, and her mood swings were under control once again. As one might predict by now, before long she was expressing the same old complaints. She couldn't stand the side effects, she felt like she was wearing a straitjacket, and so on. She began omitting the lithium for a few days at a time, saying that she deserved a "couple of days of freedom" now and then.

Dr. Stanley felt that Hannah was not facing up to the reality of her situation. Like a rebellious adolescent, she continued to see taking the medicine as something imposed on her rather than something that she was doing for herself to avoid alternatives that were even worse. Dr. Stanley did not have the ability to meet with Hannah every week. But she was confident this is what Hannah needed. As such, the psychiatrist suggested that Hannah might benefit from some psychotherapy to help sort out her feelings and change her behavioral patterns. Psychotherapy, she explained, might also be helpful with some of Hannah's other concerns, her problems with relationships, for example. The patient agreed to see a psychologist, Dr. Mark Mydland, for a consultation.

Second Year of Treatment

Hannah saw the psychologist, Dr. Mydland, for what he called "insight-oriented" therapy during the next 12 months. For the first 3 months, they focused on Hannah's relationship with her parents, spending a lot of time exploring patterns of relating to her parents that started in childhood. Hannah complained that her parents had devalued her and her problems. Specifically, she believed that they saw her mainly as a disruption to their otherwise tidy lives and fancy social concerns. She was an only child, and sometimes, she told Dr. Mydland, it seemed her parents resented her very existence. She described feeling like a burden to them, and recounted how she believed they held Hannah responsible for her manic and depressive episodes, as though somehow she was causing them deliberately. These insights were new to Hannah, and she told Dr. Mydland they were helpful.

Further discussions helped Hannah recognize how extensive her resentment of her parents had grown. Time and again, she seemed bent on retaliation, keeping her parents constantly informed of her suffering by phone calls. Also, she often would try to rub their noses in her problems by causing crisis states—for example, by omitting medication—that forced them to come to her assistance. Dr. Mydland pointed out this pattern to Hannah, suggesting that she was running her life much like an adolescent whose main goal was rebellion against her parents. Hannah considered that perhaps she needed to stop making rebellion against her parents the primary guiding force of her life.

Hannah spent the next 3 months of therapy trying to make some important changes. For example, she found a new apartment farther from her parents' home, which would cut down on the frequent impromptu visits from both sides. In addition, the patient decided to cut down on her calls and text messages to her parents, in which she would seek their advice on even minor matters. At times the telephone calls were hard to resist, but as Hannah got more used to handling simple things on her own or talking them over with her friends or Dr. Mydland instead, her parents became less enmeshed in the details of her daily life, and they became less of a factor in her thoughts and actions. Her parents had always been highly involved in helping her manage her emotions. Even as a child and teenager, they were "up my you-know-what all the time," she would tell her psychologist. With her finding some autonomy and distance from her parents now, Hannah felt confident she was making positive changes.

The next step was for Hannah to begin thinking about her own goals in life. Previously, she now realized, her parents' reactions had been such a powerful motivating factor for her behaviors that she had seldom considered her own needs and desires. Over the next 3 months of therapy, Hannah decided that what she wanted most was a "normal" life—a life uninterrupted by the manic and depressive episodes that now checkered her past. As discussions on this theme progressed, the patient acknowledged that the medication she was now taking had been the one guarantee of control over these horrifying episodes. As therapy continued, Hannah came to view the medication as the guarantor of her hopes to be a normal person rather than an instrument of parental control. Furthermore, she recognized that the medication helped her to live a truly independent life. The question was whether she could accept the trade-off that the medication required, including the loss of certain pleasures and excitement that manic periods initially produced.

Intellectually, Hannah said she felt prepared to accept this trade-off, holding out for herself the hope that one day a better medication might be found or that at some point she might no longer need medication. In the meantime, she felt that the advantages of the lithium outweighed its disadvantages.

Many bipolar treatment programs now include individual, group, or family therapy as an adjunct to medication. The adjunctive therapies focus on the need for proper management of medications, psychoeducation, improving social and relationship skills, and solving disorder-related problems (Post, 2021; Vieta et al., 2020).

The remainder of the year in psychotherapy was spent helping Hannah achieve a more gratifying existence without manic episodes. The focus was on her intimate relations, which up to now had been restricted to picking up people for casual sex while in a manic state. In her depressed state, she was less confident and more likely to avoid people. With Dr. Mydland's encouragement and coaching, Hannah began to date in a more conventional fashion, typically holding off sexual activity until the relationships progressed to the point where some true feeling developed.

The Third Through Seventh Years

By the third year of treatment, Hannah's life truly began to stabilize. She developed stability and independence from her parents, and acquired a steady partner for the first time. She remained in psychotherapy with Dr. Mydland for the next 5 years and continued to see the psychiatrist, Dr. Stanley, once a month. Throughout these years, there were occasions when Hannah would omit her medication, but it usually involved skipping only a dose or two rather than stopping completely. Whenever she was tempted to discontinue, she would recall the painful episode in Toronto.

With greater emotional stability and a more mature self-concept, Hannah was able to make greater progress in her professional life. She started applying herself more seriously to her work, took business courses, and was eventually promoted to regional manager. As she experienced the pride of professional success, the pleasures derived from manic episodes seemed less important to her. This helped her to take her medications even more reliably as time progressed.

After 7 years of treatment with Dr. Stanley, Hannah reduced her visits to the psychiatrist to just a few times per year, while continuing to consult with Dr. Mydland, the psychologist, periodically.

Epilogue

A few years later, during one of her visits to Dr. Stanley, Hannah raised the idea of taking some lithium holidays. She told the psychiatrist that she still missed some of the "normal" highs that she used to experience when not taking the drug and wanted to see if she could function without the lithium at least a few days of the week. She pointed out that as it was, she was sometimes skipping a day here and there—against medical advice—without any bad consequences. She thought it made sense to try to do this in a more regulated fashion, with the psychiatrist's supervision. Dr. Stanley was persuaded, and she worked out a plan for Hannah to begin omitting her lithium one weekend day each week.

This plan proceeded without any problems for a full 6 months, and the decision was then made to omit the lithium for the entire weekend. Once again, Hannah appeared to tolerate the omission without any difficulty. She continued to lead her stable, productive existence.

Over the next 10 years, Hannah stopped seeing Dr. Mydland but continued to see Dr. Stanley for her medication needs. In a sense they were growing older and wiser together. As the clinical field came to learn more about bipolar disorders and to develop some alternative treatments, Dr. Stanley was able to cut back on lithium and introduce a newer medication, the antipsychotic drug *aripiprazole* (Abilify). The new combination of medications allowed some of the emotional richness that she longed for back into her life—yet without heightening the risk of new bipolar episodes.

These changes were all done through a slow process of trial and error. The key to their success was that Hannah had become a wise and attentive watchdog. She always knew to call Dr. Stanley as soon as the short red dress in her closet—which she hadn't worn for years—started to look appealing again. Over the years, she obtained a business degree, advanced further in her profession, and developed a long-term romance. At last, her emotions—and her life—had indeed calmed down.

Assessment Questions

1. What event prompted Hannah's first symptoms of bipolar disorder?

2. What events may have turned her mania into depression?

3. What was the reason for her second hospitalization?

4. What medications were used in the beginning of her treatment and then several years later to assist in reducing Hannah's symptoms?

5. Why did Hannah decide to stop taking her medications, and what was the result?

6. Which of her manic behaviors became a concern to her parents?

7. Hannah suffered from delusions of grandeur. What was her specific grandiose idea?

8. Explain the concept of the physician emergency certificate. Why was this necessary in Hannah's case?

9. Why do friendships suffer when an individual is bipolar?

10. Why did Hannah decide to begin therapy with Dr. Stanley?

11. Why did Dr. Stanley choose the diagnosis of bipolar I?

12. Why did Dr. Stanley want to increase Hannah's lithium level?

13. What is meant by the term *rapid cycling*?

14. Why did Dr. Stanley suggest that Hannah see a psychotherapist, Dr. Mydland?

15. What type of therapy did Dr. Mydland use with Hannah?

16. How many years did it take for Hannah's moods to stabilize?

17. What new medication was used to replace the lithium? What are the advantages of these newer medications over lithium?

CASE 7

Mind–Body Problems and COVID-19: Somatic Symptom Disorder

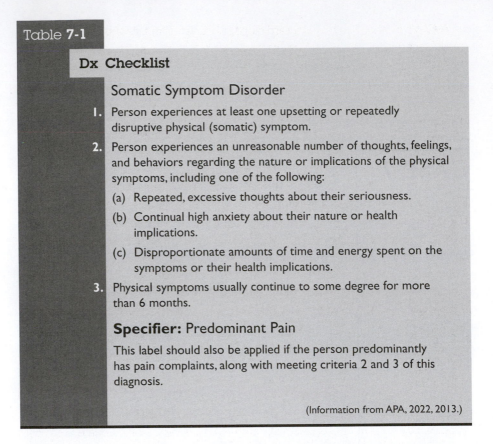

Table 7-1

Dx Checklist

Somatic Symptom Disorder

1. Person experiences at least one upsetting or repeatedly disruptive physical (somatic) symptom.

2. Person experiences an unreasonable number of thoughts, feelings, and behaviors regarding the nature or implications of the physical symptoms, including one of the following:

   (a) Repeated, excessive thoughts about their seriousness.

   (b) Continual high anxiety about their nature or health implications.

   (c) Disproportionate amounts of time and energy spent on the symptoms or their health implications.

3. Physical symptoms usually continue to some degree for more than 6 months.

Specifier: Predominant Pain

This label should also be applied if the person predominantly has pain complaints, along with meeting criteria 2 and 3 of this diagnosis.

(Information from APA, 2022, 2013.)

Although the precise prevalence of somatic symptom disorder has not been determined, research has found that it may begin at any age and is more common among women than men (Levenson, 2020).

Born into a family of doctors and nurses outside New York City on Long Island, Ashley was privileged in many ways. She was physically healthy, developmentally advanced, well-nourished with healthy foods, and had a large home protected with security cameras within a gated community. Her parents, both physicians, were disciplined hard workers earning high incomes. Their annual salaries combined, well into the seven figures range, afforded many luxuries and opportunities for Ashley and her younger sister Allie. Both girls were raised in private schools, had academic tutors, and received additional coaching and help from their live-in nanny, Carissa. The sisters were both highly intelligent and academically industrious. Driven by their parents to have multiple talents, they pursued modeling and acting gigs in addition to their studies. Between being tutored in Spanish and Carissa's directive from their parents to speak exclusively in Spanish to the girls, they became conversationally bilingual. Indeed, Ashley and her sister were born into a swift current of success in which they would never have to swim upstream.

Ashley's mother, Sarah, was a cardiologist physician-scientist who had been a successful investigator and ran a large research team for many years before becoming a full-time clinician. Now she was a senior physician in the heart center at the hospital. She mostly performed costly and complicated procedures and met with patients for pre-operative and follow-up appointments. Sarah's deceased mother had been a nurse in a pediatric intensive care unit in Manhattan. Sarah's father was a pulmonologist who died following complications from an infection he received while on a mission to provide care to remote villages in the mountains of Ecuador. All of Ashley's grandparents had immigrated to the United States from northern Europe and, as Ashley and Allie heard repeatedly from their mother growing up, Sarah's ancestry had a long lineage of people with professions in the medical field. With such a history and physician parents who would best be characterized as determined and intense, it was inevitable that Ashley and her sister would grow up thinking that they too might become doctors. Ashley joked that understanding the human body was "in her DNA," and that it was her "destiny" to follow in the footsteps of her parents and grandparents.

Ashley's father, Jerry, was an orthopedic surgeon in private practice. He was a tall muscular man who had played football in college as an offensive lineman. Jerry's parents were both doctors, but they were family medicine doctors and Jerry always knew he wanted to be a specialist. He knew how much money the primary care doctors made, and he figured if he was going to medical school, he would be sure to choose a residency program and medical specialty that would bring him a very high salary. He was a serious man, focused on his patients and his practice, and worked over 70 hours most weeks. Both Sarah and Jerry were in good health. They would wake up at 4:30 A.M. and exercise or meditate most days before eating a low-fat high-protein breakfast and arriving at work by 7 A.M. Their daughters would awake most mornings to find their parents were already out the door. Carissa, an ebullient young Columbian nanny from Miami, would get them ready for school and be there to greet them when they came home.

Ashley not only excelled in school, she was the class salutatorian her senior year. She was accepted to several Ivy League schools, but was rejected from Harvard, Yale, and Princeton. It didn't matter much to her, because she had always wanted to go to a smaller college. She decided to attend a very small liberal arts school in upstate New York known for being a women's college. By the time she was a senior in high school, Ashley had traveled throughout the world and seen many different cultures. She had grown an appreciation for how different things were in America, and she was beginning to question her long assumed dream of becoming a neurosurgeon.

Ashley COVID-19 Totally Shifts Her World

In the spring of Ashley's senior year in high school, the world was hit by the COVID-19 pandemic. Everything changed. Ashley and her sister stayed home and

As many as 60% of people confined to their homes during epidemics report substantial feelings of loneliness and sadness (Brooks et al., 2020; Ornell et al., 2020).

shifted to remote schooling. They stopped seeing their friends in person. Ashley had an acting job that was cancelled, and all prospects of modeling were postponed indefinitely. Carissa, already highly attuned to the needs of the girls and the house, became obsessive about her health and the health of the family. She rarely left the house, and when she did it was only to go to the store to buy food and other essential items that could not be delivered. Carissa became, in Ashley's mind, extremely anxious and over-protective. All they talked about was COVID — the deaths, the infections, the transmission locally, nationally, and internationally, how to prevent it, what was known, what was unknown, and so on. It was all exhausting to Ashley, but there was no way to avoid it. COVID-19 had totally shifted her world.

Sarah and Jerry were thrust onto the front lines managing patients with COVID. They worked long days and came home well into the evening most nights, their faces long with sadness and indented with red marks from hours in tightly outfitted personal protective equipment. Sarah took the brunt of it, as she had been redeployed by her department leadership to work the emergency room and intensive care unit. She listened to countless last words spoken wearily before intubation, ventilation, and, all too often, inexorable defeat to the aggressive virus. As time went on, she became increasingly despondent and helpless about the task of saving her patients and bearing witness to their lives ending without the dignity and comfort of loved ones nearby. At first, she kept this from Ashley, but eventually she decided that because Ashley wanted to become a doctor and would soon be away at college, it was time to be more open about her experiences. They started to have late night talks in the kitchen. Sarah shared with Ashley how ineffectual she believed she had become. She also disclosed how she had never felt so burned out from work. Always a woman who had been indefatigable and unflappable, she had become emotionally depleted by the daily deaths and angered by the lack of resources and endless bureaucratic processes in her hospital. One day, after noticing that she felt nothing but numbness when holding up a tablet to a patient to say goodbye to their children before being intubated, Sarah came home and broke down emotionally. She, Jerry, and Ashley talked about it in the kitchen for hours that night. Ashley held back her own tears but was upset to see her mother so badly affected. She suggested Sarah talk to a psychologist or psychiatrist. Jerry, never one to show his emotions, listened and tried to provide solutions. In a way, COVID was bringing Ashley closer to her parents. This was important to her. Seeing her mom with her hair down, transparently showing her emotions, Ashley felt especially connected to her. Allie, on the other hand, was in the basement FaceTiming her friends from the theater room, oblivious to it all.

According to worldwide surveys conducted just one month after the COVID-19 pandemic began, 73% of health care personnel had developed ongoing feelings of severe stress (N. Liu et al., 2020; S. Liu et al., 2020; Wang et al., 2020).

As the pandemic escalated into the summer, Jerry remained stereotypically masculine and stoic. "Toxic masculinity," Ashley would sometimes call it. Jerry would respond by calling her "a woke Gen-Z'er." Jerry's patient care had changed due to COVID. It shifted from elective procedures and routine visits to required and complicated surgeries. His team of nurses and technicians, usually consistent and reliable, frequently missed work due to illness or child care needs. Medical errors in his practice increased. Patient satisfaction decreased. The quality of care was eroding, and revenue was rapidly diminishing. Jerry was highly anxious about it all, but erroneously believed that trying to escape from or avoid his worries and inhibit his emotions would be the best way to cope. The whole family knew this was his go-to coping strategy. It was an open joke. Ashley and Allie, unsurprisingly, had picked up on this habit during their early adolescence. They had become experts at changing topics, deftly avoiding doing things that were unpleasant, or showing strong negative emotions.

Things at Jerry's work went from bad to worse when Ashley's favorite nurse, Consuela, contracted COVID and became seriously ill after attending an indoor family event for her aging mother. Jerry explained to Ashley that Consuela was put into a medically induced coma, and that she may or may not survive. The next day, Ashley learned that her best friend's uncle had died from COVID. Until then, as heartbreaking and devastating as it all was, death from the pandemic had not directly impacted Ashley. Now her best friend was dealing with a loss caused by COVID, and Consuela could be next. Ashley's world was turning upside down.

As the fall semester approached, Ashley chose to stay home with her family rather than live far away in a dorm, sequestered and, at some point, likely to be quarantined in a chain hotel rented by the school to prevent the transmission of the virus. She had become anxious about anyone in the family contracting COVID. This was especially true for her parents, who continued to put themselves in harm's way to take care of others. Consuela was taken off the ventilator and died, alone, in a hospital outside of her hometown and away from her family. It deeply affected Ashley, causing her to isolate herself even further. Carissa's parents in Miami had both contracted COVID, and Ashley knew many friends whose family members had been directly affected by the pandemic. Allie, a junior in high school, was becoming more and more distant from the family and alarmingly nonchalant about becoming sick with the virus.

When the fall semester began, Ashley created a new routine with online school. She kept in touch with her friends and was studious and disciplined in her schoolwork as always, out of habit or, perhaps, as a way to create a sense of normalcy. She did well in her classes but was becoming more anxious and asocial. She snapped and texted her friends but rarely saw them in person. She started questioning who her true friends were. She started seriously doubting herself for the first time in her life. Allie, on the other hand, threw caution to the wind. While her parents were at work, she would disregard Carissa's warnings about safety, leaving the house to see her friends. Ashley, now acutely aware that she was far more worried about becoming sick than Allie was, added to her list of growing worries that her sister could contract COVID. The mere thought of it kept her up

Several months into the COVID-19 pandemic, 30% or more of surveyed people had developed moderate to severe symptoms of general anxiety—symptoms that extended well beyond the specific health, economic, and family fears triggered directly by the spread of the virus (Cenat et al., 2021; Fountoulakis et al., 2021; Wang et al., 2020).

at night and caused her to send daily texts to Allie, like Carissa did, begging her to stay home, wear a mask, and stay physically distant when outside the home.

For the rest of the academic year, things stayed in a steady, stressful rhythm. Jerry and Sarah were overworked and fluctuated between emotional exasperation and emotional detachment. Jerry tried and failed to mask his misery. Sarah expressed hers more openly. Carissa obsessively kept the home going and tried to protect the girls. Allie rebelled by taking risks with her health, arguing that she was young and healthy, and even if she contracted COVID she would be okay. Ashley excelled in schoolwork but stayed socially isolated in the house, away from friends, worrying with mounting trepidation about her health and the possibility of her family members or Carissa getting sick with COVID.

Ashley A New Person Emerges at College

Once Ashley and her family were vaccinated, she became a bit less worried. Things started to look more hopeful. Her parents were less stressed and went back to their regular work routines. The family took a summer trip to Alaska. She and Allie spent more time out together doing the fun things they used to do. Still, after being away from her friends for so long, Ashley felt ambivalent about her friend group. She continued to politely avoid getting together in person, and instead spent more and more time online. Through her acting and modeling, she had a decent sized Instagram following, and she enjoyed interacting with people through direct messages, even from people she didn't know personally. In fact, she was able to connect with several people who had friends going to her college. As a result, Ashley became friendly with them, and enjoyed talking and texting with them in anticipation for the coming school year.

Ashley's parents had raised her to be open-minded and accepting of others. She was non-judgmental about other people's race, ethnicity, sexuality, and gender identity, for example. However, her childhood friends all seemed to be cisgender and heterosexual, and she had grown up in an upper-middle-class community that was predominantly white. She was excited about the prospect of meeting people from a lot of different backgrounds at college, as she always felt both privileged and, at the same time, trapped by her suburban upbringing. "We live in a bubble," Carissa used to say when they were younger. Ashley wanted to see what life outside the bubble was like. Allie, on the other hand, seemed to thrive inside her bubble. She was extroverted, confident, and fun, with a bubbly personality. She knew everyone in town, it seemed, and she thrived in this environment. As Ashley was preparing to go away to college, she sensed a coming sadness about losing Allie. She was missing her before she even left. "Pre-miss," Carissa called it, something a therapist told her years ago when she was leaving her family behind in Miami to become a full-time nanny.

At college, Ashley met many new people. She was friendly and attractive, and dressed down in order to not come across as intimidating or full of herself. She knew if she dressed up, she would get a lot of attention from men and, as she would learn, from plenty of women. And she didn't really want it now that she was so nervous about strangers and was away from acting and modeling, away from her bubble. She wore a mask everywhere, even inside when alone in her dorm room. Without a mask, she felt vulnerable, as though her safety could be easily compromised.

Through it all, she loved the atmosphere at college. Everyone came from different and unique places. They all were smart and studious, and having recently jettisoned some of the constraints and fears of COVID-19, the students she met all seemed fun, curious, and ready to cultivate new relationships. Ashley went to parties, drank more alcohol than she ever had in high school, tried cannabis gummies, and smoked marijuana. She made new friends, hooked up with a cute guy from her Bio class, and found herself endlessly receiving attention.

Despite all the excitement, Ashley was still feeling the effects of COVID psychologically. Her general level of anxiety was higher than it was before the pandemic. She had become more anxious about becoming sick, anxious about contracting COVID-19, anxious about her family and friends becoming ill, anxious about people she didn't know carrying the virus, anxious about so many things that all connected back to COVID-19. Most of the students rarely wore masks, but she refused to take hers off unless she was drinking or using drugs. To help with her anxiety, Carissa reminded her to do yoga, meditate, and exercise regularly. Her parents told her to eat well and stick to a routine. Allie told her she was overreacting to everything.

Ashley tried everything to help get rid of her anxiety yet still felt daily surges of agitation, jitters, and dread. Her worries about being infected meant that she would wipe down surfaces in the classroom, clean her hands throughout the day, and avoid people she didn't know. She had made close friends quickly, and she felt safest around them. But when they went out together, she felt a spike of overwhelming anxiety about becoming infected. To cope with this, she avoided new situations as much as possible. When she went out to new places or with new people, she would eat a cannabis gummy and drink a lot of alcohol to keep her worries at bay. This worked in the short-term and it became a new pattern for her.

One night while Ashley was with friends at an off-campus party, she was hit on by a classmate, introduced as Rachel, who she recognized from the nearby dorm. They had never talked before, but Ashley had admired Rachel's bold sense of style from a distance—Rachel rocked a short haircut dyed bright blue, a nose ring, flowery tattoos, and colorful makeup, plus a fashion sense Ashley thought of as tomboyish. They talked for hours; high and disinhibited, Ashley was surprised to find herself not only flirting, but also opening up about all of her secret anxieties.

Surveys conducted during the COVID-19 pandemic found increases in the number of children and adolescents who generally felt edgy (54%), annoyed (47%), worried (47%), sad (44%), and apathetic (54%) (Gindt et al., 2021; Zhou et al., 2020).

In turn, Rachel felt comfortable enough to open up to Ashley about identifying as nonbinary and queer and using "they/them" pronouns. Rachel had a confident, almost gruff manner, but got nervous around Ashley and stumbled over words. Likewise, Ashley found herself totally enraptured. They kissed at the end of the night, sloppy but passionate, Ashley's guard lowered by the alcohol and cannabis in her system. Normally, such close contact would have triggered her anxieties about COVID, but even the next morning, all Ashley could think about was Rachel and how she wanted to see them again.

What was going on? Ashley had gone away to college and was becoming a new person. The new Ashley was even more anxious, regularly using drugs and alcohol, and now she was making out with someone she never would have expected herself to be attracted to. And she couldn't stop thinking of Rachel. Ashley began questioning her sexuality. She had identified as cisgender and heterosexual, and had her first sexual experience with a boyfriend in high school. As a model, she had spent a lot of time around attractive women and girls since she was a child. She never had noticed any sexual interest in women before, though she admired and always found herself paying attention to good-looking women. As she thought about it, she realized that she had always found women with shorter hair attractive. She loved to look at them on the runway when modeling, and had tried unsuccessfully to befriend several similar looking models in the past.

Ashley and Rachel became close as the months went on, frequently hooking up in private, and always flirting heavily when out in public. Ashley wondered what it meant for her identity that she was dating a nonbinary person. Was she bisexual, or pansexual maybe? She wasn't sure, but she knew she felt good with Rachel. More important, she felt safe when they were together. Rachel seemed to have a balanced blend of healthy masculinity and femininity. And Ashley felt comfortable being public about their growing relationship. Her parents were supportive. So was Carissa. When she told Allie, her sister replied dismissively in an invalidating manner.

Crisis Hits Allie Becomes Sick

Although they had become distanced from each other since the pandemic, the sisters were still close. They had been tightly bonded as children, and with so much time together, it would take a catastrophic event to pull them apart. During the spring semester of her sophomore year, Ashley received a phone call from her mother that she had been dreading. Allie had become sick, contracting a mutated variant of COVID-19 that the vaccine was less than 100% effective against. She was in the hospital where Sarah worked and in serious condition. Ashley came home from school immediately and went to see her sister. Allie was sleeping, pale white and highly medicated, while rhythmic beeping sounds and vibrations from

---

Sidebar (left margin):

Dating back to the bubonic plague in medieval Europe, studies have found increases in the prevalence of anxiety, depressive, and substance use disorders in communities and nations overrun by epidemics (Ren, Gao, & Chen, 2020; Usher, Durkin, & Bhullar, 2020).

On average, the bodies of elderly persons have slower-acting immune systems than younger persons, putting older adults at a greater disadvantage when trying to overcome influenza, pneumonia, viral infections such as COVID-19, and other serious medical illnesses (Bajaj et al., 2021; Begley, 2020).

the bed and calf massager interrupted the silence every so often. Ashley was ter-rified and sat silently crying. Who was she becoming? How had her life, once so predictable, now careened off course? She looked at herself in the mirror. She looked different than before college. Her hair was up; she wore no makeup and a baggy school hoodie with loose leggings. She had a new nose ring.

Ashley had many previous nightmares about Allie or her family members get-ting sick and dying. She had worried at night, worried during class, worried all the time about her family becoming ill. Now Allie's lungs were infected, and she was having trouble breathing. What if she never fully recovered and had lifetime dif-ficulties breathing? Or worse, what if she were to die?

Thankfully, Allie was eventually discharged in good condition, and Ashley went back to school to finish the semester. She was rattled. Her anxiety about becom-ing sick increased. She reacted to every physical discomfort she had as though it could be a crisis. Pains, aches, coughing, sneezing, anything—all of it was met with scrutiny and paralyzing uncertainty. This led to a marked increase in her going to the campus health center. It also led to an increase in her cannabis and alcohol use. She became more difficult to be around socially. Rachel, who once couldn't get enough of Ashley, was now keeping some distance from her, only hanging out when partying, when it was likely that Ashley would be easier to be around and less intense.

The worst part of it seemed to be the onset of new GI problems. Ashley's stom-ach aches started soon after she arrived on campus, and worsened over time. She went to the campus health center several times to be evaluated, but they were unable to discern any organic cause each time. As a result, Ashley began a gastritis diet, avoiding red meat, acidic and spicy foods, and her favorite—caffeine. She con-tinued to drink alcohol but shied away from beer. Still, her stomach and intestines ached most days. After seeing a gastroenterologist and receiving an upper endos-copy, no acute medical problems were discovered. She was diagnosed with func-tional dyspepsia (indigestion resulting from a nonorganic source) and learned that she was at risk for irritable bowel syndrome or stomach ulcers in the future. This failed to quell her anxiety. Instead, she felt even more unpredictability and uncontrol-lability about her health. In a vicious cycle, this seemed to increase her anxiety and when she felt increased anxiety, she tended to feel greater pain. Her gastroenterolo-gist explained that, generally speaking, the mind and body are tightly connected, with each influencing the other. When Ashley asked questions, the doctor further sug-gested that the mind is not distinct from the body. What we experience and call our "mind" is neurobiological, with complex processes occurring in the brain and body influencing how and what we think, feel, and sense in our body. Ashley left wonder-ing, is my anxiety making my GI problems worse? Or are my GI problems making my anxiety worse? If there is nothing wrong with my GI system, why do I feel so much pain? She was overwhelmed and felt hopeless about what to do.

Since the start of the COVID-19 pandemic, alcohol and drug use, the number of persons displaying alcohol and drug use disorders, and the number of fatal drug overdoses have risen significantly (Niles et al., 2021; CDC, 2020a; Valinsky, 2020).

Rachel Perspective from Someone Close to Ashley

Rachel told some of their mutual friends they were wanting some space from Ashley. "I loved spending time with her at the beginning. She was fun, cute as hell, and was into me. She accepted me for who I am. She never questioned anything. Sure, she was wound up tight. But who wasn't at that time? We were coming out of the lockdown phase of the pandemic and back to school, finally. It was a weird time for everyone. I was more uptight then too.

"But after her sister got sick and recovered from COVID, Ashley seemed changed for the worse. I tried to help comfort her, but it didn't seem to matter. Unless she was drinking or high, Ashley was kind of difficult to be around. All she talked about was her health and her worries about getting sick. It was like that was the only thing she was thinking about. I love being with her, but I just can't be around all that negativity and worry. It's like, come on girl, you got this. You have everything anyone could ever want. And all you can do is think about getting sick? I'll still be her friend, and when she's cool, I'll totally spend more time with her. Honestly, truly, she's got this ongoing mysterious thing going on with her stomach. It's not something simple, like lactose intolerance. And it's always on her mind. She needs help, you know, like from a doctor or therapist, or someone."

Ashley: Help on the Way

Ashley's sophomore year spring semester grades were the lowest she had ever received: two B's and 2 A's. She was devastated. She got a B in Bio and a B− in Chem. Maybe it was from avoiding classes out of her worry she might make her GI pain worse. When she was in class, she had a hard time focusing on the lectures. Her mind raced, and she noticed every new sensation in her body. What would this mean about her chances of becoming a doctor? She had changed so much this year, and now she wondered about whether she should change her major and career ambitions. Sarah and Jerry saw how bedraggled and unsteady Ashley had become, and suggested she see a psychiatrist or therapist that summer. Ashley responded by saying she had no interest in taking medicine to deal with her worries, but that she would see a psychologist.

Sarah spoke with her colleagues in the Department of Psychiatry and came home with several recommended therapists. Ashley deeply respected her mother and decided to contact Dr. Zakir Husain, a clinical psychologist with expertise in health anxiety. She requested that they meet remotely using a telemental health approach. He agreed and they met several weeks later for an initial evaluation. After gathering biopsychosocial history information—that is, asking about her medical history, personality and coping strategies, and relationships—Dr. Husain asked a series of diagnostic questions related to anxiety, substance use, and health concerns. He learned that her anxiety began to be problematic during the height of the COVID-19 pandemic, and that the scope of her anxiety was limited to somatic concerns. Each day, she worried repeatedly about her health but was not particularly anxious about other parts of her life. He told her she likely met diagnostic criteria for somatic symptom disorder, but that he would need more information to confirm this diagnosis. He suggested she also appeared to meet criteria for a substance use disorder but believed the function of her substance use was primarily to reduce anxiety related to her overall health in general and to her GI symptoms more specifically. He wanted to target her health anxiety using an evidence-based form of cognitive-behavioral therapy called Acceptance and Commitment Therapy, or ACT for short. Ashley was saddened to hear his conclusions, but they made sense to her, and she was relieved there was a path forward. "Help is on the way," Dr. Husain said, smiling warmly, as they ended their first appointment together.

The next week, they met for their second session, and the first one using ACT. Dr. Husain asked Ashley how willing she was to try this treatment, and she remarked that she had been both excited and nervous. "Ah, ambivalence," he noted. "Notice your mind having ambivalent thoughts." Ashley ignored him and started to talk about things that happened to her in the last week. She explained how she had been feeling sick, having GI pain, worrying about her health, and volunteering at her mother's hospital. She waited for him to say something, but when he did, she was surprised. Instead of asking her to share more details, instead of reflecting and paraphrasing what she had said, instead of encouraging her to talk more about her experiences or her anxiety, instead of doing all the things she had seen in the movies and TV shows that therapists do, Dr. Husain quickly acknowledged Ashley's emotional distress and then gently requested permission to ask her several questions.

Dr. Husain:	It's normal to talk about anxiety and all the things that cause us distress. I do it. Everyone I know does it. It's common, especially in Western cultures. But consider this: What if talking about our distress in and of itself was part of the problem? What if it is not the solution after all?
Ashley:	I don't understand.
Dr. Husain:	Maybe *you* do, but your mind tells you that you don't?
Ashley:	My mind is me.
Dr. Husain:	Is it? What is your mind?
Ashley:	What do you mean?
Dr. Husain:	Literally, if you take a step back from the content of your mind, what is it, exactly?
Ashley:	I don't know. Maybe my mind is my … thoughts?
Dr. Husain:	If your mind is your thoughts, are *you* your thoughts?
Ashley:	No. I am me. Bones, organs, blood, and all the rest of my body.
Dr. Husain:	And your body creates sensations, like hunger, thirst, fatigue, and so on.

For many years, somatic symptom disorder and related problems (conversion disorder and illness anxiety disorder) were referred to as *hysterical* disorders, a label meant to convey the past belief that excessive and uncontrolled emotions underlie the bodily symptoms found in these disorders (Stone & Sharpe, 2020).

Ashley: I don't get it.

Dr. Husain: Your body produces sensations, and your brain, which is a part of your body, creates thoughts. Or at least a part of your brain does this. And other parts of your brain do other things, like helping you see, smell, hear, and so on, or keeping you breathing while you sleep, standing when you walk, and so on. Your brain has parts that enable you to think, and, at the same time, it also has the ability to observe *that* you are thinking, or to notice *what* you are thinking.

> According to research, people with higher levels of *somatic vigilance*—a general inclination to attend to one's body, and to worry about bodily arousal and discomforts—are more likely than other people to experience pain and pain-related anxiety (Burton et al., 2020; D'Souza & Hooten, 2020a).

Dr. Husain went on to provide an orientation to ACT. He explained that unlike treatments designed to help by listening only, or treatments intended to help by changing what people think using techniques like cognitive reappraisal, ACT would help her in a different way. Ashley was intrigued. She thought she was supposed to talk about her problems in therapy, and that Dr. Husain, or any therapist for that matter, would listen, support, problem-solve, and help with advice on what she should do to reduce her anxiety. Dr. Husain differentiated ACT from other versions of cognitive-behavioral therapy (CBT) by saying that in ACT, the goal is not necessarily to get rid of anxiety or have fewer worries. He had no intention of asking her for evidence to support or possibly refute the truth of her worry thoughts. Inasmuch as ACT does target cognitive processes, it is considered a type of cognitive-behavioral therapy. But it is, as Dr. Husain described, an *acceptance-based* CBT. He would help her change her patterns of behavior by guiding her to *mindfully* and *acceptingly* observe the thoughts and feelings going through her head and body at any given time, and then teaching her to replace her habitual reactions to such thoughts and feelings with responses that were more useful and "value-based." That is, although Ashley might typically accept her thoughts as "true," he would help her learn to accept her thoughts as mere thoughts, not to be conflated with unquestionable truths. Instead of playing tug of war with the truth of her worrying thoughts, he would help her let go of the rope and focus more on her daily functioning, irrespective of the worries she might be having. He used a number of metaphors, including one about falling into a hole and trying to get out using a tool that only kept her stuck and digging deeper. The session ended, and Ashley's head was spinning.

> Mindfulness techniques, which guide people to observe their thoughts and bodily sensations without judgment, were brought into the clinical mainstream by psychologist Steven Hayes and his colleagues as an important feature of their broader approach, Acceptance and Commitment Therapy.

The next week, Ashley asked for clarity about ACT. Dr. Husain answered her questions. ACT was in the family of CBTs, he said, but success was measured by how closely she was living her life aligned with her values and by how little her thinking was interfering with her daily functioning. They would assess symptoms of health anxiety periodically using self-report scales, and they would assess success with a questionnaire assessing how closely she was living day to day within her values. Ashley asked about the concept of values. Dr. Husain explained that values are learned and culturally bound, often coming from a combination of family, friends, community, and society. They are the ways we strive to live, how we want to be in different parts of our life. Ashley asked him if values were the same thing as goals, like her wanting to become a neurosurgeon. "No," he replied, "whereas goals are the things we want, values are the ways we aspire to live. Goals are *what* we want, like outcomes to acquire. Values, on the other hand, are the processes and ways that define *how* we want to live. Goals are nouns, and values are usually adjectives," he stated matter-of-factly.

They spent that session and the one after exploring and clarifying her values. They used a worksheet to differentiate her values in nine major domains of life, including, for example, how she valued being as a family member (for example, dependable, loving), friend (fun, spontaneous), partner (passionate, emotionally available), student (disciplined), and how she valued living as a community member in her school (inclusive). They went on and delineated her values about her physical health, as well as how she wanted to treat herself compassionately and nonjudgmentally. With her values now organized, Dr. Husain asked her to rate how successful she had been recently in living her life aligned with her values. They used a 0–10 scale, and Ashley realized that she had been effective in a lot of areas but was living far below her values as a family member, friend, and partner. With these areas of life now in clear view as most misaligned with her values, Dr. Husain asked her to look for ways in which her anxiety, and how she related to it, was causing or maintaining the gap between her values and actions.

The next session, Ashley began by embarrassedly disclosing that she hated the therapy homework assignment. She found it a bit easier to tell him because they were doing remote therapy. If she were in his office, she wondered if she would have had the courage to tell him. But remotely, separated by distance and with the off ramp of pressing "leave meeting" if she ever needed to, she boldly spoke up about her feelings. He was unfazed and asked for clarification. She found it aversive and shameful to think about how she herself may be causing her problems by how she copes with her anxiety. Dr. Husain asked her to notice these interpretations as thoughts and encouraged her to "thank her mind" for having these thoughts. Ashley was annoyed, but something in this unorthodox approach was compelling to her. Dr. Husain asked her to clarify which value areas were most important to her, and she quickly told him that her family was the most important area, followed by friendship, and then being a partner. "So," he said, "your family is the most important domain in your life, and it is also the area where your values are most out of touch with your day-to-day actions?" Ashley nodded. "Is this the part of your life we can prioritize for change?" Ashley nodded again.

Over the rest of that session and the next few appointments, they would aim directly together, like two archers each with their hands on the same bow, pointing the arrow toward the bull's eye of treatment outcome. The therapeutic alliance was strong. Ashley trusted Dr. Husain and respected him. She wondered about him, his family background, his training. But she feared he might experience such questions

In one survey, 73% of men and 39% of women reported that they sometimes multitask during their telehealth and/or telemental health visits, including surfing the Web, checking e-mails, and texting (25%); scrolling through social media (21%); and playing a video game (19%) (DF, 2020).

as derogatory slights asked simply because he had brown skin — communications referred to as microaggressions in academia. At one point, he shared a story about his training, self-disclosing that he was raised in the Baltimore area, but was born in Seattle.

With a clear focus on treatment outcomes and a collaborative therapeutic process, they talked about her interactions with her family, her friends, and Carissa. What thoughts did she notice? What emotions did she observe? What actions did she inhibit when she was anxious? There was so much to observe with curiosity. He helped her view her thoughts as though she were an anthropologist, observing and taking notes on what the "tribe" of thoughts had to say. He oriented her toward mindfulness and practiced with her, trying various exercises to help her become aware, in the present moment, of her thoughts, feelings, and sensations, all without doing anything to change them.

Dr. Husain explained that ACT used an underlying "hexaflex" model, in which there were actually six different psychological processes being targeted for change. Each was related to the others. They all had names that sounded like jargon or psychobabble to her, but she understood what he meant. They included (1) contacting the present moment (instead of avoiding it); (2) behaving aligned with her values; (3) engaging in committed action; (4) experiencing her self-as-context — meaning that she is not the content of her thoughts, but rather the consciousness experiencing those thoughts; (5) cognitive defusion — understanding the difference between thoughts and reality; and (6) experiential acceptance — the practice of accepting experiences and thoughts that are beyond control. At the heart of it all was the overarching treatment goal of what he called "psychological flexibility" — the ability to be responsive and effective across contexts in ways that align with her values, no matter what she might be thinking, feeling, or otherwise experiencing.

Ashley's Treatment It Begins Making Sense

Because he was using ACT, Dr. Husain frequently relied on metaphors and experiential exercises instead of the more traditional back-and-forth conversational tools common to social dialogue. To help Ashley differentiate between her thoughts and her "self," he described her thoughts as "bullies on a bus," wherein she was the driver and her thoughts, like bullies, sat in the back of the bus yelling at her, threatening her with possible catastrophes and telling her what could happen if she did this or that behavior. The bullies, Dr. Husain suggested, were used to getting their way, essentially hijacking her life by telling her what to do. Although she could, in fact, have steered the bus of her life in any way she valued, she had been too busy believing the bullies, and acceding to their demands. As a result, she had taken too many lefts and rights away from the ways she valued living, listening to the bullies as though they knew the right way to go. Under Dr. Husain's

ACT and related mindfulness-based therapy have been helpful for a range of psychological problems, including anxiety disorders, depression, PTSD, personality disorders, and substance use disorders (Jauhar et al., 2021; Zurita Ona, 2021).

Albert Einstein once said, "We cannot solve our problems with the same thinking we used when we created them."

guidance, Ashley started paying attention to these thoughts (the bullies on her bus), examining her interpretations and assumptions, and observing the ways the thoughts were directing her to live her life. She started to see a disturbing pattern: The bullies almost always convinced her to avoid people, places, or things that she wanted to approach — things that were often important to her. The bullies on her bus had been convincing her to avoid all possible risks. Indeed, as she later told Dr. Husain, she was coming to appreciate that she had been held hostage by her own thoughts. She had become fused to her thoughts — confusing thoughts with truths.

In another session, Dr. Husain tried to help her defuse from the meaning of her thoughts by having her say out loud, repeatedly with him, the word "milk." They said it together over and over: "milk, milk, milk, milk, milk, milk, milk, milk, milk, milk, milk, milk." Eventually, Ashley stopped and giggled, declaring, "The word loses its meaning when you say it so many times." This was the point, she learned. Then Dr. Husain asked her another one of his mind-numbing questions. "What if our thoughts are simply words, comprised of phonemes and arbitrary utterances made by our mouth and tongue? What if the meaning we take from our words is based on our unique learning history and the context in which we think, or talk?" Ashley was curious, and it was making sense. She stopped him, "Is this sort of like the bullies on the bus, where I can choose to make sense of and react to my thoughts however I want to? Like, I am not simply my thoughts but I can see them and choose whether to believe them or to let them go?" This time, Dr. Husain was the one doing the nodding.

As the summer wound down, they began moving toward the process of ending therapy. Dr. Husain called it "termination," then chuckled and said that he despised that word and would instead call it "ending therapy," for now. He had been consistently using self-report measures to assess Ashley's anxiety, valued actions, and tendency to try to avoid her internal experiences, or, as he called it, "experiential avoidance." On all measures she was improving significantly. Except one. She was still highly anxious, in the moderate range on a standard measure of anxiety symptoms. But her valued actions had increased, she was avoiding her anxiety less, and she was living more aligned with her values. Her GI pain had diminished only a bit, though she had learned to react without avoidance when she did experience any stomach pain. Sure, she wanted all the pain and discomfort to stop, and she continued to monitor and be sensitive to internal sensations throughout her GI tract. But it was all less impairing than it used to be.

As they moved session by session closer to the end of therapy, Ashley observed that she was noticing a lot of anxious thoughts about returning to school, about ending therapy, and, of course, about the possibility that she might become sick when she got back on campus. At the same time, she tearfully shared her insights about the useful things she had learned that summer. She had been drinking much less, rarely using cannabis, spending more time with the people who mattered most to her, and being the kind of person she valued as much as possible when with them. She made a point of spending time with Allie and her parents, appreciating Carissa more openly, and being with friends who enabled her to be her more authentic self. She also came to recognize and disclose that she was bisexual, sexually attracted to people across the entire gender spectrum. She would return to college looking for a partner with whom she could express her truest values honestly and vulnerably. Ashley noted that she had been learning to stay in contact with her thoughts and emotions, without trying to escape from them anymore. In turn, she had become more aware of the opportunities to be in the moment, increasingly defused from her thoughts even when feeling emotionally distressed, and no longer subject to the demands of the bullies on her bus. She had been psychologically imprisoned but now felt free; she joyfully told Dr. Husain that she had been "blind all the time but was learning to see." It was a lyric in a song she heard, and it rang true. "Psychological inflexibility," Dr. Husain said assuredly with a smile and subtly cocked head, "psychological flexibility."

In the final session, they reviewed her treatment progress, consolidating everything that had been learned. They planned for ways to generalize and maintain her new ways of relating to her internal experiences. They developed and wrote out a plan. In the event that her avoidance and psychological inflexibility returned, a "relapse" as he called it, she had a plan. She would complete a revised values clarification worksheet, identify where she was living most out of touch from her values, practice mindful awareness of the present moment, observe efforts to avoid or escape from her anxiety, keep reminders of what helped in her phone, and remember certain key phrases that evoked strong memories of metaphors with Dr. Husain. They scheduled follow-up video appointments each month, and she could cancel them if she wanted to. She would keep each one.

> Adults in the United States spend approximately $2 billion on mindfulness meditation programs each year. Around 14% of the United States population practice mindfulness techniques (LaRosa, 2019; Rakicevic, 2019; Ziegelstein, 2018).

Epilogue

Ashley's anxiety about contracting a serious illness waxed and waned over time. Her GI distress continued, never fully abating. She graduated with a degree in Biology and a minor in Women's Studies. Dr. Husain was available for booster sessions with her throughout college, and she met with him several more times. ACT had helped her realize she did not need to try to change what she was thinking when she became anxious. Instead, she had learned to free herself from the paralysis and avoidance she had learned in the aftermath of the COVID-19 pandemic. Her fear of others and worries about contracting a medical illness continued to a degree, but she was able to gain perspective on them. She took herself a bit less seriously, was easier to be around, and excelled socially. She even developed a lovably neurotic sense of self-awareness and playfulness about her anxious thinking. Although her previous partner, Rachel, transferred to a school in Manhattan, Ashley stayed in touch with them over the years. In time, Ashley and Rachel became close friends, and Ashley began dating one of Rachel's lesbian friends. Ashley took a job in the city as a research coordinator during a gap year before medical school applications. She was in love, felt safe, and was living fully in the city, in spite of her anxiety and periodic stomach pain. She had learned to accept the internal cognitive experiences that used to plague her. She didn't have to approve of them, but she could accept that they were happening. They were, after all, only what they were: things her brain produced, things that did not have to be taken as truths. She could accept her emotions, allow them to be present, and, in those moments, stay committed to actions that she valued. It was liberating. Though she had always dreamed of being a neurosurgeon, she wondered aloud to her new girlfriend if she might become a psychiatrist instead.

Assessment Questions

1. What were the earliest risk factors displayed for Ashley to develop somatic symptom disorder?

2. What role might the family and her family history have played in the development of her health-related worries?

3. In which ways did the COVID-19 pandemic impact Ashley's life?

4. How did Ashley change psychologically in response to the pandemic?

5. Do you think a different diagnosis, such as an anxiety disorder, was warranted? If so, could an anxiety disorder diagnosis have significantly impacted Dr. Husain's choice of treatment?

6. How do you think Ashley's anxiety impacted her GI problems, and vice versa?

7. Is Acceptance and Commitment Therapy a type of cognitive-behavioral therapy?

8. What were the targeted treatment mechanisms in Ashley's therapy? In other words, which of her psychological processes did Dr. Husain try to change in order to help her?

9. What does "acceptance" mean in this treatment?

10. What does "change" mean in this treatment?

11. What did Dr. Husain do at the end of therapy to reduce the risk for relapse in anxiety?

12. What tools and approaches were used to assess the efficacy of Ashley's treatment?

CASE 8

Prescription Drug Abuse

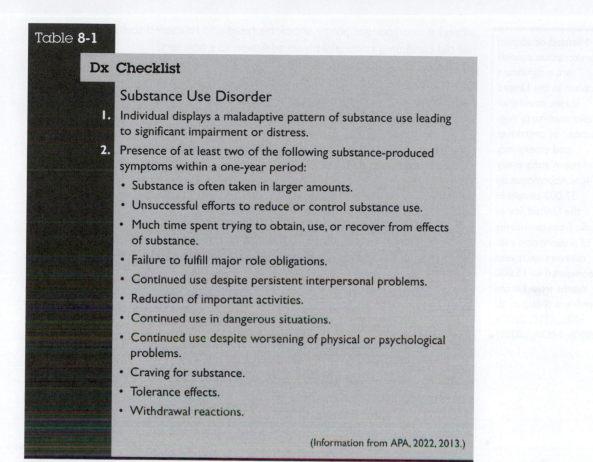

Table 8-1

Dx Checklist

Substance Use Disorder

1. Individual displays a maladaptive pattern of substance use leading to significant impairment or distress.

2. Presence of at least two of the following substance-produced symptoms within a one-year period:
    - Substance is often taken in larger amounts.
    - Unsuccessful efforts to reduce or control substance use.
    - Much time spent trying to obtain, use, or recover from effects of substance.
    - Failure to fulfill major role obligations.
    - Continued use despite persistent interpersonal problems.
    - Reduction of important activities.
    - Continued use in dangerous situations.
    - Continued use despite worsening of physical or psychological problems.
    - Craving for substance.
    - Tolerance effects.
    - Withdrawal reactions.

(Information from APA, 2022, 2013.)

Standing slouched in the back corner of a musty jail cell on charges of vehicular manslaughter and driving under the influence, Jimmy closed his eyes and said under his breath, "How did I get here?" Thinking back to his childhood, Jimmy, a 53-year-old white, heterosexual, cisgender man from rural Ohio, knew his life didn't have to end up like this. He was raised by a loving mother in a small rural town where everyone knew each other. He never moved, had decent grades in school, and had no major health problems. On account of his dad passing away when he was seven and being the oldest of two boys, Jimmy had become very good with his hands. Plumbing, electrical, engine repair—he could fix just about anything by the time he was out of high school. During high school, he worked at Hinshaw's, the local auto repair shop and, for a brief stint, as an apprentice for Mr. Buckner, the electrician in town. After graduating high school, he worked for a handyman service, where he would work for 10 years in all. Recalling the many things he did well

Misused or abused prescription opioids are a significant problem in the United States, causing an extraordinarily high number of overdoses and emergency room visits every year. Approximately 37,000 people in the United States die from overdoses of prescription pain relievers each year, compared to 15,000 deaths from heroin overdoses (Niles et al., 2021; CDC, 2020a, 2020b; NIDA, 2020a).

when he was younger, Jimmy shook his head and muttered to himself, "How the *hell* did I end up a criminal with an addiction to painkillers?"

Despite the early life factors that could have helped protect him from getting into trouble, the cards also were stacked against him in certain ways. His mother had a serious drinking problem and was often unavailable for him as a child. She was home most of the time, on disability caused by chronic pain and severe post-traumatic stress, but she generally stayed isolated in her room. Though loving and kind when sober, most of the time she was more like a dependent roommate for Jimmy and his brother. They took care of her and the house most of the time. When their mother had a boyfriend over, the brothers were subjected to physical intimidation and emotional abuse. They overheard stories about drugs, drinking, and breaking the law. They were frequently around when her boyfriend would be drunk or high on various drugs. To them, drug use and heavy drinking were normal things men in their town did. When he was a teenager, Jimmy used to think it was funny to see his mother's boyfriends and their friends acting so wild when they were under the influence of drugs. They might break things, shoot at things, or tell raunchy stories. Outlaw country music played loudly at home as the soundtrack of his youth—legends like Willie, Merle, and Johnny. Wherever he turned, the men around him talked about getting into trouble, challenging norms, and breaking the law. By the time he was 16, Jimmy and his friends would spend weekend nights at a clearing in the woods listening to music around a fire, drinking cheap beers, and smoking whatever pot they could score.

Jimmy was older than his brother, but a little less wise. His younger brother avoided using drugs after the age of 16, drank much less, and had no arrest record. Jimmy, on the other hand, was arrested for the first time at 21 for disorderly conduct after getting into a fight at the Chicken Bridge bar. At 26, he was pulled over (with more than an ounce of weed in his car) for going 64 in a 45. The ticket was expensive, but the police never checked the car for drugs. He knew he was lucky. Around these same years, Jimmy's brother went off to college and then moved to Cincinnati to begin work, knowing that he needed to escape their hometown. Jimmy, on the other hand, did one semester of community college, then quit, unable to attend class due to a conflict with his work as a handyman.

During his 20s, Jimmy spent his days working and weekends partying. At the time, he thought he was living a great life. He was unattached romantically, and had fun every weekend. He and his friends would hang out together, laughing and planning long trips in the mountains together. They would putter around the garage making or fixing things, drinking light beers and chain smoking Camels. On many weekends they would get up early and hunt small game or fish the local streams. Many nights, they would go deep into the woods to camp. If they were feeling lazy or unorganized, they would mess around in the yard behind Jimmy's place and target shoot, the rolling hills of Appalachia absorbing any drunken wayward bullets.

Whether they were in the woods or at one of their houses, there was always a fire in the evening. The guys—always Jimmy and his male friends—would drink brown liquor and light beer around the fire usually into the wee hours of the morning. Sundays they would awaken late, make jokes about missing church again, and, while battling their hangovers, find something to laugh about or plan their next trip together.

The crew was small, with several regulars. Ritchie Jr., spelled differently as part of a longstanding family tradition dating back many generations, was Jimmy's closest friend. Ritchie was twitchy and athletic, hot-tempered and quick-witted. He had been the cause of quite a few fights with neighboring kids growing up. He liked to tell people he and his ancestors were true Americans from the countryside. He was a proud American, prone to confabulating memories he recalled hearing from his grandmother—stories she had told him about how her grandma and grandpa had held off attacks from Natives Americans on their westward travels from North Carolina to Kentucky. What Ritchie did not know was that his grandmother was, in truth, part Cherokee. Her own great-grandmother had been held hostage and raped by an American soldier.

Then there was Jody. He had Irish and Scottish blood and a heavy, muscular frame. Jody's older brother used to joke that Jody fell down the stairs and hit his head when he was young. That explained, so the story went, why he was quick to make poor decisions and wasn't all that smart. Jody was a risk taker and a heavy drug user by the time he was in high school. In his 20s, Jody turned to selling drugs as a significant source of side income. He worked for the county doing service work, but made much more money dealing drugs, mostly marijuana. When Jody was in his early 30s, the local police seized 20 pounds of marijuana in a highly publicized drug bust. The sheriff's office assigned Jody's work crew to bury the seized drugs at the county landfill. Jody, having the most experience operating heavy machinery, was tasked with the job. A week after he buried it, Jody returned late at night alone and dug it back up, selling all 20 pounds to a dealer who, as it turned out, was an informant for the FBI. Jody was immediately arrested. He spent the next 18 years incarcerated before being let out on parole.

Jimmy The Car Accident

At age 35, Jimmy was single, out of shape physically, and living alone. His brother had long ago moved away. His mother died from stomach cancer when he was 30. He inherited the house he grew up in, the same as his father had when his parents had both passed. He was now working at Hinshaw's as a repair technician, a job that was unchallenging but kept him busy. After work, Jimmy and Ritchie continued their tradition of tinkering in the garage on anything with an engine. For over a year they had been working on a '78 Trans Am that Ritchie had acquired. It had

One important approach to substance use disorders is to try to *prevent* them. Drug prevention programs keep growing in number and are offered in schools, workplaces, activity centers, and other community settings, as well as on social media, the Internet, television, and radio (SAMHSA, 2021, 2019; Tremblay et al., 2020).

been in very bad shape, but Ritchie and Jimmy upgraded engine parts, cleaned up the interior, and repainted it. Eventually, after many long weekends, light beers, and chain-smoked Camels, the slick, black Trans Am was ready for the road.

Ritchie wanted to be the one to drive it first. Jimmy sat in the passenger seat. They pulled out of the driveway, turned right, and drove slowly on the gravel road, coming to a stop sign at the county road. It was a windy summer day, and the windows were down. No cars were coming in either direction. A gust of wind replaced the thick humid air for a moment. They laughed as they saw Jimmy's spent can of Bud Light from the night before blow along the edge of the highway. Ritchie turned to Jimmy and asked, "You ready boy?" Jimmy's seat was positioned high and forward. They had forgotten to shift it back after working on the back seat. Jimmy turned to Ritchie and smiled, then took his right hand and moved it from his lap to the front of the window frame. He slapped the windshield with his palm three times, then said, "Let's do it!"

They had retrofitted the engine to boost the horsepower and acceleration. Ritchie spun the wheels in neutral, then jolted the engine into gear, fishtailing left onto the old county road. The Trans Am lurched forward, and Jimmy clamped his hand hard onto the front windshield and the metal frame separating the door from the windshield. Ritchie squealed and yelled, holding the wheel with both hands. The Trans Am sprinted and growled.

It only took a few seconds for the accident to happen. As the car launched from stop, Jimmy instantly knew by the sound that their engine work had paid off. He felt proud. It was the result of nearly a year of work and an impressive accomplishment. Unfortunately, before driving away, they had forgotten to secure the latch to the hood. It only took a few seconds for the car to hit 65 miles per hour. It was at that speed that the hood violently slammed backwards. Jimmy's right hand had no chance. His fingers were smashed by the impact. Ritchie stopped the car and started anxiously laughing. Somehow the windshield was not damaged. Jimmy held his hand to his chest, wincing and screaming in severe pain. Ritchie drove back to the house and took Jimmy in his truck to the local emergency room, located 45 minutes away. By the time they arrived, Jimmy's right hand was significantly larger than his left hand. It was swollen, purple, and disfigured, fingers twisted and mangled.

In the emergency room, the medical personnel immediately gave Jimmy an intravenous painkiller. He stayed at the hospital overnight and was discharged the next day. Ritchie picked him up and drove him home. Jimmy was given oxycodone pills to manage the pain and instructions to keep his hand elevated and immobile. He received surgery soon after, and he was unable to work with his hands or drive for months.

At home, Jimmy took his pain medications as instructed. The pain was intense without the medications. He experienced sharp pains when he moved his wrist

Prescription drug abuse can happen to anyone who has an injury and is prescribed oxycodone or similar opioids, but certain risk factors further increase the chances of such abuse, including certain genetic predispositions, unemployment, and problematic personality factors (Duncan, 2020; NIDA, 2020b; Thomas, 2020).

or fingers and dull throbbing pain at other times. It was all frustrating as well. If he couldn't work with his hands, what good was he? It was the only work he knew. He felt relief every time he took his medication, and he quickly came to think of it as his lifeline. When his pain increased, he would take an extra pill. Take more as needed, the doc had said. It didn't take long to learn that oxycodone was the only thing keeping him from utter misery. He had never taken oxycodone before, so he didn't worry about becoming addicted. His brother was worried, however, and routinely checked on Jimmy. Ritchie and friends came by after work most days. Most of the time they would make jokes about Jimmy being high on "oxy," or ask him if they could have one of his pills. Jimmy thought it was funny but noticed that he was beginning to feel possessive over his pain pills. He even snapped at Ritchie's friend Shannon, who picked up his prescription bottle and held it up to read the label. "That ain't yours, Shannon. Put it down!" he said urgently. Like hell would any of the guys get their hands on his oxy.

Months later, Jimmy had recovered and was back to work. He had successfully tapered off oxycodone. From then on, he joked about how "good that stuff was" and how he might get himself into another accident sometime. "Just sayin'." It would be another 10 years before his next accident, and it was not intentional.

Déjà Vu Another Accident, More Oxycodone

By age 45, Jimmy had become highly skilled as a welder. He had helped build bridges and worked in several nearby manufacturing factories. He was confident as a welder and often did welding projects alone in his garage. He had recently begun to take pipes and car parts and fuse them into strange angular shapes. He made one for fun while high on pot one night, and when he showed his friends, they suggested he make a few more and try to sell them. "City folks will buy anything they think is original art from the country. Charge 'em up, brotha. Make 'em pay." He did exactly that, and the artwork sold. He started an online store on Etsy and figured this could be an easy side hustle. One night, while alone and drinking heavily, Jimmy decided to cut a large steel pipe in half as part of a new project. He hoisted an end of the pipe onto his sawhorse table, pulling the other end up on an angle until it rested awkwardly on top, both ends hanging over the much smaller wooden platform. It must have weighed over 100 pounds. Sweat dripping from his forehead, Jimmy grabbed another beer and took a few large swigs. It was the last of the six pack he had bought earlier in the day. He figured he would switch to bourbon and call it a night after he made some progress on the new pipe art.

Jimmy lit the torch and began cutting the pipe. As the flame cut through, Jimmy realized he had not properly clamped down the pipe. It was too late. The pipe split in half, both sides dropping to the floor and making a hideous clanging sound.

Jimmy's right foot was instantly broken by the force of the pipe. It didn't matter that he had shoes on. He knew right away he needed to go to the emergency room. It felt like déjà vu when he called Ritchie and his friend arrived to take him, 10 years later, on a familiar ride to the local hospital.

After his previous accident, Jimmy was prepared for what was to come. He asked for oxycodone as soon as he was greeted by medical staff. They did an X-ray and quickly administered a pain killer with a name he didn't recognize. Like before, the medicine was instantly relieving. And, like before, after discharge and subsequent surgery, Jimmy was given a prescription for oxycodone.

Jimmy Trouble Brewing

In the year following the emergence of the COVID-19 pandemic, the number of persons with opioid use disorder rose to new heights—a rise attributed to pandemic-related factors such as losses of employment, decreases in social interactions, declines in drug testing, and reductions in in-person treatment (Niles et al., 2021).

His recovery from the broken foot did not go smoothly. Compared to when he broke his hand 10 years earlier, Jimmy was in worse physical shape. In addition, he was single and unable to hold a steady relationship with a woman. He didn't have anyone to help him around the house. His friends had all gotten married and had kids. As a result, even before breaking his foot, Jimmy had become lonely and hopeless about his future. He usually tried not to show it to his friends, but he wished he could be young again, free to camp and hunt and fish, free to fix cars and ATVs and motorcycles. He longed for those days but knew they were over. His drinking had become worse too. He drank a six pack on weekend nights, and often drank on weeknights while working in the garage. Now he was home for months again, out of work and in pain, wishing he could get rid of both his physical pain and emotional misery. For the first time in his life, he started to think about what could happen if he killed himself. They were only fleeting thoughts, and he tried to get rid of them by thinking of other things. But still, the mere presence of occasional suicidal thoughts was a sign. He knew he was not doing well.

The orthopedic surgeon at the hospital told Jimmy at his surgical follow-up visit that he needed to lose weight and decrease his alcohol use. He warned Jimmy about the problems that would happen if he drank alcohol while taking oxycodone. He counseled him about the risk of addiction, explaining that he could become dependent on oxycodone. It was an opioid, he explained, like heroin or morphine. It had a similar chemical structure. It produced similar effects. It was legally prescribed but commonly misused or abused, causing many deaths and emergency room visits due to overdose. Jimmy listened and nodded, but he had heard it all before. He wasn't worried. He could handle it. He knew why the doc was telling him these things. He had experienced the effects of oxycodone 10 years earlier. He knew how much better it made him feel, how well these pills could take away his pain. But he told himself that he wouldn't become addicted.

Eventually, Jimmy began tapering down the oxycodone under the physician's orders. He felt confident, and his pain was less severe than it had been. His foot would be in a cast for more time, but he decided he would try to go back to work. When he arrived, his boss took one look at his cast and crutches, then shook his head. "No, sorry Jimmy, but you can't come back to work like that. You'll need to wait until you are able to walk without a cast or crutches. Sorry." Jimmy was devastated. He wanted more than anything to get out of his house and back to work. He was lonely, depressed, drinking, and still taking oxycodone. "Come on, boss, for real?" Despite his pleas, he was turned away and went home. He wasn't supposed to be driving yet, but he did anyway. Jimmy stopped at the ABC store for some liquor, then went to the Walmart for groceries and beer.

His old friend Jody was now out of prison and back in town. They saw each other in the Walmart parking lot and talked. As much as he knew hanging out with Jody was risky, Jimmy wanted to do something to escape from his mental anguish. Jody said he would come by later that evening with another old friend, Frasier. "Shoot, you seen Frasier?" Jimmy said. "I ain't seen that man in years. Bring him by, I'm still at the same place." Jimmy felt a surge of excitement.

Late that night, Jody and Frasier arrived. The three caught up, laughing about old times and drinking in the garage. Jody asked Jimmy what pain medications he was taking. "Oh, you on oxy?" Jimmy chuckled, knowing where the conversation would go next.

At the end of the night, Jody whispered to Jimmy that he could get more oxy if needed. He knew a guy who had a friend with a diversion scheme from a rural urgent care clinic. Oversight was loose, and the guy had gotten ahold of enough oxy to sell to Jody. Plus, Jody knew a friend whose mother had a prescription for oxycodone that her son kept refilling and diverting, giving his mother half the dose she was prescribed and selling the rest. Jimmy knew he would soon be running out of oxy, so he told Jody he'd call him if he needed to. When Jody left, Jimmy wondered if he would ever feel the need to call him.

When his prescription ended, Jimmy went to get a refill. The doc told him that he could not justify another refill, that Jimmy was supposed to be tapering his dosage as directed, and that the pain should have subsided by now. Jimmy didn't realize that he could be refused a prescription. He was stunned. Anger surged, and he exploded at the doc. He demanded that he be given a refill, raising his voice and getting the attention of a nurse outside the clinic room. "Everything okay in here?" she asked. The doctor responded, "Everything is okay, thanks." Jimmy left the clinic feeling shocked. He didn't feel intense pain in his foot, but he did still have some pain, and the oxy was the only thing that worked. When he didn't take his oxy on time, he would start to feel increased pain. He didn't get it. Why couldn't he have another refill?

He called Jody and later met up with him. Jody sold him oxy at a discounted price. "Friend rate," he said with a serious face and businesslike tone. Jimmy couldn't believe how expensive the friend rate was, thinking it was a rip-off compared to

Surveys suggest that 0.7% of adolescents and adults in the United States (around 2 million people) display opioid use disorder in a given year (SAMHSA, 2021, 2019). Approximately 75% of them are addicted to prescription pain relievers and 25% to heroin.

what he paid for the prescription. Still, he was angry and feeling worked up from the doctor's visit, so he said nothing about the price and immediately took a dose twice what he had last taken the day before. "I need to catch up," he told no one as he drove away. He drove home and went to sleep, drifting away and feeling like he was floating on a cloud, held up in the air by tiny balls of electricity that touched him all over, creating a warm buzzing sensation. His pain was gone. His anger and depressed mood were things of the past.

The next week he gradually took more and more of the oxycodone. As he neared the end of his supply, he began to feel anxious about whether he would need more, or if he would need to call Jody. Sure enough, he met up with Jody and bought another week's worth—then another the next week, and another the following week, and so on. He was taking more and more in order to get the same effects. By this point, he knew he was becoming addicted and felt ashamed. He was more alone than ever before, out of work, depressed, and socially isolated. Worse, he felt desperate whenever his pain would increase. When that happened, he could be irritable, petty, and reckless with his decisions.

Since he had inherited his house, Jimmy never had to pay mortgage or rent. As a result, he had saved quite a bit of money over the years. It was quickly being whittled away by his oxycodone addiction. As the months went on, his foot healed and he was able to work again, but he still felt emotional and physical distress most days, and oxy was the antidote, bringing him relief from misery each time. After missing work multiple times due to sleeping in after a night of drinking, Jimmy was fired. His boss had noticed a change in his behavior since the foot injury. "He just isn't the same person anymore," he told his wife the night before letting Jimmy go. Now without a job or a family, and seeing his friends infrequently, Jimmy felt more depressed than ever. To feel better, he drank more and more and smoked more marijuana and cigarettes than he had in years. He didn't have a car payment, and without kids he had no other significant expenses. He filed for disability and began receiving monthly payments, enough to help temper the loss in his dwindling savings account.

Over the next few years, Jimmy slowly deteriorated. He ate less, lost weight, became even more isolated socially, and spent increasing amounts of time planning how he was going to acquire oxycodone. When Jody had no oxy, Jimmy bought morphine or fentanyl. On several occasions, he bought heroin. All of these drugs had the same general effect. Jimmy would be feeling physical pain and discomfort, then take an opioid, then feel better. He learned that injecting opioids was the fastest way to feel better, and he began using needles to shoot up whenever possible.

Jody was Jimmy's main source for drugs, but Jody was known by the police. After getting pulled over doing 55 in a 25 mile per hour zone while high on opioids, Jody agreed to become an informant in order to avoid going back to prison. This led to an unfortunate turn of events for Jimmy. One night, Jimmy was waiting across the

One of the most powerful prescription pain relievers is *fentanyl*, which is more than 20 times stronger than heroin (Niles et al., 2021; CDC, 2020a, 2020b; NIDA, 2020b).

street from the ABC store parking lot for Jody, eager to buy another week's worth of oxy or whichever opioid Jody had on him. Jody pulled up and walked over to another vehicle parked nearby. It was his supplier. Rather than wait, Jimmy got out of his car and ambled over to Jody. When he arrived, Jody was already talking to his supplier, Perkins. Jody introduced the two of them, but then sternly told Jimmy to leave. "I'll give you a call in a bit," he ordered. Jimmy was in a bad mood and told Jody not to talk to him in that tone. "I can buy this stuff from someone else, Jody. I don't need you. I'll buy from Perkins directly. I've got the cash." Jody paused, then shook his head. At that moment, three undercover police cars suddenly appeared. "On your knees, all of you! You are under arrest."

Jimmy spent his first ever night in jail feeling withdrawal effects. By the second and third nights, he was screaming in agony, holding his stomach and balling himself up in the corner of his cell. He begged for pain medications, telling anyone in earshot that he was on disability due to pain and needed his medications. He felt worse than the worst case of stomach flu he had ever experienced. It was excruciatingly painful.

Ritchie posted Jimmy's bail, and he was released. The first thing Jimmy did after coming home was frantically look for oxy pills he may have hidden previously. He didn't find any, but he did find several *benzodiazepine* pills — antianxiety medications that would take the emotional edge off. The pills helped him feel better, but he decided to acquire more opioids. He called Frasier and met up to buy heroin and fentanyl. About a week later, Jimmy again met with Frasier for yet another drug buy, this time in an unfamiliar alley in a neighboring town. Jimmy didn't feel safe. He didn't know Frasier like he used to, and after everything he had been through recently, he was suspicious, almost paranoid, about whom he could trust. They made the drug exchange, more like two strangers in an emotionless business arrangement than two childhood friends.

On the way home, Jimmy reflected about how sad it was that his relationship with Frasier had changed. They used to camp, hunt, and fish as teenagers. They had spent many late nights and weekends together, and even gone on a camping trip to the Red River Gorge in Kentucky one time. It reminded him of how much his relationships had changed with all the guys in his crew. He became tearful and pulled his car over. He injected himself with the heroin he had just bought, put his head back in a blissful purge of sadness for a few minutes, then started driving again. After several miles, Jimmy was pulled over. He had been right to be suspicious. The police were following him. He was arrested for possession and went back to jail, where he would stay until he agreed to become a confidential informant to help the police. The deal meant he could stay at home with an ankle bracelet monitoring his location, bound to his house unless permitted to leave on assignment for the police, and, in turn, he would have his court case postponed. Who knows, a prosecutor said, maybe Jimmy would never be sentenced. Additionally, he had to agree to begin treatment for opioid dependence. If he stopped going to treatment, he would be sent to jail.

Treatment Intensive Outpatient Care

Jimmy had never been to therapy before. The idea of talking to someone seemed unhelpful and unnecessary. What could they say or do that would help him? He preferred taking medications for treatment, and, as his luck would have it, the mandated treatment approach included both medication and psychotherapy at a local treatment center. He had been prescribed an opioid replacement medication, *suboxone*, which was actually a combination of two drugs, buprenorphine and naloxone. Suboxone was a newer alternative to *methadone*, a long-used opioid replacement medication. Within the suboxone, the buprenorphine component acts as a so-called drug *agonist* by attaching to opioid receptors in the brain and thus reducing the patient's urge to use opioids, whereas the naloxone component works as a drug *antagonist* by blocking the desirable effects that taking an opioid would otherwise produce. It was a smart medication, and Jimmy was willing to take it as prescribed.

The clinic was nearly 45 minutes from his house. He would need to attend an intensive outpatient program, also called an IOP, for several months. The IOP required him to attend *individual therapy sessions* two times each week, where he would receive treatment based on a type of cognitive-behavioral therapy called *dialectical behavior therapy skills training*. He also was required to attend *group therapy sessions* four times each week in the evening. Two of those group sessions per week were like classes, where Jimmy would learn to monitor and manage his cravings to use substances by developing skills at reducing the negative stimuli in his life, tolerating distress, regulating his emotions, and improving his interpersonal behaviors and choices. The other two groups per week were designed to be fellowship-based support groups—a place where substance users could share their stories and support each other through the difficult process of recovery. In total, he would need to drive to the treatment center six times each week. Three of those times each week, Jimmy was also required to provide a urine specimen, so that the treatment team could routinely and objectively assess whether he tested positive for a wide range of substances. Because it was an *abstinence-based* treatment program, if Jimmy tested positive for any substance, he would be removed from the IOP and would have to return to jail.

His first week of treatment went well. Jimmy was feeling better now that he was taking suboxone. He didn't have the urge to use or buy anymore, and as a result he felt less emotionally distressed. He knew that he was lucky not to be incarcerated and was grateful to be given a second chance. Jimmy also knew that he had a problem with opioids. He admitted it to his brother, his friends, and the

Rural settings often lack access to certain evidence-based interventions for addiction, such as *suboxone*. Suboxone can be an expensive medication, limiting its use; however, research indicates that it is efficacious and helps reduce the risk of both fatal and nonfatal overdoses (Grinspoon, 2021).

police. When treatment began, Jimmy felt cautiously optimistic. On one hand, he was feeling more hope and readiness to change than ever before. He wanted to stop using, and he had felt helpless on his own. On the other hand, he was anxious and relatively unmotivated to go to therapy. True, he didn't really understand what was involved in therapy, but he had heard stories. Would they make him interpret those weird-looking inkblots, talk about his childhood traumas, or try to interpret his dreams? In his mind, the suboxone was a godsend. The rest of it he could do without, but he would go through with it anyway because he didn't want to go back to jail.

Despite his reservations, Jimmy complied with the IOP requirements. To his surprise, he even liked his individual therapist. Her name was Peggy, and she was a middle-aged woman with a degree from a masters' program who openly talked about her own past history of addiction. Her last name was O'Neill, and Jimmy asked if he could call her Peggy-O, since he had recently had a one-night stand with a drug-addicted woman named Peg and wanted to associate his counselor with a different name. Peggy-O helped Jimmy learn to pay attention to the people, places, and things that were associated with his substance use. For example, he came to recognize that Jody, Frasier, and the ABC store all were associated with his use of opioids. They were, as Peggy-O called them, *classically conditioned reminders*, also known as *triggers* for cravings and substance use; because Jimmy had used opioids in the presence of those people and places, his brain associated them with the pleasurable effects of opioids, and so they increased his cravings.

Peggy-O also taught him about the basics of addiction—tolerance, withdrawal, and dependence. He understood these concepts intuitively, but it was helpful for him to have names for his experiences. He learned that *tolerance* happened when he needed to use more opioids to get the same effect. The physical pain he felt when he wasn't using was his primary *withdrawal* effect. Jimmy learned that for most people this was the worst part of addiction to opioids and a primary reason to continue using. Peggy-O called it *negative reinforcement*. The relief Jimmy would experience whenever he took an opioid during a withdrawal reaction was so powerful that it increased the probability of him using again in similar circumstances. Instead of using the word *addiction*, Peggy-O called the pattern *dependence*, and she helped him recognize that he had become dependent on opioids, unable to function in his daily life without them.

In group skills training therapy sessions, Jimmy learned about how to make changes to his home environment to reduce the probability of drug cravings. He threw away all of his drug paraphernalia. He ceremonially destroyed all of his old pill bottles. He removed Jody and Frasier's numbers from his phone. As the weeks went on, he learned how to assertively ask for what he wanted or to say no effectively, how to regulate his emotions better, and how to tolerate physical and emotional discomfort without using drugs. Such cognitive-behavioral

Once persons with opioid use disorder begin *opioid replacement* medications, they may need to take such medications for many years, if not the rest of their lives (Seligman et al., 2021; Strain, 2021b).

Although opioid use can cause intense sensations of pleasure, many researchers believe that the opioid drug's removal of withdrawal-produced physical pain often plays a major role in the development of opioid dependence and associated problems such as crime, shared use of needles, and high-risk sexual behavior.

interventions were, as mentioned earlier, all part of the dialectical behavior therapy skill training program. The skills training took place in two-hour groups of around 10 people. In the first hour of the group, two co-therapists would go around the room to each person and review their efforts at implementing recently learned skills. In the second hour, the group members would be taught new skills. Members took notes while they learned new ways to cope with life's stress and the challenges unique to substance use. They sat around a large round table. They shared their homework with the group. It reminded Jimmy more of school than what he had imagined therapy would be like. In one session, this is what happened:

Therapist 1:	Who would like to start by sharing their homework practice?
Patient 1:	I'll go first. I tried to use the worksheet you gave us about emotion regulation, but I didn't get very far.
Patient 2:	(laughs) I didn't try it at all. You did better than me.
Patient 3:	Me too.
Therapist 1:	Let's look at what you did. Start at the beginning. We are on Emotion Regulation Worksheet 3, the one titled "Addressing Myths about Emotions."
Patient 1:	So I tried, like I said. I circled number 3 and number 6 on the worksheet. Two myths, or whatever you call 'em. Then I tried to challenge them like the instructions say to do. The first one says "negative feelings are bad and destructive," and I challenged it by writing in "negative feelings are just a part of life." They ain't bad or good. Know what I mean? Just real. I also wrote down that when I get mad or upset about stuff, it can get me motivated, and I can use it to help me to communicate if I need to."
Therapist 1:	That's terrific, you did great.
Therapist 2:	I agree! Those are really helpful ways to challenge that myth.
Therapist 1:	Can anyone else relate to this myth or how he challenged it?
Patient 2:	I really don't like feeling any emotions. It's why I always used drugs. Know what I mean?
Therapist 2:	(looking at Patient 2) That's a common reason to use… to deal with emotions. (Looking around to everyone else) I'm wondering if any other group members can relate to the myth and how he challenged it in his homework?
Patient 5:	I struggle with this one.
Patient 6:	Oh this one is impossible for me.
Therapist 1:	It's really common for people in this group to struggle with this myth that negative emotions are necessarily bad and destructive. We hear about it a lot. And this skill and worksheet can help you learn to actively identify and challenge the myth when it emerges. The myth is

kind of like a general way of thinking that can influence how you react to a situation.

Patient 1:   Yeah, and I have always thought feelings are bad. Matter of fact, I remember being told directly by my parents growing up that it's good to keep your emotions in check. Even better not to have them at all.

Patient 7:   It makes sense to me. I had the same thing growing up. Why do our parents do this to us?

Therapist 1: We live in a culture where it is common to learn to inhibit your emotions, to keep them inside, and to try not to have them at all. It's no wonder that drugs and alcohol are so often abused, because they may help people avoid or escape from feeling emotions, especially negative ones. Let's see how others did with their homework. Thank you so much for sharing (turning to Patient 1). Let's go around the room (looking to Patient 8 who is next to Patient 1) and continue sharing the homework.

In his fellowship-based support group, Jimmy listened to story after story of others and their problems with substance use. He was surprised to hear a common theme. Most people reported that they began using legally prescribed drugs, like oxycodone, only to develop problems with tolerance, withdrawal, and dependence after a period of prolonged use. Some of them, like Jimmy, turned to heroin and other street drugs. Others continued to misuse prescription opioids or benzodiazepines. Whether legal or not, the stories were remarkably similar. Jimmy listened quietly, and he shared his story when it was his turn to talk.

Jimmy completed the IOP successfully. He managed to stay abstinent, testing negative for all substances over the course of treatment. Moreover, he felt confident that he would be able to stay off opioids. In the meantime, he was staying at home tethered to his ankle bracelet. Ritchie came over now and then to drop off food and drinks, work on cars, and drink by the fire pit, the same as they always had done. After Jimmy's successful treatment and his helping the police with information about a regional drug supplier, the ankle bracelet was eventually removed. Jimmy felt a new lease on life. He was healthier than he had been in a long time, and the suboxone helped ensure his cravings were held at bay. He stayed on disability, but spent more time being social with old friends and neighbors.

Other kinds of interventions for people with various substance use disorders are *self-help* (or *mutual-help*) groups and organizations, which are developed and led primarily by persons with substance abuse histories rather than by clinicians—for example, Alcoholics Anonymous, Narcotics Anonymous, and Cocaine Anonymous. Still other intervention programs are live-in *therapeutic communities* and *residential treatment centers* (Peavy, 2021; Saitz, 2021; Farrell et al., 2020).

Ritchie A Friend's Perspective

"I just felt bad for the dude. I've known Jimmy my whole life, and he is my best friend, not including my wife of course. We did everything together as kids. I seen him go through a lot and be strong. His daddy dyin'. His momma's old man used to be hard on Jimmy. He treated him like a dog sometimes. It got scary. And then his momma gettin' cancer. It was real bad too. She was in a lot of pain. Jimmy was tough, man. He was a rock. Helped his little brother more than that ingrate appreciates. His brother leavin' town hurt Jimmy somethin' fierce. I get it, going to make more money in the city and all, but it just ain't right leaving Jimmy without any family around. And he never came back. Never was there for Jimmy when he broke his hand or his foot. My man needed help and his own brother, not even two hours away, couldn't get off his ass to come back to his roots to help out. Anyway, I think this hit Jimmy pretty hard.

Jimmy never seemed to be able to hit it off well with the ladies, so he never had a long-term girlfriend. Most of his women were short-term, like one-night stands or maybe a couple of weeks. Jimmy never seemed to want to be serious about women. So he was alone for a long time. I got my wife and kids, so when I would leave Jimmy's place, I'd go home to a family. Jimmy? He would go to bed alone, wake up alone, and had no one. To tell you the truth, I always felt bad for him.

So it wasn't a surprise that he got mixed up on oxy. Yeah, looking back, I guess you could say that we could see it comin'. But man did he change after the foot injury. He was real quiet, stayed away from people, seemed like he was becomin' a different person. Not gonna lie, it was a real tragedy. A real tragedy. I'll always be there for him. He's my friend. But I ain't gonna let him around my kids or family, I'll tell you that. Nah, I'll keep goin' to his house. Some of our best times we spent in his garage. I miss those days."

Relapse, and Worse

After his intensive outpatient care program, Jimmy was abstinent for several years. He ate healthier, smoked and drank less, and maintained a healthy weight. He was proud. He tapered his suboxone dose down low. He did weekly outpatient therapy, "counseling" as he called it, with his therapist Peggy-O from the IOP. He spent time with Ritchie in the garage. He sold industrial art on Etsy. He never did return to work, but between his art, disability checks, and savings, he had enough money to get by.

He even started dating. The first few dates he went on didn't pan out, but then he met Tammy, a short, redheaded middle-aged divorcee from Bear Creek, an even smaller town 20 minutes away. She had a thick country accent and a sturdy determination to live healthy. Her kids were grown and independent. She was emotionally stable, had a job, and had a tender, loving way about her. She was unlike any woman he had known. Just what he needed. She was devoted to her church and faith and wouldn't put up with any nonsense from Jimmy on Sunday mornings about skipping church. Jimmy found church surprisingly tolerable, and in time, he even liked it.

Tammy refused to move in together unless they were married. Jimmy wanted to propose to her, but he was nervous and kept delaying. After more than a

---

Relapse rates are high even in the most efficacious treatments for opioid use disorders, suggesting that new and more effective treatments are needed (Strain, 2021a, 2021b).

year, Tammy started to distance herself from him. She no longer immediately answered when he called or texted. She was sweet and kind to him when they were together, but it seemed she would give all sorts of reasons that she couldn't spend time with him as much as they used to. They still went to church, but she was increasingly distracted and aloof with him there. Sometimes after church, she would talk to everyone except him outside, leaving him alone for long periods of time. Why was she changing, he obsessively wondered. Jimmy had no experience in dealing with relationship conflicts like this. As a result, he simply resorted to avoidance. He stopped calling Tammy as much. His texts were shorter, less warm, and less frequent. After church, he would go to his truck and wait for her while she talked to her friends. Even when he saw her from afar talking to other single men, he stayed in the truck, unsure what to do. He started to feel hopeless about their future together.

When Tammy broke up with him, Jimmy became so depressed that he hardly left the house or spoke to anyone. He was empty on the inside, angry at himself, at a loss for what he would do next with his life. Now in his 50s, Jimmy was starting to think about the next phase of his life. His father had died at the age of 48 and his mother at 57. Suicidal thoughts crept into his head on nights when he drank too much. Having these thoughts worried him, although not like the first time he had them. He had stopped seeing Peggy-O for counseling, and rarely saw Ritchie anymore. Spiraling deeper into depression, Jimmy felt worse and worse.

Tammy may have been gone, but Jody and Frasier were back in town, both out on parole. In addition, Frasier and Shannon stopped by Jimmy's place, letting him know Perkins was around and could hook them up with whatever they needed. They called him Perk, and Jimmy thought that was an appropriate nickname. Jimmy hadn't seen these guys in a long time. Crestfallen and dejected, Jimmy was glad someone—anyone—wanted to see him. "Sure, I'll go with y'all to see Perk."

Given his depressed state of mind and the re-emergence of such profound negative influences, Jimmy's life took a fairly predictable turn from that point forward. Using, as it always had, brought instantaneous escape from his emptiness. He felt like his psychological weight vaporized with each pill or needle. It felt like freedom. Though he still remembered the negative consequences of his last bout with dependence, those memories felt insignificant compared to the urgency of his current feelings of emptiness. This time, he resigned himself to this as his way of life. He met a bunch of new people—friends of friends. They used together. He was no longer alone at home all the time. He still saw Jody and Frasier some nights, and Shannon or Perk on other nights. He went back to making art in the garage, believing that while high his creativity would kick into high gear. At first, he had tried to apply some of the techniques he had learned in therapy

> Depression and substance dependence commonly co-occur. It is not always clear which causes which. The two conditions can interact and intensify each other, with increasing substance use making depressive symptoms worse and increasing depression putting one at risk for more substance use.

to keep from becoming dependent again, but eventually, he talked himself into thinking that using was, in a way, good for him. It gave him more friends, more energy, fewer negative emotions. Ultimately, it would end a life as well. But, as it turned out, not his own.

It was late one fall night, near the fairgrounds by town, when Jimmy first saw the police following him. Already riding a buzz of heroin and alcohol, Jimmy decided to drive over to the ABC store to get more bourbon. Shannon and Frasier were coming over, and he wanted to have some brown liquor to share. The police car turned in each direction that he turned, keeping a distance. Jimmy pulled into the ABC store lot, and the police car kept driving. Jimmy went into the store and stocked up—Bulleit, Jack, and his favorite Buffalo Trace. Sitting in his truck, he texted Shannon and Perk, "Where y'all at?" He waited a minute for their response, taking in the brisk air and flickering stars. Inhaling deeply and feeling devoid of emotions, he pulled out of the lot. There were no police. Jimmy sighed.

Passing by the fairgrounds he was taken by the lights and people. He saw parents with children eating cotton candy, teenagers flirting and laughing, carnival barkers, and rides—oh, the lights of the rides! The Gravitron spun like a UFO planted into the earth, swirling lights blinking rapidly. The Salt and Pepper Shaker flipped people in rickety metallic cabins upside down and right side up, alternating back and forth with increasing tempo. Gleeful screams could be heard with each vertical drop. His car slowed, and he let a woman and two children walk by. He stared out the window, then closed his eyes, feeling like he was floating, in a dream, or perhaps in the slice of time between sleep and awakening. He remembered being at this same state fair when he was young. He closed his eyes and saw his mother holding his hand, and his father walking in front of them to get a turkey leg and deep-fried Snickers. Sounds were muffled and disjointed. He couldn't tell if they were his memories or the sounds outside his truck. It didn't matter. He smiled and opened his eyes.

Pulling away impulsively, Jimmy pressed down on the accelerator without looking to see if anyone was crossing the street. His truck jumped forward, lurching, belching at the fairgrounds with its loud upgraded exhaust. A teenage boy darted in front of the truck, running at high speed from his friends, who were chasing him playfully. The boy had no chance. His back was turned as he was running backwards, pointing and hollering at his friends. It happened quickly. Jimmy was looking up and into the clouds, which swiftly moved under a full moon. He felt a thud, then a bump, like there was a speed bump. But it was only on his right side, and it was the back wheel. People yelled and shrieked, and he stopped his truck. Within seconds, he knew what he had done. He looked into the rear-view mirror, watching as a gaggle of teenage boys and girls covered their mouths and circled the boy's lifeless body.

Epilogue

Jimmy spent 10 years in prison before being released. While incarcerated, he completed substance abuse treatment and managed to remain abstinent from all of the temptations of drugs smuggled into the prison. He read, took community college classes, and stayed out of trouble. Ritchie came to visit once a year, on his birthday. His brother never did come to see him but sent him cards and remained in touch. It turned out that substance use treatment in prison was helpful, and being incarcerated ensured that he was less likely to use. As his cravings to use subsided, Jimmy became less depressed. He knew what he had done, and he felt terrible. At the same time, he knew he had no other option but to continue to improve himself. He couldn't give back the life he took. He couldn't fix all of the relationships he had broken. So he devoted himself to the only thing possible—moving forward. When he was released, now a man in his 60s, Jimmy contacted the family of the young boy he had accidentally killed. He apologized deeply, and they graciously accepted his apology, but they would forever be scarred because of his actions, and Jimmy knew it. He spent the remainder of his life making welded art, staying abstinent, and going to church. When he died of a heart attack at the age of 66, he left all of his savings and home to the family of the boy.

> According to some studies, the mortality rate of persons with *untreated* opioid use disorder is 63 times the rate of other persons (Strain, 2021a).

Assessment Questions

1. What were the protective and risk factors for Jimmy in childhood and adolescence?

2. How did the boyfriends of Jimmy's mother influence him when he was younger?

3. What principle of reinforcement did oxycodone have on Jimmy's drug use behavior?

4. What social and cultural factors may have played a role in the development of Jimmy's prescription drug dependence?

5. How was the experience in the IOP different from what might be expected in usual outpatient therapy?

6. How did Peggy-O define addiction?

7. What was the main symptom of dependence that Jimmy experienced?

8. What psychological factors likely contributed to Jimmy's early drug use?

9. What is the difference between medications with *agonist* and *antagonist* effects? Was suboxone an agonist, antagonist, or both?

10. What factors led to Jimmy's final relapse?

11. Do you think treatment in judicially mandated programs can work? If so, why? If not, why not?

CASE **9**

Bulimia Nervosa

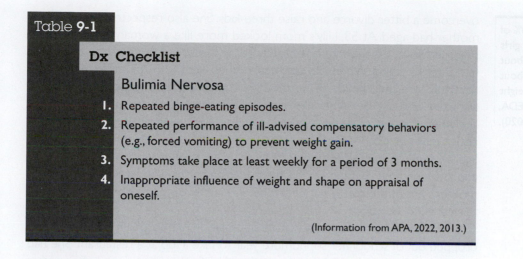

Table 9-1

Dx Checklist

Bulimia Nervosa

1. Repeated binge-eating episodes.
2. Repeated performance of ill-advised compensatory behaviors (e.g., forced vomiting) to prevent weight gain.
3. Symptoms take place at least weekly for a period of 3 months.
4. Inappropriate influence of weight and shape on appraisal of oneself.

(Information from APA, 2022, 2013.)

Lilly was a young woman who worked as a hostess at a modern farm-to-table local cuisine restaurant. She was born and raised in Southern California, in a small tourist town in the hills near Santa Barbara. Her childhood was not a happy one. Her parents divorced when she was 12 years old. She and her two older brothers remained with their mother, who often seemed overwhelmed and unable to run the household effectively. Lilly recalled her childhood as frenzied, chaotic, with little sense of control over week-to-week activities. Sometimes, she would tell her friends at school it seemed as if no one were in charge.

Despite these challenges, Lilly persevered with tenacity and poise. When her brothers went away to college, Lilly began high school, and alone with her mother and their cats Reuben and Cherise, the household was manageable. During those years, she developed a close relationship with her mother, indeed too close, Lilly would later come to realize. Her mother seemed like her closest friend, at times the entire focus of her social life. When her AP Psychology teacher described helicopter parenting, parents who hover all around their children's lives, it felt like an exact description of her relationship with her mother. They relied heavily on each other for comfort and support, which interfered with Lilly developing close friendships with girls her own age. They spent an excessive amount of time together, shopping, going out to eat, or running errands here and there. Lilly's mother was obsessed with keeping her appearance as young, thin, and fashionable looking as possible. She would talk to Lilly about the most recent fashion trends, "how important it is to look good and be put together," or how people wouldn't pay attention to you if you looked old, out of shape, or dressed matronly. Lilly loved her mom dearly and respected how she had managed to overcome a bitter divorce and raise three kids. She also respected how well her mother had aged. At 53, Lilly's mom looked more like a woman in her 30s. She practiced yoga, ate a strict plant-based diet, and kept her brown shoulder-length hair carefully styled. When Lilly and her mother went to restaurants, men would routinely turn their heads at her mother when she walked past them. She was attractive, and Lilly saw in her mother what she imagined she would strive to look like when she was older. So Lilly didn't mind when her mother gave her advice about makeup, clothes, or fitness. She knew her mother loved her, and mostly figured she just wanted the best for her. But her mother also was quite critical and judgmental of Lilly and her brothers, leading her to wonder sometimes if her mother's attention to Lilly's appearance was a way of telling her that she didn't think she looked good.

Lilly attended a nearby state university, majoring in hospitality. However, she dropped out of school her sophomore year to take a job at a restaurant. She had begun working in the restaurant part-time her freshman year and after a year was offered the position of daytime manager. It was a well-paying job, and since her interest was hospitality, Lilly figured it made sense to take this job, knowing it would add to her resume and that she might learn more on the job about hospitality than she could in the classroom. Her mother was unhappy about her decision to leave college, and let Lilly know about her displeasure. Lilly reassured her that she intended to go back and finish up after she had worked for a while and saved some money.

Soon after she started at her full-time job, Lilly began dating Stephen, a man she met at work. He also worked in the restaurant business and was introduced to her by a coworker. Her mother liked him at first, but after several months she began to turn on Stephen. Lilly was in love by then, and her mother couldn't hide her growing contempt for him. She openly criticized how he looked in front of others, commenting on his receding hairline and his "dad bod." She told Lilly that she could "do better." Lilly and Stephen met her mother for lunch one day. Stephen brought them both a rose from his garden. Lilly clasped his hand and kissed him on the cheek, thanking him. Her mother smiled with disdain, then began complaining about the weather and the table location at the restaurant. Lilly became agitated and told her mother she had had enough. "Why do you always ruin my day? He brought you a rose and you can't even be nice enough to thank him!" Her mother clapped back, "He isn't good enough for you dear, and everyone knows it. Sorry, Stephen, but it's true." Lilly grabbed his hand and stood up, tears streaming down her face, and left with Stephen.

Lilly and Stephen dated for another year, eventually becoming engaged. Everything seemed to be going well until Stephen began to behave differently. He went from being dependable and emotionally stable to being unpredictable and prone to emotional outbursts. Lilly would soon learn that he had developed a problem with alcohol and legally prescribed but misused painkillers. He was drinking at work, lying to Lilly about it, and taking oxycodone that he would buy from customers at his restaurant. Lilly was doing everything she could to hold it all together. She was working full-time, taking care of the apartment they shared, exercising and walking their dog every day, and staying close to her girlfriends. But she couldn't control Stephen's drinking and use of pills, and when he was admitted to an addiction treatment center, Lilly knew she may need to end their relationship. He was discharged and soon relapsed. Lilly felt like her world was spinning out of control, and she decided to end the engagement. She felt sad and angry, and she resented that her mother had been right about Stephen. It was time to pick up the pieces and go on without him.

A period of psychotherapy helped ease her grief and her adjustment following this tragedy, and eventually she was able to move on with her life and to resume dating again. However, serious relationships eluded her. Lilly knew that she was a moody person—she judged people harshly and could be irrational and critical of herself or others easily—and she believed this discouraged potential partners. She suspected that her employees didn't like her for more reasons than the fact that she was the boss, and she found it hard to make new close friends.

Lilly Fundamental Concerns About Weight and Appearance

Throughout her adolescence, Lilly had always been sensitive to people's opinions about her appearance and weight, particularly the opinions of other women. She recognized that this sensitivity likely came from the not-so-subtle messages from her mother about her appearance. She can still remember the day they went to a local pool with friends when she was 12 years old. She overheard her mother talking to the other mothers, telling them that she wondered if Lilly was going to have "hormonal problems" because she seemed to be chubbier than all of the other girls. Lilly didn't initially think of herself as chubby, but socially she always seemed to fall in with a group of women who were equally preoccupied with dieting and weight control. To Lilly, their preoccupation seemed to be based not on vanity but on anxiety. They lived under a cloud of concern that their weight and eating might somehow grow out of control. Typically, her acquaintances did not have significant weight problems, nor were they unusually vain or intent on being popular. In fact, most of them had serious academic interests and career goals. Thus she found it almost ironic that they in particular were so focused on their physical image. But focused they were, and Lilly became no exception.

From age 14 to 21 she always tried to keep her weight between 115 pounds and 118 pounds, a standard that began in the ninth grade after she thought she

Body dissatisfaction, depression, and self-reported dieting are important risk factors in the development of eating disorders (Cooper & Mitchell, 2020; McElroy et al., 2020).

had a slightly overweight period. She would rigidly follow what she called her weight watcher plan, although she had never actually gone to the program of the same name. The eating plan consisted, when she was being "good," of a breakfast of toast with avocado and water, a lunch of salad with quinoa or lentils, and a low-fat, high-protein meal at dinnertime. On some days, when she was being "bad," it also included a couple of candy bars or two large gourmet chocolate chip cookies. She tried to keep "bad" days to a minimum, but there were probably three or four of them each week. Lilly felt she could tolerate such days, however, as she was a regular exerciser, attending spinning classes at the gym or doing Pilates at home at least 3 nights per week. During a particularly "bad" week, however, she might go to the gym a couple of extra times to exercise on her own.

In addition, she developed the habit of weighing herself several times a day to reassure herself that the reading did not exceed 118 pounds. When the scale showed that her weight was at or below 118, Lilly felt enormous satisfaction, similar to what other people might feel if their bank statement showed a comfortable balance. Lilly saw her 118 pounds as the well-earned reward for sustained and concentrated effort. And like a miser who counts her money over and over, she would get on the scale frequently to recapture that feeling of satisfaction, especially when other aspects of her life felt less than satisfying. One evening at home, when she saw that her weight was 114, she returned to the scale a dozen times to experience the pleasure at seeing that number.

> Repeatedly engaging in body-checking behaviors (for example, weighing oneself, checking in the mirror, comparing one's body to that of others, measuring body size with clothes or other instruments) has been found to be a maintaining factor of eating disorders.

At the same time, the frequent weighing had its downside. Sometimes she would weigh 120 or more pounds and have a very negative reaction: Even though this was still a very healthy weight, she would feel fat and bloated and would resolve to limit her eating to a much stricter version of her weight watcher plan. In addition, she might throw in extra exercise sessions for good measure. In the meantime, to avoid anyone seeing her "fat" body, she would hide it under bulky sweaters and other concealing clothing. This way, at least other people would not gossip about her.

The more she felt upset about her body, the more she tended to check her body shape and size. She would try on different-sized clothes from her closet to see how they fit. She had one pair of "skinny jeans" that she fit into a few years prior, but only for a short time. She saved them, swearing that she would fit back into those again one day. She would stand in front of the mirror and suck her stomach in as far as she could and see if that made her feel any better. It tended to make her feel worse, but it did give her more motivation to have a really "good" day the next day.

Lilly Caught in a Binge–Purge Cycle

When she was 23, Lilly's eating habits became a major problem. She began to binge eat, sometimes two to three times per week. Typically she would become aware of the urge to binge in the afternoon while at work. Because she restricted her food intake during the day as much as she could, she would become very hungry, and the food in the restaurant at work would smell delicious. As the afternoon progressed, the urge would build into a sense of inevitability, and by the end of the workday, she knew she would binge that night. She would then start to fantasize about the foods she would bring home from the restaurant.

Lilly's binges usually included food that she had labeled as "bad"—foods that in her mind should never be eaten if she had any hopes of maintaining proper weight. On one binge day, for example, she got off of work and order a cheeseburger and fries to go. She said goodnight to her coworkers, then drove immediately to buy several scoops of ice cream with Oreo, Heath, and Kit-Kat toppings, all in her favorite chocolate coated waffle cone. The final stop was the grocery store, where she bought a box of donuts and bag of chocolate bars.

Once home, Lilly locked the door behind her and put her phone on silent. Something about the secrecy, the single-mindedness, and what Lilly called the depraved indifference of her binges made her feel as if she were committing a crime. Yet once the eating began, she felt powerless to stop it. After the first mouthful, the binge was destined to run its course.

On this particular evening, Lilly tore into the cheeseburger first while she sat in her kitchen checking Instagram, TikTok, and Snapchat on her phone. She ate rapidly, without pause, taking little notice of the stories or photos. After the cheeseburger and fries came the ice cream. Lilly changed out of her work clothes, then proceeded to the donuts and chocolates. This she ate in her living room at a slower, more leisurely pace while she watched a reality dating show on TV. Within about an hour and a half she eaten everything. In fact, within a 3-hour period, Lilly had consumed more than 4,000 calories.

The young woman often felt as though she were in a changed state of consciousness during such binges. Nothing else in the world seemed to matter when she was eating like this. She would avoid answering texts or responding to social media posts. She didn't think about her mother or her difficulty dating. It was like a drug, she sometimes thought, that could take her away from her miseries for a short while, a time-out from the quotidian emotional distress of daily life.

Although Lilly viewed her binges with disgust in hindsight, she couldn't deny there was some pleasure in it when they were occurring. It was the only situation in which she could eat foods that she loved. Under normal conditions, eating was not a source of pleasure, because she would restrict herself to unappetizing foods. For her, normal eating meant dieting—avoiding all foods that she enjoyed. She was convinced that if she regularly ate foods that she did like, she would set in motion a process that she couldn't stop. And now, indeed, her binges seemed to be bearing this theory out.

Once each binge ended, the next step, in Lilly's mind, was to repair the damage caused by the amount of calories consumed. Even though her binges started out

A *binge* is defined as consuming an objectively large amount of food during a relatively short time (less than 2 hours), a behavior accompanied by a feeling of loss of control.

Surveys find that adolescents and young adults who spend more time on social media and on fashion and music websites are more likely to display eating disorders, have a negative body image, eat in dysfunctional ways, and want to diet (Ioannidis et al., 2021; Latzer, Katz, & Spivak, 2011).

feeling like a rush of adrenaline and could temporarily keep her from having to think about or deal with stressful things, by the time they ended she felt disgusted and sick. Physically she would feel bloated and heavy. The rest of the night she would feel gastroesophageal reflux from the volume and fatty content of what she had eaten. The blow to her sense of self was even more pronounced. Binge eating was so inconsistent with her usual style of behavior that she wondered if she was developing some sort of split personality: the competent, striving Lilly versus the irresponsible, out-of-control Lilly. She was becoming concerned for her mental health. Her mother would be very upset with her if she knew.

Most important, the binge posed a severe threat to the one area of life which, in her mind, had become a measure of her success and worth as a human being: her weight. After a binge, she felt that if she didn't do something about it, she might see a 5-pound weight gain on the scale the next morning. During her first 2 or 3 months of binge eating, she would attempt to avoid weight gains by trying to fast for a day or two. Then she saw a documentary on YouTube featuring women with bulimia that examined purging behavior at length. The message of the documentary was to avoid this fate at all costs. However, with her binges becoming more extreme and her weight reaching an all-time high of 124 pounds, Lilly saw purging as the solution to her problem: a way of eating what she wanted while avoiding undesirable consequences.

She started to purge at home several times a week. She would stand over the toilet, touch her finger to the back of her throat, and throw up as much of the binge food as she could. The first time Lilly tried this, it was not so easy. Indeed, she was surprised at how hard it was to stimulate a gag reflex strong enough to bring up the food. Eventually, however, she often didn't have to use her finger at all; the food would seem to come up almost automatically as she bent over the toilet.

In the early stages of her disorder, Lilly's purging felt gratifying. It typically brought an immediate sense of release, as though some terrible wrong had been set right. The bloated feeling would go away, and Lilly would avoid seeing a weight gain the next day. But over the next few months, the need to purge grew and grew. Even after eating normal meals, Lilly would feel fat, and she couldn't get the thought of purging out of her mind.

Beyond purging, the young woman would try additional practices to undo the effects of binge eating. For example, she tried hitting the gym to exercise each day. Before going, however, she had to follow a particular ritual in front of the mirror. She had to convince herself that she looked thin enough to appear in a gym environment. She put on her workout clothes and inspected herself in the mirror from every angle. Lilly's weight was within the normal range: she was 5 feet 5 inches tall and weighed 125 pounds. Her body mass index (BMI) was 20.8, which was at the lower end of the normal range of 18.5 to 24.9. Anyone would have described her as slim. However, there were aspects of her body that caused

---

Typically, binges are followed by feelings of extreme self-blame, guilt, and depression, as well as fears of gaining weight and being discovered (APA, 2022, 2013).

People with bulimia nervosa often have inaccurate and disturbed attitudes toward their body size and shape. Compared to individuals without an eating disorder, people with this disorder have a tendency to overestimate their body size in a laboratory setting (Artoni et al., 2020).

her repeated concern. She felt that her center of gravity was too low, meaning she was heavy in her hips and thighs. If, after surveying herself in the mirror, she believed that she looked dumpy, she would abandon her plan to go to the gym. She just couldn't face going there "looking fat."

Usually, however, if Lilly spent enough time in front of the mirror, she was able to convince herself that her appearance was not entirely repulsive. Sometimes to do this she had to change outfits, moving to more concealing clothing. She would spend at least 2 hours at the gym, alternating between jogging on the treadmill and doing high intensity interval training. Going to the gym achieved two things in her mind. It burned calories and it kept her away from food. When she returned home, usually at about 9:30 P.M., she drank a couple of cans of coconut water and tried going to bed. Unfortunately, the long workout often left her ravenous, and frequently she found herself getting up again to binge and purge.

When she was not bingeing or skipping meals, Lilly would try to follow her diet plan. Sometimes she would allow herself a snack of fat-free cookies or vanilla frozen yogurt. When eating in this way, she felt she was in an odd harmony with the universe. The restrictive eating gave her a sense of control, competence, and success. She felt more worthy as a human being, and more at peace.

Unfortunately, the controlled feeling could not be sustained. Eventually, she would give in to periodic binges. And after bingeing she felt compelled to begin the cycle all over again.

> Most cases of bulimia nervosa begin during or after a period of intense dieting, often one that has been successful and earned praise from family members and friends (NEDA, 2020).

A Friend's Perspective Piecing Things Together

Even as Lilly's pattern of bingeing and purging at home was increasing month after month, she was able to keep it under control at her job. She sensed that allowing the pattern to enter her work life would mark the beginning of the end of her promising career. To be sure, there had been some slips. One afternoon, for example, she ate a whole order of lasagna in the break room. The full feeling that resulted was so intolerable that Lilly went to the employees' bathroom and purged. However, afterward, she felt horrified at the idea of someone observing or finding out about her purging, and she promised herself that she would try with all her might to limit the practice to home. It was not easy to do, but for the most part, she was able to keep her bingeing and purging out of the workplace.

That is not to say that Lilly's problems totally escaped the notice of people at work. Coworkers were increasingly able to tell that something was amiss, and some began to piece things together. Caitlin, a 22-year-old server and friend, was one such individual.

Working under Lilly in the restaurant for the past year, Caitlin had developed a cordial relationship with her manager. Although the two of them were not close friends outside of work, they had gone out after work to get a drink a number of times together. In recent months, however, Caitlin noticed that Lilly had become more distant and withdrawn at work, and she became concerned for her coworker's well-being. "I always knew that she wasn't the happiest person in the world and that she was certainly unhappy about not having any boyfriends," Caitlin later told another manager at the restaurant.

Of course, that was true of a lot of people, so at first I didn't give it much thought. However, after a while I started to notice a troubling pattern in Lilly. She would be very cheerful and friendly—for her—when I'd first arrive for my shift around 11:30 A.M., but as the day wore on her mood would turn distant and sour. From about 3:00 onward, she would hardly talk to me or anyone else, and she often seemed to be staring into space as though she was thinking about something far away.

Not long after this started Lilly stopped making plans to see me outside of work. Since we didn't get together all that often, at first it didn't seem that unusual. She was always "busy," too busy to spend time with me outside of the restaurant. A couple of times, I asked her what she was so busy with. Not that I was prying, but I was curious about what she was up to, since I really didn't think she had anything going on besides work. But when I would ask her, she would suddenly seem nervous and say something like, "Oh, just a few things I'm working on. Stuff for friends, you know."

I didn't know, but her tone made it clear to me that I shouldn't pry further. After about 2 months of this, it was apparent that she didn't want to spend any time with me outside of work. She never had any time to get together. And if I said, "Well, we really should find time to get together soon," she would brush the whole issue aside. Her moodiness at work was getting worse, too, and I wasn't the only one who noticed it. Of course, we all knew that she's not the most jovial of managers, but now she seemed totally distant and nervous at work. And she always was in a tremendous hurry to get out of the restaurant at the end of the day. I kept wondering what was going on in her personal life—what was she so desperate to get to after work—and why she wanted to shut me out of her life altogether.

Her appearance was also suffering. Her skin started to look dry and irritated, and her hair was damaged and frizzy. Her face, especially around the eyes, seemed kind of puffy, like she wasn't getting enough sleep. Her eyes were also red. It looked as if unhappiness was showing in her face. She also seemed very tired at work. I knew something was wrong, but I was afraid of asking her what was going on.

Finally, I decided that I was worried enough about her to go ahead and ask what was going wrong, regardless of what her reaction was. It seemed more important than maintaining our friendship. So I just asked one day, "Lilly, I can tell that you're very upset about something. You seem like you're very unhappy and secretive all the time, and you don't look very healthy. Is there something you want to talk about

Individuals with bulimia nervosa are more likely than other people to have symptoms of depression, including sadness, low self-esteem, shame, pessimism, and errors in logic (ANAD, 2020; Cooper & Mitchell, 2020; McElroy et al., 2020).

with me? I am worried about you. You know, I do consider you a friend, whatever you think of me, and I do care about you."

She just looked at me very coldly and said, "I don't know what you're talking about. You have some tables to bus." But her coldness led me to believe that she knew very well what I was talking about. Then I noticed that her weight, while generally on the increase, seemed to be going up and down every few days. I started to suspect that there was some kind of eating disorder going on. Of course, I'm no expert, but I had a feeling that maybe she was so depressed about something that she'd taken to binge eating or something. I knew that this was dangerous, but what could I do? She was uninterested in pursuing our friendship or in responding appreciatively to any offers of support. Eventually, her responses to me became downright nasty. So finally I decided that I had no choice but to wash my hands of the whole situation and stop trying to lend my hand. I had done what I could.

Lilly in Treatment Gaining Real Control

After 6 months of bingeing, Lilly found that she was falling further and further behind. As the binges and snacking had become more regular, she gradually gained weight, "ballooning," as she called it, to 133 pounds. She had never been this heavy before, and she felt desperate to lose the weight. All the purging, dieting, and exercise was failing. Her mother had noticed and commented multiple times that Lilly had gained weight and looked unhealthy.

Lilly was becoming increasingly worried that she might resort to more extreme measures, such as purging at work, to lose weight. Ironically, her only temporary relief from these anxieties was achieved through bingeing. But after the binge and purge were over, Lilly would often find herself sobbing. Overwhelmed, she contacted the eating disorders clinic at the local university hospital. They suggested she come in for an evaluation. She was ambivalent, but after reading online about the clinic, she decided to begin treatment. She figured she could always just go once, and if she didn't like it, she could decide to stop whenever she needed. Now resolute in her decision, she clicked on the link for new patients at the eating disorder clinic Website.

After waiting a few days for a response and not receiving one, she called the clinic. The person answering the phone sounded so young, she thought, a young woman with a high-pitched voice. Lilly was anxious. She felt exposed. Feelings of helplessness emerged. She answered some basic questions about name, number, and so on, and was gearing up willingness to tell her story. The woman on the phone finally asked the question. "What are you hoping to get out of treatment in our clinic?" Lilly took in a breath, and readied herself for her story. After what seemed like only a few sentences, the woman on the phone gently interrupted, her voice squeaking a bit as she said thank you, that is all we need to know for

Approximately 1% of all individuals meet the diagnostic criteria for bulimia nervosa in their lifetime. Around 75% of cases occur in women and adolescent girls (NIMH, 2021b, 2017e; ANAD, 2020).

now. Something about having a lot more time when she comes in to tell the therapist more details. Lilly felt an uncomfortable mix of relief and agitation. She wrote down the date and time of the clinic appointment. She was going to meet with Dr. Nancy Weinfurt, a nationally renowned expert in eating disorders and director of the eating disorders program at the clinic.

During her first interview with Lilly, Dr. Weinfurt concluded that her eating behavior and related attitudes about food and weight fit the DSM-5-TR criteria for a diagnosis of bulimia nervosa. First, Lilly reported recurrent episodes of binge eating, over which she felt little or no control. Second, she engaged in inappropriate compensatory behavior in response to the binges—mainly purging and occasional fasting, but some inappropriate exercising as well. Finally, Lilly's self-concept was largely influenced by her body shape and weight.

> In most cases, bulimia nervosa begins in adolescence or young adulthood, most often at age 15 to 20 years (NIMH, 2021b, 2017e; ANAD, 2020).

Many therapists tend to use a combination of approaches in the family of treatments called cognitive-behavioral therapies (CBTs) to treat persons with this disorder, and, indeed, this was Dr. Weinfurt's approach to treating Lilly. The treatment plan had two main components: (1) changing Lilly's bingeing and compensatory behaviors and (2) changing her distorted thinking patterns—her assumptions, interpretations, and beliefs, for example—about weight, body shape, and other concerns that might cause distress and lead to bingeing. The techniques she would use from CBT included educating Lilly about her eating disorder, helping her perform more appropriate weighing and eating behaviors, teaching her how to control binges and eliminate purges, and leading her, through cognitive interventions, to identify and change dysfunctional ways of thinking.

Session 1 Lilly framed her problem mainly in terms of the bingeing. She stated that the binges were increasing in frequency and were causing her to gain weight. What was most upsetting, she didn't seem to have any control over the binges at this point. Her weight was inching up, and she felt helpless to stop it.

Dr. Weinfurt listened sympathetically and expressed optimism that Lilly's problem could be solved. She then showed the client a diagram that depicted a model of bulimia nervosa (see Figure 9-1), explaining to Lilly that although bingeing was her main complaint, it was really just one element in a system of interconnected parts. That is, the bingeing was the result of such elements as unpleasant emotions, concerns about shape and weight, and strict dieting. Furthermore, in a vicious cycle, the bingeing was also helping to intensify these other parts of the system. Similarly, it was both causing and being caused by purging, another element in the system. To stop a bingeing pattern, treatment had to bring about changes in all of the system's elements. It could not focus on bingeing alone.

Dr. Weinfurt then outlined the treatment approach. First, she explained that certain steps usually help to reduce the urge to binge. Chief among these is structuring eating in a manner that keeps physical and behavioral deprivation to

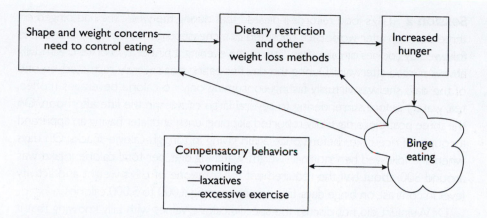

Figure 9-1

Cognitive-behavioral theory of the maintenance of bulimia nervosa

a minimum. In addition, the therapist noted, it is usually helpful to develop certain measures for heading off binges should the urge arise. Finally—and this is where Dr. Weinfurt felt it advisable to tread lightly initially—it is usually helpful with this kind of problem to become less preoccupied with eating and weight matters. She explained that when people have a problem with binges, it is sometimes because such matters have assumed a greater role in the person's thinking than is desirable.

The psychologist also told Lilly that she would like her to start keeping track of her eating and related stresses. Dr. Weinfurt allowed Lilly to choose whichever method felt most comfortable to her: using one of the apps that she recommended, keeping detailed notes in her phone, or writing everything down on a record form which she could then scan and e-mail to Dr. Weinfurt. Lilly expressed some reluctance about such record keeping. She explained that she had tried keeping records of her eating in the past and had not found it helpful. If anything, it had increased her focus on her eating. Dr. Weinfurt acknowledged that Lilly's past record keeping might not have been helpful but suggested that it would be used more constructively now. Now the record keeping would be part of an overall strategy, and clinical experience showed that it was quite important. It would allow the therapist to understand Lilly's eating better and help the young woman make appropriate changes.

Dr. Weinfurt did acknowledge that, as Lilly suspected, the record keeping might initially increase her preoccupation with her eating and weight but said that such increases would be temporary. Over time the client would become less focused on the whole problem. Lilly agreed to download the recommended app and give it a try for the coming week.

Around 43% of those with bulimia nervosa receive treatment (NIMH, 2021b, 2017e).

Session 2 Lilly's food records indicated that during the week, she had binged on three evenings after work. Each consisted of a cheeseburger or hamburger and fries followed by cookies or cake; then, later in the evening, a pint or two of ice cream. Lilly always purged afterward. During the day, her eating was severely restricted; on one of the days she was virtually fasting, consuming only no-calorie beverages (coffee, tea, water) before surrendering to several large cookies in the late afternoon. On the three post-binge days, Lilly reported skipping lunch and later having an apple and a couple of rice cakes before once again giving in to high-calorie snacks. On days when she followed her "normal" weight-watching diet, her total calorie intake was around 800, about half the requirement for someone of Lilly's weight and activity level. In contrast, on binge days, Lilly was consuming 4,000 to 5,000 calories.

Dr. Weinfurt did not discuss the specific calorie values with Lilly, knowing that it can be counterproductive for patients with bulimia to monitor calories too closely. It creates a dieting mentality that the treatment is trying to discourage. Instead, the psychologist simply noted that soon they would begin the process of trying to fashion a more regular eating pattern for Lilly, one that might lower some of her urges to binge.

They spent most of the session reviewing basic facts about weight and eating. Dr. Weinfurt explained that it would be important for Lilly to recognize first that her current weight of 126 was not considered excessive according to standard criteria and second that the deprivation needed to maintain the very low weight of 115, her "ideal" weight, could in fact lead to physically overpowering food cravings.

Lilly said she understood that 115 was on the low side but voiced strong reservations about accepting anything higher, particularly 126, as a weight for her. Dr. Weinfurt suggested that there was no need to decide on an appropriate body weight for Lilly now, only to recognize that her assumptions about proper body weight might call for some reexamination sooner or later.

The psychologist then recommended that the client stop weighing herself more than once per week, explaining that frequent weighing was fueling Lilly's preoccupation with her weight. Moreover, frequent weighing gives false feedback, as day-to-day scale fluctuations often reflect water retention or a particular state of the excretion cycle rather than true weight gain or loss based on body fat. Lilly replied that this would be a big change for her, but on the other hand, she liked the idea of not feeling chained to the scale.

Dr. Weinfurt made one additional recommendation, that Lilly stop skipping lunch at work, a habit that she had developed. The therapist said she understood Lilly's motivation—concern about weight gain—but explained that skipping meals ultimately produces overeating.

> The weight of people with bulimia nervosa typically stays within a normal range, although it may fluctuate markedly within that range.

Lilly: I just don't see how I can do what you're proposing. If I don't skip some meals, I'll become huge. I don't need lunch anyway. I am usually too busy at work. Sorry, not to be too critical of you—I hate it when people do this to me—but wouldn't it make more sense for you to tell me to stop bingeing?

Dr. Weinfurt: Yes, I could tell you to stop bingeing. But bingeing is probably the thing that you have the least control over right now. Instead, it's better to focus on something that you have more control over, such as whether you eat lunch or not. I know you feel that skipping lunch is helping you to maintain your weight, but skipping meals actually produces the urge to snack or binge. Not skipping meals will eventually help you to stop overeating.

Lilly: It makes me nervous to think of eating lunch every day.

Dr. Weinfurt: I know this will take some getting used to. But let's try it out this week, and we'll review how you feel about it next time.

Lilly: OK, I'll try it.

Dr. Weinfurt closed by giving Lilly three main instructions for the week: (1) continue to keep the food records, (2) weigh herself only once, and (3) eat lunch every day.

Session 3 Lilly's records indicated that she had had two binge nights during the preceding week. As instructed, she had made an effort to eat a lunch every day, which for her was still one of her routine diet meals that was low in calories and left her vulnerable to overwhelming hunger pangs in the evening. In addition, the client had limited weighing herself to only once during the week. Dr. Weinfurt asked how Lilly felt making these changes.

Lilly: To tell you the truth, it's making me very nervous. I feel I must be gaining weight. Not only am I still snacking and bingeing, but I've added regular lunches.

Dr. Weinfurt: What does the scale say?

Lilly: 125 pounds.

Dr. Weinfurt: So your weight is basically the same. Even if it were higher, it wouldn't mean that you were necessarily gaining weight. As we've discussed, one week's weight reading doesn't tell much about the overall trend.

Lilly: Well, it just feels wrong not to skip lunch occasionally.

Dr. Weinfurt: I know how difficult this must have been, and I appreciate the effort you've made. However, you will eventually benefit from this change. I'm afraid, though, that what I'm going to ask you to do next will not be any easier. However, I think you're ready for it, and it's important that we keep moving forward.

Lilly: Don't tell me you want me to start eating even more!

Dr. Weinfurt: Yes. That's exactly it. As we discussed in the beginning, your calorie intake on your so-called normal days is too restricted and is therefore producing binges. You need to start consuming more calories in the course of your regular meals.

When researchers place normal-eating human and animal subjects on very restrictive diets, they develop a tendency to binge. This finding seems at least partly related to increased stress as a result of caloric restriction.

Lilly: But how do I do it? I have no idea what else to eat. I've been eating this way for so long.

Dr. Weinfurt: One way is to match your eating to what others eat, perhaps even take your cue from friends, coworkers, or even recipe books. Right now you seem to be having half of a salad for lunch. As you probably know, most people eat the whole salad. I'd like to ask you to do the same. For breakfast, many people have something like cereal, fruit, or eggs in addition to toast, so you could add more of those foods as well.

Lilly: I hate this idea. But you are the expert. I guess I could try it. But if this doesn't work I am going to tell you.

Session 4 Lilly reported having made the suggested meal changes, adding cereal to her breakfast and eating a whole salad with protein for lunch, although complaining that eating that much made her feel fat for the rest of the afternoon. Dr. Weinfurt praised the client for these changes and reminded her that there was a difference between feeling fat and actually gaining body fat. The psychologist suggested that Lilly relabel the feeling that she got after a regular meal as feeling full, which has nothing to do with a true weight gain. She taught her to notice those sensations were important signals her body produced to let her know she was full, but that her interpretations and attributions borne from these sensations were not grounded in fact. She was not fat because she felt full, she was learning. Fat and full were not the same.

Lilly's food records during the week indicated two episodes that the client labeled as binges, each consisting of two slices of pizza and a pint of ice cream. This amount of food was less than in her past binges, yet she still described them this way because of the frame of mind she had been in at the time: She was focused only on the eating and afterward felt the usual guilt and shame, only to purge as a matter of routine and habit. Dr. Weinfurt observed that, nevertheless, eating somewhat more during the day had seemed to promote less ravenous eating in the evening.

The psychologist now suggested a two-pronged approach, in which Lilly would further normalize her meals and would also develop some strategies for eliminating binges at night. With respect to meals, Dr. Weinfurt observed that Lilly was still limiting herself to very little or no dinner in the evening. She suggested that instead she start to have a regular dinner: protein with rice or potatoes, plus vegetables. It had been a while since Lilly had prepared a regular dinner, and so she was concerned that the sheer effort might force her back to her old habits. In turn, the therapist suggested that she prepare her dinners on Sunday afternoon for the evenings that week. She could make and store in the fridge her meals of rice with chicken and green beans, turkey sausage with potatoes and corn, and the like. It may not be a long-term solution, she realized, but in the short term Dr. Weinfurt believed this could be a way to develop new habits.

Next, Lilly and Dr. Weinfurt discussed some measures for avoiding binges should the urge arise. First, the psychologist advised that she plan an evening activity at least three nights a week: a movie, a dinner out, or a moderate exercise class. Second, Lilly should buy all of the food for the week in one or two shopping trips, preferably on the weekend; she should shop from a list and go to the store on a full stomach. Third, Lilly should change her route home from work so as to bypass the stores in which her binge foods were usually purchased. Finally, she agreed not to bring home any food from the restaurant.

Finally, Dr. Weinfurt said she thought the time was right for Lilly to start refraining from purging. The client's better eating habits had already reduced the severity of her binges, and so she was better off just accepting the full caloric consequences of those binges, as opposed to purging. The psychologist emphasized that purging was actually helping to produce bingeing by making Lilly feel that she could protect herself from the consequences of a binge. In other words, knowing she could purge, she was feeling freer to binge. Rejecting purging, on the other hand, would help Lilly to try to control her bingeing. Dr. Weinfurt also pointed out that if Lilly retained the calories from the binge, she would be less likely to feel deprived afterward, thus reducing the need to binge later.

Lilly expressed agreement with the goal of not purging, saying it made her feel disgusting. But once again she was concerned about gaining weight. Dr. Weinfurt reminded the client that the proposed measures did not, according to experience, cause people to gain weight. That is, the increased calories that might result occasionally from not purging would be offset over time by a reduction in overeating. This could be verified by keeping track of Lilly's weight. Lilly said she would do her best not to purge.

Session 5   Lilly reported that she had followed the new meal plan, eating a regular breakfast, a whole sandwich for lunch, and on most nights, a complete dinner — sometimes a meal she had preprepared and other times one she prepared in the evening. Snacks consisted of fruit and rice cakes. Also, as advised, the client had scheduled activities for herself on several nights.

Still, there were two episodes that Lilly described as binges: a pint of ice cream on one night and a couple of large chocolate doughnuts on another night. The quantities of these "binges" were not really extraordinary — it now appeared that her more regular meals were holding down her cravings — but Lilly considered them intolerable, and she purged on both occasions.

She said that she had decided to purge because she just felt so fat after eating those foods. Still, she asserted, "I really want to stop purging," and she asked for another chance to try during the coming week. Dr. Weinfurt encouraged the client to try again but asked that she bring some so-called bad foods to the next session. The psychologist explained that they could do a practice exercise

> Vomiting fails to prevent the absorption of half the calories consumed during a binge. Similarly, the use of laxatives or diuretics largely fails to undo the caloric effects of bingeing (Mitchell, 2021).

in which Lilly would eat the foods with Dr. Weinfurt and then practice tolerating the feeling of fullness.

Session 6 Lilly reported having purged after two episodes of "overeating" at home in the evening. In one case, she purged a box of gourmet chocolates; in another, she purged two pieces of triple cream carrot cake. She had intended not to do any purging this week, but once she ate those foods and felt as if she had gained weight, she couldn't stand it.

Dr. Weinfurt asked the client whether she had brought any "bad" foods, as advised. Lilly at first stated that she had forgotten, but then admitted that she had deliberately not brought the foods in the hope of avoiding the eating exercise. The psychologist, having anticipated this complication, informed Lilly that she had brought some chocolate doughnuts to the session herself. The client reluctantly agreed to do the eating-without-purging exercise during the session. She said she might as well get it over with, as it appeared she could not do the exercise on her own right now.

Dr. Weinfurt brought out two large chocolate doughnuts and suggested that they each eat one. Lilly balked, saying she hadn't expected the doughnuts to be so large, and she asked whether she could just eat half. The psychologist explained that the exercise would be of no value if Lilly restricted her eating to an amount that felt safe. "I know," Lilly replied, "but I'm afraid of gaining weight."

Dr. Weinfurt then asked Lilly to estimate how much weight she would gain by eating the doughnut. "I don't know; 2 pounds?" she guessed. In response, the psychologist gave Lilly some facts on eating and weight gain. First, the doughnuts themselves did not weigh more than 3 ounces each, so ingesting one of them could not increase her weight by more than 3 ounces. Moreover, like all foods, some of the doughnuts' weight reflected their water content, which would be excreted eventually; most of the rest would be burned off in the natural course of events. Dr. Weinfurt suggested they conduct an experiment in which the client would weigh herself on the office scale just prior to eating the doughnut and then immediately afterward.

Lilly agreed to eat the doughnut, first weighing herself on the office scale; her weight was 132. She then ate her doughnut slowly, as if taking a bitter herb, but at the same time she admitted that she liked it. After finishing, the young woman remarked that she felt really fat and had a strong desire to purge. The psychologist suggested that she return to the scale. Lilly discovered that her weight did not show any increase. Dr. Weinfurt used the finding to make the point that feeling fat after eating and actually being fat or gaining weight are not the same. The therapist also noted that sometimes eating a large quantity of food will indeed produce a considerable weight gain immediately afterward, but most of this gain is water and will be excreted eventually. In order to get used to this, however, Lilly would have to stop purging.

> The behavioral technique that requires clients to confront their fears by eating taboo foods to show that eating can be harmless and even constructive is similar to the *exposure and response prevention* therapy used in cases of obsessive-compulsive disorder (Mitchell, 2021; Butler & Heimberg, 2020).

For the remainder of the session, Lilly and Dr. Weinfurt focused on other matters, reviewing Lilly's meal plan, binge control strategies, and evening activities. All three areas seemed to be going smoothly. At the end of the session, the psychologist asked Lilly how she felt about having eaten the doughnut. The client replied that she still felt fat, but not as much as before. She said it had been a long time since she had let such a feeling stand without purging afterward. Dr. Weinfurt repeated the importance of Lilly's not purging after she left the office or undertaking any other compensatory measures. The young woman indicated she thought she could comply.

Finally, the psychologist asked Lilly what the prospects were of her refraining from all purging during the coming week, should she get the "fat" feeling after eating. Lilly replied that she thought the prospects were better now. If she could keep this doughnut down for the rest of the night, she thought the experience would help her resist purging on future occasions.

Session 7 Lilly reported that she had gone the full week without purging. There were a couple of occasions when she had been sorely tempted—once after she ate a whole pint of ice cream at night and another after eating a couple of large chocolate chip cookies. When she first selected those foods, she had in fact planned to purge afterward. However, she later willed herself not to do it, recalling her success in the therapist's office.

Dr. Weinfurt praised Lilly for this accomplishment and said she wanted to help the client lock in these gains by once again eating some "bad" foods together. Today, the psychologist explained, she had brought some large chocolate chip cookies. "I was afraid of that," Lilly replied, but she was clearly more willing to conduct the exercise this week.

Once again, they ate together and Lilly agreed not to purge either these cookies or any other foods in the coming week. As usual, she was to continue eating regular meals, observing the binge control strategies, and scheduling activities at night.

Sessions 8 to 11 During the next four sessions, Dr. Weinfurt and Lilly continued to eat foods that the young woman would normally have avoided—potato chips, pizza, and cake—and again Lilly refrained from purging. In fact, she succeeded in not purging throughout the 3-week period, despite several occasions when she ate "bad" foods at home.

During this period, the combination of regular meals plus the lack of purging seemed to be naturally reducing the client's desire to binge. By the 11th session, she reported bingeing only occasionally, and the quantities were actually rather modest.

Also during this period, Dr. Weinfurt had Lilly add some taboo foods to her diet. By the 11th session, the client was deliberately eating such items as pizza or a

---

Cognitive-behavioral treatments for bulimia nervosa produce moderate to substantial improvement in as many as 75% of clients (Mitchell, 2021; Cooper & Mitchell, 2020; McElroy et al., 2020).

sausage-and-peppers hero for lunch, chips or candy bars for afternoon snacks, and barbecued chicken for dinner.

Throughout this whole period, Lilly worried about gaining weight, but the scale indicated that her weight was remaining the same—123 to 126 pounds. Still, she complained that this eating pattern made her feel fat.

Lilly: I know the scale says my weight is the same. But when I eat such large meals during the day, I feel fat and bloated. My clothes are tight, and I know that people can tell I'm fat. Before, I didn't have this feeling. I miss that feeling of being in control.

Dr. Weinfurt: How were you in control before?

Lilly: By dieting … By … I don't know. I just felt like I had everything under control.

Dr. Weinfurt: But what about the binges?

Lilly: Well, except for the binges.

Dr. Weinfurt: I don't think you can separate one from the other. Your pattern of eating was causing binges. Besides, the term *control* doesn't really describe what you were doing. You weren't controlling your food, you were being controlled by a vicious cycle of ineffective eating patterns, bingeing and purging.

Lilly: Well, I had a feeling of control most of the time. It made me feel good—like I was accomplishing something.

Dr. Weinfurt: You seem to be equating control over food—or what you thought was control—with accomplishment.

Lilly: Well, maybe it's not the control part. I mean, I can see that the idea of controlling food is sort of dumb by itself. It doesn't make you accomplished or anything. It's more my weight that matters. Maybe I wasn't going about it in the best way, but 125 pounds is fat as far as I'm concerned, and nothing in the world is going to convince me not to lose that weight.

Dr. Weinfurt: What's wrong with 125 pounds?

Lilly: It's more than I should be weighing.

Dr. Weinfurt: But we've seen that 125 is normal for your height.

Lilly: I don't care. I *am* fat at 125.

Dr. Weinfurt: I'd like you to consider the possibility that your thinking on this matter is part of the problem. For example, what evidence do you have to support the idea that you're fat?

Lilly: I feel fat.

Dr. Weinfurt: Fat isn't a feeling. It's a thought. An interpretation, really. We're trying to see if that thought is justified. If we were to take a look at the evidence or facts, together, what evidence would we have?

Americans spend more than $72 billion each year on weight-reduction foods, products, and services (Business Wire, 2020, 2019).

Lilly:	Well, I used to weigh less—that's evidence—but I suppose you would say I used to be too thin. How about the fact that my love life is non-existent? I haven't had a date in months.
Dr. Weinfurt:	What was your love life like when you weighed 115 pounds?
Lilly:	Not that great either, I suppose. People don't want to go out with me because I'm so miserable more than because I'm fat.
Dr. Weinfurt:	But you still believe you're fat.
Lilly:	Well, I guess I'm not actually obese. I just look heavy at this weight compared to what I used to look like.

This discussion seemed to shift Lilly's view of her weight slightly: She moved from certainty she was fat to thinking that maybe she just looked heavier than she used to. Still, Dr. Weinfurt felt that her client's thoughts had not yet shifted far enough. It was critical that she arrive at a more neutral view of her weight.

The psychologist asked Lilly to consider all the ways in which her current behavior differed from the way she had behaved at 118 pounds. Lilly noted that at her current weight she tended to (1) turn away friends who wanted her to go out and meet people, (2) check her body shape for extended periods in a full-length mirror before leaving the apartment, (3) wear concealing clothing, (4) spend most of her time alone outside of the restaurant, avoiding her mother who she knew would comment on her appearance, and (5) rarely respond when guys would ask for her Instagram handle at work or the gym.

Dr. Weinfurt explained that these actions were actually all serving to strengthen Lilly's belief that she was overweight and undesirable. The therapist thus suggested behavioral exercises to help Lilly change such behaviors, and they agreed to devise the first set of exercises at the next session.

Sessions 12 to 15   Lilly and Dr. Weinfurt devoted the next four sessions to planning and carrying out behavioral exposure exercises and cognitive reinterpretation exercises to help eliminate Lilly's fear and avoidance of various activities. In these exercises, Dr. Weinfurt systematically guided her client to perform and reinterpret those activities that, according to the previous week's list, Lilly had been avoiding or eliminating from her life.

The first exercise was for the young woman to remove her sweater at work and venture around the restaurant for a minimum of 1 hour—later 2 hours—each day. When she carried out the plan initially, Lilly felt enormous anxiety. As instructed, the client recorded her negative thoughts and then tried to refute them in writing. In one instance, for example, Tia, a "slim" coworker, had seen Lilly in her form-fitting blouse and had done a double take when she walked by. Lilly's first impression was that Tia must be thinking that she had grown fat. As part of her written exercise, Lilly also considered contrary evidence—for example, that Tia had not actually said anything about her appearance. Lilly then produced an alternative

Research indicates that individuals with bulimia nervosa are extremely focused on weight matters and virtually define their self-worth in these terms (Cooper & Mitchell, 2020; McElroy et al., 2020).

interpretation of her interaction with the coworker—namely, that Tia looking at her twice as she walked by could just as easily have been a meaningless glance or a reflection of some other concern.

At first, such counterarguments didn't feel very convincing to Lilly. But after continued written thought exercises, coupled with the behavioral exposure, her thinking and feelings started to shift. In fact, after 2 weeks of not concealing her shape, Lilly was no longer feeling very self-conscious in this activity. She still had thoughts from time to time that people might be judging her appearance, but she had become skilled in identifying and challenging these thoughts, rendering them less distressing and impairing.

The client's anxiety was also reduced following repeated exposure to other activities, coupled with the thought exercise. By the 15th session, she no longer felt the need to wear concealing clothing at work or at the gym, and she was leaving her apartment with just a quick glance at the mirror. Lilly had even gone swimming several times at her gym in front of others and felt pretty comfortable doing so.

Lilly:	By doing these things over and over I'm getting used to them. I'm back to doing normal things in spite of my weight. People don't really seem to view me any differently. More likely, they simply don't care one way or the other. I guess I need to consider why I care so much.
Dr. Weinfurt:	What thoughts do you have?
Lilly:	I guess I've been equating my weight with some sense of worthiness, like I don't deserve anything unless I'm thin. Where do you think I got that?
Dr. Weinfurt:	I don't know, but obviously our culture promotes that concept to some extent. One possibility, from what you have told me, is that your mother's excessive focus on how she looks and her criticism of your appearance could have contributed. You also have been raised in a culture where everyone is online and most online platforms don't show raw or unfiltered moments. Instead, the messages you have internalized may be that there is a certain standard of beauty that is expected in you, that what you see on the outside for others in filtered social media posts is what you should strive for everyday, all the time. It's hard to know what the causes are, but it is likely that the world around you shaped you into these patterns. In any case, the important thing is to recognize that whatever the causes were, you now have solutions.
Lilly:	Yeah. That all sounds right. I think these exercises have helped to some extent. But I can't help feeling that being successful or worthwhile is tied to being thinner.

Dr. Weinfurt had Lilly consider arguments both for and against the belief that thinness is a sign of success. Lilly concluded that being thinner might be desirable from an appearance standpoint, at least to some extent. To further explore this, the psychologist had Lilly carry out a new exercise. The client agreed to survey the appearance of women whom she considered attractive or successful, particularly at the gym and the swimming pool. Lilly was to attend specifically to the flaws in body shape they might each possess. Such observations would help her recognize that she might have given her own flaws in body shape unfair emphasis.

Sessions 16 and 17   By the 16th session, Lilly had been almost binge-free and purge-free for 8 weeks. She was continuing to eat regular meals, including formerly forbidden foods. And she had eliminated most of the behaviors that had been inspired by anxiety over her weight and shape.

By the 17th session, she had spent 2 weeks carrying out the exercise of noticing other women's body shapes. She noted that the exercise was very different from the way she normally directed her attention to other women. Usually, she would focus on their most flattering attributes. If one had a small waist, she would focus on that; if another had toned legs, she would look at them, all the while making unfavorable comparisons with herself. With this new exercise, she was forcing herself to do the opposite, and it was quite an eye-opener. She learned, for example, that Tia, the coworker Lilly had always considered the epitome of thinness, was actually quite thick in the calves and had large feet. Similarly, she noted that a woman at the pool, one Lilly had consistently admired, had one breast noticeably larger than the other. These observations, in combination with the ongoing behavioral exposure exercises, were helping her to see her own situation in a different light. She was starting to consider that maybe her dissatisfaction with 125 pounds was overblown. Although she still would prefer to weigh closer to 120, she was now thinking of postponing any further weight loss; the effort might not justify the result.

Dr. Weinfurt was very supportive, suggesting that it would be best to put the whole weight loss question on hold for at least several months. This would give Lilly time to lock in her more realistic views on weight and body shape. Then the client could consider the question of weight reduction objectively.

Sessions 18 to 22   The next five sessions were devoted to the consolidation of Lilly's behavior and attitude changes and to relapse prevention. During this period, she had been instructed to stop her daily food records and behavioral exercises. In addition, the sessions were spread more and more apart to give the client practice in functioning for longer periods without supervision. All continued to go very well, and treatment ended after the 22nd session. In the final session, Dr. Weinfurt advised Lilly to keep on the lookout for any signs of slipping into old habits: for example, skipping meals, avoiding many foods, excessive weighing, and of course purging. If she were to detect any such signs, she was to counteract them right away; if this proved too hard to do on her own, she was to contact Dr. Weinfurt for booster sessions.

Relapse may occur, even for people who respond successfully to treatment for bulimia nervosa. As many as one-third of those who recover may relapse within 2 years (Engel et al., 2021; Mulheim, 2020).

Follow-up studies, conducted years after treatment for bulimia nervosa, suggest that as many as 75% of individuals had recovered, either fully or partially (Engel et al., 2021).

Epilogue

Four months after the final session, Lilly contacted Dr. Weinfurt. She said that she had successfully maintained her progress, although there had been one occasion, about 2 months after the treatment ended, when she purged. Lilly said she regretted the purging immediately afterward and had been purge-free for the past couple months. She continued to follow a regular meal plan, although she had to admit that her old eating habits were often tempting. Her weight remained about the same throughout this period.

Her main reason for getting in touch, she told Dr. Weinfurt, was that she was not doing well in her dating relationships: On more than a few occasions, she had driven off guys by being too critical and moody. She told Dr. Weinfurt she was worried she was acting like her mother and would be unable to have a successful marriage and family one day. She asked for the name of a therapist who was experienced in interpersonal problems. The psychologist suggested a colleague and asked Lilly to continue to keep in touch. Dr. Weinfurt was sorry to learn she was still struggling with relationships, but she was very pleased with her continued success in the realm of eating and appearance. With those problems under control, Lilly's chances of addressing her interpersonal problems, or any other problems for that matter, were greatly improved.

Assessment Questions

1. What was the concern that Lilly had, along with many others who have bulimia nervosa?

2. Describe Lilly's eating plan, including her "good" and "bad" eating habits. Do you think her eating plan was reasonable?

3. When did Lilly's eating behaviors begin to become pathological?

4. What prompted Lilly to decide to purge after her binges?

5. What was Lilly's nonpurging activity to lose weight?

6. According to the information provided in the text, how do individuals with bulimia generally perceive their body size compared to control subjects?

7. How did Lilly's eating disorder affect her relationships with her coworkers?

8. Why did Lilly finally decide to seek treatment?

9. Describe the cognitive-behavioral theory of the maintenance of bulimia nervosa.

10. Dr. Weinfurt asked Lilly to keep a record of her eating behaviors. What did Dr. Weinfurt see as advantages to this exercise, and why was Lilly reluctant to participate in this assignment?

11. At what age do most cases of bulimia begin?

12. From reading about Lilly, list all of the reasons you think she developed bulimia nervosa.

CASE 10

Alcohol Use Disorder and Marital Distress

Table 10-1

Dx Checklist

Alcohol Use Disorder

1. Individuals display a maladaptive pattern of alcohol use leading to significant impairment or distress.

2. Presence of at least 2 of the following within a 1-year period:

   (a) Alcohol is often consumed in larger amounts or for longer than intended.

   (b) Unsuccessful efforts or persistent desire or to reduce or control alcohol use.

   (c) Much time spent trying to obtain, use, or recover from the effects of alcohol.

   (d) Failure to fulfill major role obligations at work, school, or home as a result of repeated alcohol use.

   (e) Continued use of alcohol despite persistent social or interpersonal problems caused by it.

   (f) Cessation or reduction of important social, occupational, or recreational activities because of alcohol use.

   (g) Continuing to use alcohol in situations where use poses physical risks.

   (h) Continuing to use alcohol despite awareness that it is causing or worsening a physical or psychological problem.

   (i) Craving for alcohol.

   (j) Tolerance effects.

   (k) Withdrawal reactions.

(Information from APA, 2022, 2013.)

One-quarter of middle school children admit to some alcohol use. Around 29% of high school seniors drink alcohol in a given month and 2% report drinking every day (Johnston et al., 2020).

Randy was a heavy drinker from the first time he tried alcohol. He began drinking as a freshman in high school and immediately consumed large amounts at parties with his friends. Throughout high school, he limited his drinking mostly to weekends. He and his friends would use their fake IDs to get a case of beer and bottles of cheap vodka or rum, and then drive to a wooded areas in the suburbs. There they would turn on music, sometimes make small fires, and sit outside or in the back of their pick-up trucks, drinking heavily into late hours of the night.

Randy generally returned home from drinking after his parents fell asleep, so they never fully appreciated the extent of his drinking. They themselves were weekly social drinkers, and it never occurred to them that their son's drinking could be a problem. They would sometimes reason that they had drunk alcohol when they were younger, and they turned out okay. It was all socially acceptable for kids their age, his parents would tell themselves and their friends. Besides, Randy and his friends never got into any trouble as a result of their drinking—none, at least, that his parents knew about.

Randy Drinking Becoming Worse

In college, Randy joined an off-campus fraternity known for partying, and he continued his high school drinking pattern. But without the structure of home and high school, and within the culture of the fraternity, Randy's drinking became more regular. Almost every Friday and Saturday night, the fraternity brothers would hold keg parties where the booze would run heavy and long into the night, usually until the wee hours of the morning. Some of his fraternity brothers drank as much or more than Randy, helping him normalize his own drinking and leading him to conclude that at least he didn't drink as much as *they* did.

Three years after graduation, Randy married Kelly, who he had met in college while she was in a sorority and used to come to his frat parties. Kelly herself enjoyed an occasional drink but always stopped at one, since she did not like the sensation of feeling light-headed or being out of control. She knew Randy drank heavily, but she assumed that all guys his age drank this much and expected his pattern would change as he got older and took on the responsibilities of a family and a career. The pattern did later change. But rather than drinking less, Randy began drinking more.

Randy had a good job in sales. His job was remote, allowing him to work from home and while on the road, affording him an opportunity to drink most days. When he traveled for work, he regularly drank during lunch meetings with colleagues and customers. In addition, he would "reward" himself after each workday by drinking expensive vodka and Venezuelan rum at home. Within a few years of joining the work world after graduating college, he was averaging 8 to 10 drinks daily. This pattern continued for the next 17 years.

In spite of his high level of drinking, Randy received positive work evaluations and promotions throughout the 17 years. He had no legal problems due to drinking. Although he regularly drove with a blood alcohol level over the legal limit, he had not had any accidents or arrests. He was a high-functioning alcoholic with a good career and family.

Kelly Becoming Increasingly Concerned

What Randy could not ultimately avoid was the toll his drinking took on his marriage. For the first several years, Kelly tolerated her husband's drinking, not

When people consume 5 or more drinks on a single occasion, it is called a *binge-drinking* episode. Thirty-eight percent of full-time college students binge-drink each month, one-third of them 6 times per month (NIAAA, 2021a; SAMHSA, 2021, 2019).

Alcohol plays a role in one-third or more of all suicides, homicides, assaults, rapes, and fatal automobile accidents in the United States (NSC, 2020a; Orpana et al., 2020).

recognizing it as a problem. A man with a serious drinking problem, to her way of thinking, was someone who couldn't hold a job, got into fights, stayed out all night in bars, or beat his wife while drunk. Randy, however, talked to her every night when on the road traveling, and when in town working he had a quiet dinner with her either at home or at a restaurant. Sure, he always drank one or two at dinner and a nightcap after, but he seemed to be able to be one of those people who could hold his alcohol without having any problems. Or at least this is what she told herself for many years, until the problems began.

During the first 5 years of their marriage, Kelly worked full-time in a consulting firm. She worked long and hard hours but felt fulfilled and enjoyed the high salary. They were able to save for their future, and she was proud to make more money than her husband at such a young age. However, when she gave birth to their daughter, she worked part-time from home and made significantly less money. After several years like this, their son was born, and Kelly stopped working full-time to focus on raising a family. She had helped them save a lot of money during her time as a consultant, and Randy was happy to see her take less time to work and more time to take care of the young children and the home.

When their children both entered school full-time, Kelly began to work remotely in consulting again. Although it was demanding, she enjoyed the work, and the infusion of extra money felt great. However, after a while, she began to feel the effects of Randy's drinking, as he was unable to provide much companionship or assistance in the evenings. She realized it had been this way for the past few years, but she had attributed this to the kids and the need to attend to their needs every night. By the time they were both in bed, Kelly was exhausted most nights and would go to sleep before Randy. Now, with more routine and less stressful days at home, she wanted to connect with him at night after the kids went to bed. But he wasn't emotionally available. He would sit in his basement "man cave" watching sports while responding to e-mails and drinking. Kelly didn't feel welcomed in Randy's man cave. She always felt ignored when she tried to join him. As a way to have more social contact, Kelly began joining volunteer organizations in her community. Before long, she was going out some weeknights and weekends with new friends to attend volunteer functions. Randy told her it didn't bother him but responded by withdrawing into his drinking even more.

Alcohol Use Disorder and Marriage Don't Mix

At age 40, Randy seemed to be the picture of success—on the surface. The father of a 9-year-old daughter and a 5-year-old son, he was vice president in charge of sales for his company, earning a high salary and regular bonuses. He had worked for the same company for a long time and worked his way up from sales associate to manager and now to an executive role. He was near the top of the organizational chart and was respected by his colleagues. He arrived at work consistently before 8:00 A.M., rarely missed an important meeting, and usually met his deadlines and sales quotas.

At the same time, Randy was continuing his long-term pattern of daily drinking, mostly vodka or rum, but sometimes bourbon or whiskey too, along with a few beers. He usually took his first drink of the day at lunch, when he went out to eat with colleagues or clients. To start off, the businessman would have a couple of vodka and waters while waiting for his meal. When his food arrived, he would order a beer to go with the meal. Longer meals meant another round of beer. Randy was under the impression that he was drinking no more than his lunch companions. However, he was actually doubling their consumption — not that they took special notice of his drinking. Although outgoing and gregarious at these lunches, Randy's general behavior didn't differ much from that of the others. His heavy drinking over the years had caused him to develop a tolerance to alcohol, so his three or four drinks over lunch affected him no more than one or two drinks might affect someone else.

At least 2 days a week, Randy had another work-related drinking opportunity. This was at a private club where his company entertained important clients. The club had an open bar, with waiters who took drink orders and automatically brought refills as soon as an empty glass was detected. It would be hard not to drink in such a place, Randy reflected. And of course he had no intention of making any such effort.

The purpose of the parties was to entertain visiting clients. The idea was to build relations with them on a personal as well as business basis. Randy's company was looking for every edge possible, and if this meant spending several hundred dollars on a party that would help to secure accounts worth millions, it was considered well worth the investment.

Randy was acutely aware of the pressure to be friendly, jovial, and well-liked at these parties. In fact, the parties were a trial for him. There were high expectations for him to be entertaining, and each time, he was doubtful of his ability to carry it off. The alcohol took an edge off his anxiety, loosening him up and allowing him to mix freely. It took at least three drinks for him to reach this point and at least another two to keep the feeling going for the rest of the party.

Once home from work, whether on a party night or not, Randy felt the need to unwind. One Tuesday evening was typical. He came home and had a couple of rum and Diet Cokes before having dinner with his wife and their two children. He had planned to drink nothing more, aside from two beers with dinner, for the rest of the evening. But as usual, things went well beyond that. After dinner, Kelly had to go to a PTA meeting, and when she left, Randy felt bored. He knew that his wife would like him to do the dishes or entertain the kids while she was gone, but looking at the pile of pots and pans in the kitchen did not inspire him. Anyway, the

> **DSM-5-TR does not have separate diagnoses of substance abuse and substance dependence. Rather, the separate criteria for abuse and dependence found in past diagnostic systems have been collapsed into one set of criteria in DSM-5-TR (APA, 2022, 2013).**

kids seemed perfectly satisfied watching television in the living room. He made a half-hearted effort to ask them if they wanted to play a game or listen to a story, but they barely looked up from their show.

Feeling he had done his duty, Randy poured himself a drink and went out to the back deck to relax and listen to music. He sat there surfing the Internet on his phone for the next hour and a half, pouring himself another couple of drinks along the way.

When Kelly returned, she found a quiet house and felt resentful. The dishes in the kitchen were untouched, and the kids were still dressed and nowhere near ready for bed. And as usual, Randy was in his favorite spot in the basement drinking. Some nights, Kelly would just ignore the situation, get the kids ready for bed herself, and do the dishes. But that night she yelled at her husband, telling him he was lazy, irresponsible, and self-centered. Randy seized on the "self-centered" part and told his wife she should try applying the label to herself. She was the one who was out every night pursuing personal interests. Kelly asked what point there was in staying home to sit around doing nothing with a drunk. For his part, Randy denied he was drunk, saying he had every right to have a couple of drinks to unwind. What did she care anyway, since she wasn't even home?

Then the phone rang and Kelly went to answer it. It was one of Randy's colleagues. Kelly didn't even consider turning the phone over to her husband; she carried out her usual policy of shielding him whenever he got calls this late in the evening and this deep into his drinking. She simply told the caller that he was out visiting a friend. After hanging up, she decided just to drop the whole matter and get on with things. Why waste any more time banging her head against a wall?

Arguments such as these left Kelly feeling increasingly unhappy with their life together. Indeed, she and Randy now barely had any life together. In the evenings, they went their separate ways. On weekends, they—mainly Kelly—did household errands. For recreation, she would attend activities tied to her volunteer work; he would watch sports on television or sit outside listening to music while looking at his phone and cooking meals on the grill, drinking himself into isolation. The children would either tag along on Kelly's errands or hang around the house, receiving only limited supervision from Randy. Over time, Kelly began to consider leaving him.

The End of Normalcy

Randy and Kelly sat down one evening to do some paperwork for their taxes. As usual, Randy had been drinking throughout the evening, but he was still quite alert and had no problem in sorting receipts, organizing records, and carrying out calculations. It was a 2-hour project, and the couple actually worked effectively together, chatting and even joking throughout the task. It was one of their rare periods of togetherness; how ironic, Kelly thought, that it should come over an activity like taxes. They got the whole job done that night, and both went to bed in good humor.

The next morning, however, Randy said something that floored his wife. He asked her when she wanted to get together to do the taxes. She stared at her husband in disbelief but soon realized he was absolutely serious; he had no recollection of having completed the paperwork the night before. Kelly told Randy that they had already done the taxes, and he didn't believe her. "How could I forget doing taxes?" he asked. At this, Kelly ran to get the evidence, the paperwork from the night before. Randy was shaken. Kelly was right. He had done the taxes, but for the life of him he could not remember it. It was as if somebody else had done the whole thing for him.

Truly upset, Randy decided that from then on he would have no more than a couple of beers in the evening. However, after a few days, his determination broke down and he returned to his usual pattern of drinking.

After the incident with the taxes, Kelly took to quizzing Randy routinely about events from the day before, and it soon became clear that the tax affair was not an isolated event. There were many mornings when he could not recall details from the night before. Kelly finally persuaded her husband to seek professional help with his drinking problem. She had seen an advertisement describing a community clinic that specialized in treating alcohol use disorder and related marital problems through the use of marital therapy. Kelly called for information and then, with Randy's agreement, arranged an appointment for them.

Randy and Kelly in Treatment A Marital Approach

While interviewing Randy and Kelly, it became clear to Dr. August West, a psychologist who had been in practice for over 20 years, that Randy had alcohol use disorder. The client had developed a tolerance to alcohol. He often drank larger amounts than he intended; he had a persistent desire for alcohol; he drank to intoxication on a daily basis and had done so for many years; he neglected household obligations because of his drinking; and he continued his drinking despite realizing that it was possibly causing memory difficulties.

Dr. West was trained in cognitive-behavioral therapies and for problems with alcohol, he usually used a behavioral model, called the SORC model, as a framework for his interventions. The acronym SORC stands for the chain of events—stimulus, organism, response, consequences—that lead to a given pattern of behavior. In the SORC model of alcohol use disorder, *stimulus* refers to external situations that prompt drinking, such as being at a bar, being with certain friends, or having an argument with one's spouse. *Organism* denotes events that take place within the individual, such as thoughts, emotions, or withdrawal

> When people develop tolerance to a substance, they need increasing amounts of it to keep getting the desired effect.

symptoms. *Response* refers to the specific drinking behaviors prompted by stimulus events and organismic states. And *consequence* refers to the results of drinking behavior, such as the reduction of anxiety or reduction of productivity.

According to the SORC model, each instance of drinking is a response to stimulus events or organismic states, and drinking is maintained because the consequences are in some way reinforcing. Correspondingly, to eliminate excessive drinking and to help people develop more adaptive behaviors, therapists must try to change each element in the SORC chain.

Whenever a client's drinking was destroying their marriage, Dr. West would conduct treatment within a couples' therapy format, in which he would use a combination of cognitive and behavioral techniques, applying them in three stages. In the first stage, he would teach the drinker skills for reducing and eliminating excessive drinking. In the second stage, he would help the spouse to see their role in the partner's drinking, both as a trigger and as a consequence. In the third stage, he would offer communication and problem-solving training to help improve marital functioning. Throughout treatment, he would use the language and principles of the SORC model.

> Some of the most common problems to arise between partners when one of them abuses alcohol are marital conflict, infidelity, domestic violence, marital stress, jealousy, and divorce (NIAAA, 2021b; Watkins, 2021).

Session 1   After gathering a complete picture of Randy's problems and of Randy and Kelly's marital difficulties, Dr. West explained to them the logic behind his treatment approach. Specifically, he presented the SORC model, noting that drinking can be viewed as a behavior that an individual carries out in response to certain situations or feelings, which the psychologist labeled *triggers*. Sometimes the drinking may occur out of habit; other times it may be a means of coping with the triggers themselves. For example, the drinking may be a way of coping with feelings of anxiety, loneliness, or the need to be sociable. The psychologist explained that the goal of treatment was for Randy to develop alternative ways of responding to these triggers.

Dr. West also noted that sometimes the triggers themselves should be changed. That is, certain situations, be they marital or work situations, may have some undesirable features, in addition to promoting drinking. The psychologist pointed out that although it would be important for Randy to learn to respond to such circumstances without drinking, it might be equally important to eliminate or reduce some of the undesirable features themselves. For example, if Randy was drinking because he was lonely, it might be helpful to see what could be done to decrease his loneliness. If he was drinking because of habits in certain places every night, he could change his behavioral patterns to avoid those places or the things that served as cues to increase the chances that he drinks.

As they talked, Kelly voiced concern that she was being blamed for Randy's drinking. She stated that if her husband were lonely, he had only himself to blame. It was hard enough dealing with Randy's drinking—and for her to be considered responsible was the last straw. And she explained that she had tried to move any triggers for drinking before, but there simply too many of them in the house. She became incensed: "He has drunk so much for so long that to remove his triggers would mean we would have to literally move to a new home!" Randy put his head down and rubbed his temples in frustration. The therapist felt frustrated too, but with his experience he knew how difficult it can be to remove all triggers for alcohol use. This would only be one part of the overall cognitive-behavioral approach to treatment for Randy.

Dr. West clarified his point, explaining that the person with the drinking problem should be viewed as entirely responsible for their drinking. At the same time, the psychologist noted, it would be important for both Randy and Kelly to examine the changes that each was willing to make to help him avoid alcohol. Under no circumstances, however, would Kelly be asked to make changes that she felt were unfair.

Next, the psychologist explained the behavioral monitoring that would be used throughout treatment. Both Kelly and Randy would complete a monitoring record each day. Both Kelly and Randy had smartphones, and they agreed that the easiest method to do the monitoring would be to use a self-monitoring app that would provide a daily alarm prompt to complete the form. On his app, Randy was to record any urges to drink, the intensity of the urges (on a 1-to-7 scale), the type and amount of drinks consumed, and his marital satisfaction that day (also on a 1-to-7 scale). On her app, Kelly would record her perception of Randy's urges to drink, the level of drinking she perceived that day, and her level of marital satisfaction.

Also, Dr. West instructed Randy to complete a trigger sheet (see Figure 10-1) during this first week, both to assess his drinking in SORC terms and to help him see the triggers and consequences of his drinking. Because Randy was so shaken by his memory lapses and concerned about his health in general, Dr. West felt that his motivation to stop drinking was strong. Nevertheless, he gave the client an additional homework assignment that involved listing both the advantages and disadvantages, as Randy saw them, of continued drinking versus abstinence.

> In a given year, 5.4% of all adults in the United States exhibit a pattern of alcohol use disorder (SAMHSA, 2021, 2019).

Session 2   Dr. West, Randy, and Kelly examined Randy's drinking in detail, based on the records of the past week. The client's trigger sheet indicated that there were three main circumstances in which his drinking occurred: business lunches, business parties, and watching television in the evening. During the business situations, the following thoughts often occurred:

"Everyone always drinks."

"I need to drink or else I will stand out in a negative way."

"If I don't drink and others do I will feel left out."

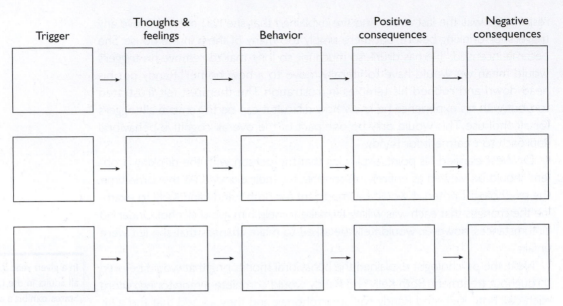

Trigger		Thoughts & feelings		Behavior		Positive consequences		Negative consequences
	→		→		→		→	
	→		→		→		→	
	→		→		→		→	

Figure 10-1

"Triggers" sheet used by Randy (from McCrady et al., 2022; McCrady, 1990)

According to the trigger sheets, his drinking in these situations had two positive consequences: the thought that he was doing what was expected of him and the ability to socialize well with clients. Although Randy was unable to cite any negative consequences, Dr. West noted one that he could see: By drinking consistently in business situations, Randy kept himself from ever learning whether his assumptions about the need to drink were valid. Perhaps Randy was overestimating the external pressure to drink at business functions. Dr. West suggested that he test this possibility by observing the drinking of others—not just the heavy drinkers—to see if everyone was drinking as much as he.

According to the trigger sheets, two thoughts often occurred in the other major drinking situation, watching television at home when Kelly was out: "I need to decompress from everything" and "I work hard and deserve a break." Randy also noted that a positive consequence of drinking at home was a feeling of comfort and relaxation, while negative consequences included his failure to do anything constructive with his time, distancing himself from his children, and upsetting Kelly.

Dr. West suggested that for the coming week Randy begin reducing his drinking in either the business or home circumstances. Randy volunteered to reduce it at home. He agreed to try to limit his home drinking to one drink before dinner. In fact, he stated that he felt guilty about neglecting his household responsibilities, and

Around 27 million children in the United States have a parent with alcohol use disorder, a situation that can produce much family conflict for them (AAMFT, 2021b).

he hoped that cutting back his drinking at home would bring him and Kelly closer together. Kelly was relieved by her husband's wish to improve their relationship. She volunteered to stay home every evening if this would help him in his effort. It was decided that she would still go to one monthly PTA meeting.

Dr. West noted that with these changes in the home, some consideration should be given to the evening's family norms structure. If Randy were simply to follow his usual pattern of watching television by himself after the kids went to bed, Kelly would feel neglected and become resentful, leading him back to alcohol in short order. Thus, it was decided that Randy would not watch any television on his own during the coming week. Instead, after dinner, the couple would do the dishes together. Then Randy would help their daughter with her homework. After that Kelly would give the kids their baths, and Randy would read them bedtime stories. With the kids in bed, the couple would do any remaining household tasks or read or watch television together until bedtime. This would virtually guarantee that he would drink less alcohol at night while at the same time spending more time with Kelly and feeling less guilty about shirking his parental responsibilities. It was worth a try.

Session 3 The couple reported that Randy had successfully limited his drinking at home to the one drink before dinner. In addition, the two of them had followed the new evening schedule. Kelly was very pleased with her husband's progress, especially with the renewed sense of togetherness that the new evening routine was producing.

At the same time, Randy expressed some areas of concern. Although his drinking had decreased, his urges to drink remained frequent and intense, perhaps more intense than ever. Indeed, his records showed that on most days he was rating the intensity of his urges as 5 to 7 on a 7-point scale. He was worried that he would not be able to keep up the new pattern.

Dr. West explained to Randy that these intense urges were a common and predictable result of his reductions in drinking. The psychologist pointed out that when people habitually use a drug under certain circumstances, they can develop a craving for the drug whenever those circumstances arise. If the craving is not satisfied with drug intake—in this case, having a drink—then the craving will rise and may become intense. This is what Randy was now experiencing in the evenings. On the other hand, Dr. West emphasized that if Randy continued to resist drinking, the urges would gradually weaken.

Toward the end of the session, Randy also mentioned that he had decreased on his own the amount of drinking during business lunches. As directed, he had observed the drinking behavior of his colleagues at lunch and was surprised to see that he was drinking much more than the others. He was above all surprised to learn that one of his most respected colleagues abstained from alcohol entirely during lunch. In turn, he decided to start having only one scotch before lunch and only one beer with the meal.

Between home and the business lunches, Randy had lowered his daily average from 12 drinks to 4. Since the change was so large, Dr. West did not press for any further reductions for the coming week.

> Research suggests that including the spouse in some aspect of the treatment of people who abuse alcohol increases the probability of a successful outcome (AAMFT, 2021a).

Session 4   The couple reported that things were continuing to go well with the evening routine. Randy continued to limit himself to the one drink before dinner, and the couple was dividing up the household and child care tasks. With Kelly continuing to stay home each evening, Randy was starting to feel that he had his wife back; with Randy remaining sober and sharing household responsibilities, Kelly was starting to feel that she had her husband back. The rewards produced by the new routine seemed to be locking in the couple's commitment.

Randy also reported that he had reduced his drinking even more. He was now going without drinking at lunch. With this reduction, he was now averaging only about two to three drinks per day—a significant reduction, but there was still more to do.

The client expressed concern about his ability to reduce the drinking further. So far, he had made no attempt to change his drinking at business-related dinners and cocktail parties, which would occur 2 to 3 days a week. He continued to have four or five drinks at each event. Reducing his drinking in these circumstances seemed like an impossible task, he said. Randy noted that his colleagues and clients drank heavily at these functions and expected him to join them. If he didn't drink, they might perceive him as less friendly—and he might truly be less sociable without alcohol.

Dr. West encouraged Randy and Kelly to work together to develop a solution to this dilemma. He suggested that they draw on their experience in treatment so far, as well as on ways in which each had coped with other difficult situations in the past. Randy noted that he usually favored a logical approach, breaking a problem down into specific goals and then proposing individual steps to help achieve those goals. Kelly noted the importance of emotional support from friends and family.

Thus, Randy first identified the goal at hand: to attend his business functions without drinking, while remaining friendly. He considered that perhaps he could hold a glass of club soda in his hand throughout the evening, but he seriously doubted whether he could socialize effectively without alcohol. He just knew it wouldn't be the same.

Dr. West: How do you know it wouldn't be the same?

Randy: I need the alcohol to feel comfortable in those situations. There's a lot of pressure on me to be a regular guy; you know, to entertain the clients and keep them happy. I need to be able to be funny, work the room, and talk to everyone.

Dr. West:	Have you ever been to one of these events without drinking?
Randy:	No.
Dr. West:	Then there's no way of knowing for sure whether your sociability would suffer if you didn't drink.
Randy:	I suppose that's true. But …
Dr. West:	Also, you seem to be assuming that the mood and actions you achieve through drinking is the only acceptable mood at these parties. Is it possible that you don't have to be as outgoing as you think?
Randy:	I don't mean to be rude, but you have to understand … It's very important to be outgoing at these events. A lot of money is on the line. Our quarterly goals are high, and I have a lot of pressure to help the company meet them.
Dr. West:	I get it. And I don't mean to suggest any of this is easy. But let me ask—is everyone as outgoing as you?
Randy:	No, not everyone. My boss is kind of a quiet guy. He's the relaxed, confident type. The guy just exudes confidence but doesn't have to say a lot. You know, talk softly but carry a strong stick. Isn't that the saying? Something like that?
Dr. West:	Do you think that clients are put off or offended by his behavior?
Randy:	No. In fact, I think he puts the clients at ease. I could never be that way, though. I'm the guy who entertains everyone. I bring energy to the room. Always have. It's just how I am.
Dr. West:	Perhaps there is some middle ground between your boss's quiet style and the style you usually display.

Randy agreed to conduct an experiment of sorts. He would try keeping a glass of club soda in his hand and observe whether abstaining from alcohol hurt his behavior at business functions. If he did experience strong urges to drink, he would deal with them by reminding himself of the experiment.

Kelly added that in the past, she had rarely attended these business functions, as she had long since decided not to link her social life with Randy's. However, in listening to Randy's plans, she felt that carrying them out successfully would be a tall order for him without some support. Accordingly, she thought she should start accompanying him to these functions. Her husband welcomed this offer.

Dr. West complimented them on having arrived at a strategy on their own. He made one additional recommendation: that before each party Randy and Kelly decide the specific length of time that they would spend there. This would help keep their task more limited and manageable. They used a code word to extract themselves from situations where they may have a hard time ending a conversation. This way either one could approach the other and say the word in a sentence, and they would know it was time to leave.

Among individuals with alcohol use disorder, men outnumber women by at least 2 to 1 (SAMHSA, 2021, 2019).

Session 5   Randy reported that he had remained abstinent for the two business parties he and Kelly had attended this week. He said that the urge to drink had been intense at both parties, but with Kelly distracting him and reminding him of his goals, he had been able to keep on track.

Randy noted that carrying the club soda around had relieved him of any awkwardness. Also, contrary to his expectation, he found that he was nearly as outgoing without the alcohol as he had been with it. He described feeling anxious and excitable at the events, and said he used that anxious energy to behave fairly similarly to what he normally would do. All this time, he had been assuming that his social skill at these parties was due to the alcohol. Now he realized that he was able to act the way he always had whether drinking or not.

With all the reductions Randy had made—at home, at lunch, and at these two business parties—his total intake for the week was only 10 drinks, an average of about 1.5 drinks per day. Also, his urges to drink were less frequent, although the intensity of those urges remained high. Finally, he and Kelly felt that things were continuing to go well at home, as they had developed a regular routine for sharing household responsibilities.

Based on this success, Dr. West asked whether Randy was ready to consider total abstinence. The client responded, "I don't know. It seems like too big a step." Kelly, however, pointed out that in numerical terms her husband wasn't that far from abstinence, especially considering how far he had come. Randy said he realized it was just a matter of eliminating the remaining drink or two each day, but somehow taking that added measure seemed too extreme; he said he'd feel like he was losing his safety valve.

Kelly replied that she felt Randy was still not facing up to the full seriousness of his drinking problem. She appreciated all the effort he had made thus far, but she thought he was kidding himself if he thought he could maintain a safety valve. What he was describing was not a safety valve but an open pit.

After some thought, Randy said that what really bothered him was the personal statement he would be making by becoming totally abstinent, practically "branding [himself] an alcoholic." Kelly responded that he was getting too hung up on terminology. If it made things any easier, she suggested, why not view himself as having an allergy to alcohol: Alcohol simply didn't agree with him, in the same way that some people can't tolerate dairy products. In the style of Dr. West, she even suggested that Randy view abstinence as an experiment. Why didn't he just try it out? He could then find out through experience whether complete abstinence was as difficult or stigmatizing as he feared.

Her suggestion seemed to strike a chord with Randy. Once again, viewing a new step as an experiment seemed to enable him to move forward; it no longer seemed like such a leap. Thus, he devised a plan. He was scheduled for a knee operation in the next week, which would force him to spend a week at home

One of the most debated areas in the clinical field is whether persons with alcohol use disorder must become abstinent to overcome their disorder or whether they can learn to keep their alcohol use under better control. Research suggests that controlled drinking and abstinence may each be a useful drinking goal, depending on the person and on the nature of their particular drinking problem (van den Brink & Kiefer, 2020; von Greiff & Skogens, 2020).

recuperating. This, he felt, would be an ideal time to see what it was like to stop drinking entirely.

Under Dr. West's guidance, the couple worked out the details. First, they would remove all the alcohol from the house the day before the operation. In addition, Randy would buy some spy novels to keep him entertained during his recuperation. And Kelly volunteered to cut down on her child care work that week so she could spend more time with her husband.

Dr. West further recommended that Randy treat himself to a special reward during this period, since complete abstinence would represent a major loss of gratification. The client decided to buy a new high-end grill that he had been wanting.

Session 6   Randy reported that he had remained abstinent during the entire period. He found that total abstinence was less difficult than he would ever have imagined 6 weeks ago, when he started treatment. Of course, the skills that he had been learning for managing his urges and cutting down on his drinking had set the stage for this accomplishment. At the same time, he recognized that the triggers encountered during this 1-week abstinent period had been limited and that the challenges would increase when he returned to his regular routine at home and at work.

Dr. West agreed. However, he repeated the principle that Randy's urges to drink would continue to weaken—extinguish—as long as the client continued to resist drinking in various situations. The psychologist explained that treatment from now on would follow a relapse prevention mode, meaning that Randy must always be looking for ways to maintain abstinence. Whenever urges to drink occurred, he was to view them as signals to devise alternative ways of coping with a situation, not as signs of weakness. In addition, Dr. West cautioned both Randy and Kelly not to react with alarm if a slip occurred. They should simply view such slips as indications of a need to be more watchful under certain circumstances and to develop better coping skills.

Sessions 7 to 9   At session 7, Randy reported on his first week of normal activities as a nondrinker. As expected, his urges to drink had increased, but not as much as he had anticipated. One bit of welcome relief had occurred during lunchtime, when he had his first business lunch without drinking. He had been concerned that ordering a club soda would be ridiculed by his colleagues. Instead, no one seemed to notice. The others just ordered their drinks as usual, without paying attention to Randy. The second time that he ordered a club soda, one colleague did ask him if he had given up drinking. Randy replied, "I've decided alcohol really doesn't agree with me." The colleague accepted this as perfectly reasonable, although to Randy it felt like a momentous revelation. He was stunned when the conversation went on as usual after his proclamation.

> The self-help program Alcoholics Anonymous has more than 2 million members in 118,000 groups across the world (AA, 2020).

In sessions 8 and 9, he reported that both the frequency and intensity of his urges to drink had declined quite a bit. He was now feeling only about two distinct urges to drink per day, and these were only moderately strong. In addition, he was continuing to devise new methods of coping with urges. He found, for example, that urges to drink often arose at parties when there was a lull in the social action. Previously, he would go refill his drink under such circumstances; now, however, he was using the urge as a signal to go talk to Kelly or someone else, and he was finding that this allowed the urge to disappear. Another strategy he found helpful was avoiding excessive hunger; if he ate more evenly during the day, he was less likely to feel strong urges to drink.

> About half of treated couples say they are "happily" married at the end of couple therapy (Lebow & Kelly, 2020; Wampler, 2020).

Sessions 7 to 9 were also devoted to a more direct focus on Randy and Kelly's relationship. Over the course of treatment, Dr. West had concluded that the relationship was basically loving and supportive, but because of Randy's drinking, they had little positive interaction. To help reestablish more positive feelings, the psychologist recommended that they set aside a couple of periods each week to do fun activities together, such as play a game, go for a walk, or go out to dinner. The couple agreed to do this. At first, the activities seemed forced to them, but after doing them a few times, they started to look forward to them and sought out additional opportunities to do things together.

The next exercise that Dr. West proposed seemed even more artificial to the couple at first. He had them designate a specific day each week on which they would go out of their way to please each other. For example, if Randy thought that Kelly would be particularly pleased by his making the bed, he was to make the bed; if Kelly thought that Randy would be pleased by her making him a cup of coffee, she was to make the coffee. The goal of this exercise was to lead each spouse to focus more on the needs or perspective of the partner, as well as to increase the number of positive interactions between them.

Sessions 10 to 15　The final 6 weeks of treatment took three main directions: (1) cognitive therapy to help Randy manage his negative emotions more effectively, (2) communication training to help Randy and Kelly get better at resolving marital difficulties on their own, and (3) relapse prevention.

Cognitive Strategies　Periodically, Randy would brood about failings or mistakes he believed he had made at work. For example, he might become excessively worried about a client's long delay in returning a phone call. Typically he would think that he had somehow bungled the original phone call and offended the client, and he would consider the dire consequences of losing the client. Before long he would also be worrying about losing additional clients, as well as his job and his income.

When Randy brought up one such incident, Dr. West guided him to recognizing the errors in his thinking. First, the psychologist encouraged the client to consider the evidence both for and against his negative conclusions. He also encouraged Randy to consider alternative interpretations of the troubling event. Upon carrying out this exercise, Randy recognized that he had done nothing deliberate that could have offended this client. He also allowed that the client might have been delayed in returning his phone call because he (the client) had been busy, sick, moody, or just plain slow. Finally, Randy recognized that it wouldn't make much difference in the overall scheme of things even if the client were to take his business elsewhere. Cognitive reviews of similar incidents brought similar results.

Dr. West also had Randy regularly write down the irrational thoughts that he had when alone and produce alternative, more balanced interpretations of the events in question. Randy found that this exercise suited his logical way of thinking and improved his moods.

Communication Training for Marital Difficulties Although making good progress, Randy and Kelly still had a few basic issues to settle. One of these was the question of the consulting work Kelly was doing. Currently, she was working full-time, and the work was starting to wear on her. She was constantly busy from morning to night. Even with Randy's help, she barely had time to relax, let alone do something enjoyable outside of the things they were doing as part of Randy's treatment, and she didn't want to resent him for this.

Randy had become much more aware of the burden his wife was under since he had taken over more responsibilities in the evening, so the couple was able to come to a quick agreement that 2 days a week of child care should be the limit for Kelly. However, Kelly's desire to go back to some of her volunteer activities was not so easily worked out. She said that in spite of being much happier with Randy's companionship, she needed a periodic change of scenery and wanted to explore some more meaningful interests.

> In 60% of married-couple families with children in the United States, both of the parents have jobs (BLS, 2021).

Randy:	What do you mean, more meaningful interests? What could be more meaningful than your family? I thought we had made progress with this?
Kelly:	Sweetheart, we have. But I just need to get out. You spend 10 hours a day away from the house at your job. I need to get out, too.
Randy:	I work that job to support us. Imagine where we would be without that job?
Kelly:	I get it. But you are gone most of the time, and I am home all of the time. I have to have a life too, Randy. It's not all about you and your needs.
Randy:	You're saying I am selfish?
Kelly:	You have a problem, Randy. Alcohol use. And we are trying to solve that problem but I have to get some change in my life too. For us to have a healthy marriage, I have to have my needs met too. I don't understand what is so hard to get here, Randy?
Randy:	So what are you saying, that we don't have a healthy marriage? Are you saying what I think you are about staying married?

Dr. West interrupted to highlight out how far the two of them had strayed from the issue. They had begun with the question of Kelly's doing more volunteer work and had ended up questioning whether to remain married.

The psychologist pointed out that each of them had a tendency to view any statement of dissatisfaction from the other as an attack that required a counter-attack. When, for example, Kelly seemed to compare Randy's work to having outside interests, he quickly defended himself rather than trying to understand Kelly more. She then became upset with him not understanding her. This led her to trying to be understood and Randy, in turn, making assumptions and interpretations about what she may have been implying.

Dr. West proceeded to teach them a communication strategy that might help avoid such misunderstandings and conflicts. Before expressing their own feelings, Randy and Kelly were to try summarizing the meaning of the other person's previous statement, allowing the partner to verify or deny the accuracy of the summary. So, the psychologist explained, when Kelly said, "You've got your job; I need to do something outside the house too," Randy could first try to summarize Kelly's meaning before responding.

Randy said, "I guess your main message is that you find it harder to be tied down to the house than I realize. You feel that my job involves certain social opportunities that I take for granted. I guess that could be true."

The psychologist then asked Kelly to summarize the meaning of Randy's statement, "I worked that job to support us when you were home with the kids." She replied:

Kelly:	I guess you seem to think that I'm not recognizing the importance of your job to our family. I didn't mean to imply it's not important. I know you work hard and it's not for your entertainment. But your work also gives you meaning apart from making money. You get to socialize and have fun with people. I want the same kind of thing.
Randy:	Is family is not meaningful enough?
Kelly:	My family *is* the most meaningful thing. I think it is for you, too. But that doesn't mean we can't have additional interests. You like to cook on the grill and watch sports, for example. I wouldn't ask you to stop doing that just because it's not family-related.
Randy:	I see what you mean. I do get satisfaction beyond making money from my job, and I suppose you're looking for something else besides your work and the family at home. I think I would go nuts if I was at home all day every day.

The couple eventually agreed that Kelly would spend one night out a week doing volunteer work or with friends. They continued to practice summarizing each other's meaning whenever they found they were starting to argue.

Relapse Prevention   In preparation for the end of treatment, Dr. West placed special emphasis on relapse prevention. The most important task was for both Randy and Kelly to be alert to warning signs of relapse, particularly indications that Randy might be at risk for drinking. The psychologist divided the warning signs into behaviors, cognitions, and moods. An example of a behavioral sign was Randy's taking a longer-than-usual business lunch; a cognitive sign was Randy's thinking that his drinking problems were over and he could easily stay sober; a mood sign was Randy's becoming increasingly worried about things at work. For each of these warning signs, the psychologist had the couple discuss strategies for managing the situation. They also agreed to call and arrange for a therapy session if Randy had a drink. In addition, Dr. West scheduled four follow-up sessions: for 1 month, 3 months, 6 months, and 1 year after the final treatment session.

Finally, toward the end of treatment, the psychologist had Randy and Kelly enroll in a group for couples who had completed the same type of therapy. This was not a treatment group but a group for couples with a history of drinking problems to meet and discuss ongoing concerns and support one another. It was led by a couple who themselves had once had drinking problems but who had been abstinent for over 10 years and had undergone training as lay counselors.

Epilogue

By the end of 15 sessions, Randy had not had a drink for more than 2 months, and he remained committed to abstinence. In addition, he and Kelly reported they were communicating better and working out their problems more effectively.

Dr. West saw them four times over the next year. Randy continued to be abstinent throughout the year and reported having only a few urges to drink each week. Moreover, the couple's marital satisfaction remained high. They continued to attend the couples group once a week as part of Randy's relapse prevention strategy. Kelly was able to find meaningful and fun things to do outside of home each week, and Randy was supportive. Overall, life without alcohol was better than Randy ever could have imagined before beginning therapy. As Randy would often say, he had put the monster back in the bottle and along the way had rediscovered his wife, his children, and the many pleasures that life could bring.

> The rate of alcohol use disorder is three or more times higher in the close biological relatives of individuals with alcohol use disorder (Duncan, 2020; NIDA, 2020c, 2019).

Assessment Questions

1. What are the statistics for American high school seniors and their consumption of alcohol?

2. When did Randy's drinking develop into pattern drinking?

3. Do you think Randy developed a tolerance for alcohol? Give a reason for your answer.

4. Why did Randy's wife, Kelly, not think of Randy's drinking as a problem?

5. When did Kelly begin to realize that alcohol use disorder and marriage don't mix?

6. What prompted Kelly to realize that Randy needed professional help with his drinking problem?

7. Describe the SORC model that Dr. West decided to use with Randy and Kelly.

8. Why did Dr. West feel it was important for Kelly to participate in the therapy with Randy?

9. Describe the five components of the triggers sheet that Randy used.

10. What are some of the alarming statistics that result from alcohol use and abuse?

11. What are key areas under debate regarding the use of alcohol once a person has developed alcohol use disorder?

12. What are some of the activities necessary to keep a couple together during therapy, with one family member suffering from alcohol use disorder?

13. What are some of the key features for relapse prevention?

14. What was the final outcome for Randy?

CASE 11

Sexual Dysfunction: Erectile Disorder

Table 11-1

Dx Checklist

Erectile Disorder

1. For at least 6 months, the individual finds it very difficult to obtain an erection, maintain an erection, and/or achieve past levels of erectile rigidity during sex.
2. The individual experiences significant distress.

(Information from APA, 2022, 2013.)

Sexual dysfunctions are a group of disorders in which persons cannot respond normally in key areas of sexual functioning, making it difficult or impossible to enjoy sexual intercourse.

Bryce was a 53-year-old heterosexual, cisgender, married man and financial editor of a nationally renowned online news service. He had been raised in a West Texas town near El Paso. His parents were strict and conservative socially and politically, themselves both the products of disciplinarian fathers who preached the value of God, faith, and family. Bryce's father was a local sheriff known for being tough on crime. His mother, who didn't work outside of the home, was a serious woman who made sure Bryce and his siblings understood the value of education. She wanted the best for her children and was unwavering in her determination for them to get as far as possible in school while also becoming upstanding law-abiding citizens. It was a serious house to grow up in, with rules, order, and discipline threading the fabric of family functioning.

Bryce wasn't as interested in sex as most of the boys around him during adolescence. Between the small conservative ranching community and the messaging he received from his parents, he just didn't spend much time trying to date or have sex during his teen years. Being raised before the advent of the Internet and ubiquity of access to online pornography, he had seen very few images of naked women as a teenager. His parents didn't let him watch anything with nudity, and there were no books or magazines like that in his home. He wasn't interested in hanging out with the guys in his town who had stashed away paper copies of *Penthouse*, *Hustler*, or the other harder porn magazines sold behind the gas stations in El Paso — he figured nothing he might see would be worth risking the wrath of his parents. After high school he joined the army with the hope that later he would receive a college education paid for in part by his service. The guys in the army were always talking about sex. It was totally different from what he was used to. He was a virgin, and his new army buddies talked about their sexual experiences and desires like they were experts. He felt embarrassed, and he took the first chance he had after basic training ended to have his first sexual experience. It was with a long-haired brunette woman, a sex worker who worked from a motel outside the base. She had no idea he was a virgin, and he acted as if he knew what he was doing. When he returned to base, he was proud to tell his friends about what happened. Feeling emboldened and wanting to have sex again, he continued a couple of times each month to go to the motel, sometimes with his buddies from base, and other times alone. He tried dating local women as well and had sex with several of them, usually after at least two nights out. Bryce was young at the time and was enjoying experimenting with different woman while dating. Over time, he stopped having sex with sex workers, believing that his mother would never let him come home to see her again if she ever found out.

Bryce and Mary

After serving in the army, Bryce went to college and majored in economics. There he met his first long-term girlfriend, Allison, an attractive and extroverted woman with sandy blond waves of hair, hazel eyes, and a flirtatious streak that Bryce found impossible to ignore. Allison was from Arizona, the daughter of a local gold miner and, so it was said, great-great-granddaughter of the famous outlaw Clay Allison. Their relationship was fun, free from too many rules, and full of sex both routine and spontaneous. He had fun with Allison. She had a wild spirit and zest for life. But after 4 years it became apparent that neither of them wanted to spend the rest of their lives together. Eventually they broke up. After that, Bryce became more serious about whom he dated. He focused more on his professional development too, deciding to pursue an interest in journalism and then, over time, securing positions of greater and greater responsibility in the newspaper business. Because of his knowledge of economics, he eventually covered financial news.

During this time, he continued to date and had a few short-term relationships. When he met Mary Jones, he was 31. She was 26. Mary was different from the other women Bryce had been dating, who tended to be, in his words, "more the wild type." She was demure and serious, reminiscent of his own mother, with a career as a financial analyst in a local hospital. They met through a mutual friend at a Cinco de Mayo party. They dated for a year before Bryce proposed to her. Their first child, a girl, was born about 2 years later, followed by another girl 18 months later and a boy 2 years after that.

As Bryce later would explain to his doctor, he and Mary did not have significant sexual problems during the first 20 years of their marriage. At first, he did sometimes ejaculate quickly, but this was typical for him in adjusting to a new partner. After a few weeks he was able to continue sex with Mary until she had been brought to climax, and then, feeling good about his ability to hold off until that point, they would finish intercourse with Bryce having an orgasm. Mary was less sexually adventuresome than his earlier partners. She hinted at wanting to have

As many as 30% of men worldwide ejaculate early some of the time; 4% of men meet all of the criteria for a diagnosis of *premature ejaculation* (Snyder & Rosen, 2020).

sex but was more likely to let Bryce initiate, even if she was the one who was more interested.

He loved Mary. She was giving, kind, and thoughtful in the little ways that most women Bryce had dated were not. She had brown eyes and a rounded face with full lips. Her skin had a light caramel undertone, probably from her Native American and Mexican ancestry. She was from Big Foot County, near where Bryce had grown up. She had an upbringing similar to Bryce's. Her dad was a rancher who made whiskey, and, according to Mary, he made it well. Her mother raised Mary and her older sister until, one night when she was young, Mrs. Jones was in the barn when a snowstorm came in quickly. The roof caved in. Mary and her sister were left to be raised by their father, and in his grief, he was never the same again. He turned to the bottle, and when he drank heavily, he became angry, his rage sometimes spilling out where Mary and her sister were left to witness. Mary had grown up terrified of her father and bereft in the wake of losing her mother. Bryce understood how being raised by Mr. Jones had impacted her attitudes about dating, men, and ultimately sex. But he loved her, and he respected how much she had overcome to get to where she was in life.

Mary attended parochial school through high school. After graduation, she went to college and earned a bachelor's degree in finance. Her first sexual encounter was with a guy she met in a psychology class in college. They became serious after a few weeks, but the relationship didn't last long, as Mary became increasingly dissatisfied with his lack of focus and direction in life. Even though they were still in college, she expected a man to have drive and ambition. After he chose to take a summer internship in Washington, DC, Mary decided to end the relationship. She dated a few other men but had few sexual partners until she met Bryce. Even after they were married, Mary did not consider sex to be a key element of their marriage. Although she enjoyed sex with Bryce, most of the time it was not something she cared to initiate on her own.

The Unfolding of a Sexual Dysfunction

As many as 90% of all men with severe depression experience some degree of erectile dysfunction (Rosen & Khera, 2021; Snyder & Rosen, 2020; Yang et al., 2019).

During his 53rd year, Bryce was under extra pressure at work because of the downsizing of the editorial staff in his department. Although he was not affected directly, some of his junior colleagues had been laid off, and Bryce now had to work hours that he had not put in since he was a night reporter on the city beat, back before online news had largely replaced print journalism. He was feeling more tired than he had in years, and he also felt some degree of job apprehension. Although told that his own job was safe, he had been in the news business long enough to know the score. On top of all that, his financial responsibilities had increased, with two children in college and a third to be entering soon.

Partly because of Bryce's preoccupation with his job, he and Mary began to go to bed at different times. He would stay up later on many nights, anxiously catching up on e-mails and reviewing copy. As work became more stressful, he was more and more tired. And, naturally, he had less energy. He and Mary began to have sex less frequently—sometimes only once a month. However, one night in February, Mary was decidedly in the mood, and she was uncharacteristically unwilling to take no for an answer. As she made sexual overtures, Bryce tried to dissuade her, telling her he was too preoccupied with work. However, she became extremely insistent. To help him relax, she poured him a large glass of wine and sat with him at his computer. He still did not want to pursue things, and instead talked to her about all of the problems with the article he was reviewing. She feigned deep interest, offering responses to his outrage that mirrored his own, though she didn't have the same depth of feeling as he did about the topic. They sat together talking. After drinking a second glass of wine, Bryce was prepared to put his preoccupations aside and attend to Mary. They went into the bedroom together, and she disrobed in front of him. Looking into his eyes across the bed, she reached out and began to touch him, first on the stomach, then outside his underwear on the head of his penis. Bryce was starting to get aroused.

Usually, sex with Mary followed a formula. They would watch the evening news in bed on Saturday night, and if Bryce was feeling amorous, he would turn toward Mary and start kissing and fondling her. If Mary was similarly inclined, she would respond by relaxing her limbs and returning Bryce's kisses. After a few minutes of foreplay, Bryce would move into the missionary position, on top of her until intercourse was completed.

That night, however, Mary was acting much more dominantly. As Bryce lay on the bed, she continued to touch him, ultimately pulling down his pants once she noticed his penis beginning to enlarge in response to her touch. She continued stimulating him manually, removing his underwear, until he was almost fully erect. She moved her head toward his abdomen and kissed it a few times, then used her mouth and tongue to please him orally for a few minutes. He became fully erect. She lay back on the bed and urged Bryce to initiate intercourse. He was very interested.

As Bryce positioned himself to enter his wife, he found, unbelievably, that his erection was starting to go soft. Completely bewildered, he tried to reposition his penis to enter her from a different angle. He tried again several times, at one point using his thumb and forefinger to firmly stick the head inside of her. He could not get firm enough to continue. All the while, Mary continued to urge Bryce on in a manner that he found enticing. However, the more he tried, the more he became aware of the flaccid state of his penis, and the less he succeeded. Finally, Mary asked Bryce what was wrong, and he said he didn't know, but that he was probably too tired and stressed from all of the things going on at work. They were working on a new Website build, revamping the layout, taking on a new strategic approach to the way financial news is written. He was in charge, he explained, and

According to surveys, half of all men experience erectile difficulty during intercourse at least some of the time. Around 16% of men worldwide qualify for a diagnosis of erectile disorder, including 8% of men in their 20s and 37% of men in their 70s (Snyder & Rosen, 2020).

he felt overwhelmed by it all. Mary wanted to believe all of this, but at the same time she wasn't sure she could. Why now? What is wrong with him? Bryce was wondering the same things, but he didn't say them. They moved to their respective sides of the bed. Both of their minds raced as they closed their eyes and anxiously tried to fall asleep.

At work the next day, Bryce was in a state of confusion. His interest in sex had not been high recently. But the night before he had failed to achieve an erection with Mary, and he didn't understand why, especially with how interested she was and how she had been the one to initiate. He wondered whether he would be able to stay erect the next time and decided he would initiate sex with Mary later that night.

Their evening followed a familiar rhythm, and they headed upstairs to watch the late news. As they watched television, Mary gave no evidence of the desire she had displayed the night before. Just as well, Bryce thought, as he didn't need any additional pressure in what he was about to attempt. As the news concluded, he leaned over toward his wife and began stroking her in the usual fashion. She relaxed, and Bryce continued fondling her. He was pleased that this encounter seemed to be following their routine, but there was nothing familiar in his thoughts. The whole time, he was paying attention to the condition of his penis and whether he seemed to be showing enough responsiveness. About 5 minutes into the encounter, he realized he was only partially erect, and for the life of him he couldn't remember whether or not this was normal for him during foreplay. He decided to end his suspense by proceeding to the main event. However, as he did so, his erection only got softer, and within a minute he concluded that all efforts at penetration were hopeless. He felt embarrassed again, and rather than talking about what had just happened, this time he tried to play it cool, shrugging his shoulders and moving his head between her legs to stimulate Mary to orgasm, all the while turning over in his mind the question of why he had failed once again.

Mary, sensing his frustration afterward, tried her best to be understanding and to take the pressure off Bryce. She told him to let the issue rest for a while. Maybe he was too stressed right now to be interested in sex, and she had been wrong to force the issue the other night. By the same token, he should avoid forcing the issue now.

But Bryce could not simply let it go. Each night in the coming week he tried initiating sex with Mary, always with more or less the same results. He would become semi-erect during foreplay, but at the moment of penetration he would be acutely aware of any sign of difficulty, and this very awareness seemed to deflate him further.

Finally, he took Mary's advice and tried to let the matter rest for a while. Curiously, he found he could get normal erections when masturbating alone. He wondered whether this meant that he and Mary were becoming sexually

If a man is able to have an erection in certain circumstances—for example, when masturbating or with certain partners or when asleep—then it is generally concluded that psychological factors are at least partially responsible for his erectile disorder.

incompatible but then dismissed the idea as absurd, knowing that they had had a good marriage and sex life for over 20 years.

In the next couple of months, things became only slightly better. Bryce attempted intercourse with Mary on average about once a week. On a couple of occasions he succeeded in getting hard enough to enter her, but his frantic efforts to achieve an orgasm before getting soft seemed almost to guarantee that he could not maintain the erection. Moreover, each new attempt at intercourse had become an unbearable trial. After each disappointment, Bryce brooded over the experience and its implications.

Throughout this period, Mary tried to soothe Bryce, telling him that it wasn't important and that things would get better. However, Bryce could tell that she herself was beginning to wonder what was happening. Once she hinted that maybe he needed to take a vacation—or see a doctor.

What Mary didn't know was how much this sexual problem was beginning to carry over into the rest of her husband's life. At work Bryce had become painfully self-conscious about his predicament. He felt like a weakling, less than a normal man, and also felt certain that others, if they knew about his difficulties, would mock him or think of him as pitiful. In meetings with male colleagues, he now felt a sense of distance and inferiority that he hadn't known since his days as a college intern, when he was awed to be in the presence of the gruff, competitive newspaper types. He felt like a fraud who didn't belong with the grownups.

After 6 months of disappointing results, Bryce decided to seek medical assistance. As it happened, the television and Internet frequently had advertising for medicine offering "effective treatments for erectile dysfunction." Bryce waited a month until his annual physical exam with his long-time primary care doctor. At the appointment, the doctor told him that his experience was common, surprisingly so, among men past the age of 50. Bryce felt somewhat reassured but still wanted help. He asked for a referral to a urologist, but his primary care doctor instead suggested that he be seen in a specialty clinic by a multidisciplinary team of providers. Bryce was embarrassed about the prospect of being seen by a whole team.

"Can't I just see a urologist? I thought they were the experts," he said. "I don't know how comfortable I am with the idea of talking to a team of different people. I think I should be seen by a urologist, ideally a man, if you don't mind."

His doctor reassured Bryce. "I totally understand how this could feel uncomfortable. A lot of men feel that way. At the clinic, you will be seen by a urologist, but it is possible you also will be seen by others, including a psychiatrist or psychologist. The team would work together to determine if the problem you are having is organic, psychological, or both." Bryce had always trusted his primary care doctor, and he deferred to him. "Okay, let's get on with it then," he said sheepishly. The doctor handed him a piece of paper that simply read "Deer Creek Clinic."

Most cases of erectile disorder result from an interaction of biological, psychosocial, and/or sociocultural factors.

He turned to the computer and entered the referral order into the electronic medical record with Bryce still in the room. "There," he said calmly, "the referral has been made, and you will hear from them soon to schedule an appointment. You should expect your first appointment to be with a urologist, possibly followed by visits with other members of the team."

Several weeks later, upon checking in to the Deer Creek Clinic, Bryce was greeted by a young male staff member. He felt relieved it was not a woman. He completed self-report measures of sexual functioning, physical health, relationship satisfaction, and anxiety on a tablet in the waiting room. A male medical assistant then called his name and greeted Bryce politely as they walked back to a clinic room. After being weighed and having his blood pressure and heart rate measured, the medical assistant turned to the computer, entered his information into the electronic medical record, and told Bryce that the doctor would be with him shortly. Again, Bryce felt somewhat relieved. So far, everything felt familiar, like a normal trip to the doctor for any problem. Soon, a male urologist named Dr. Brant entered the room. After briefly exchanging pleasantries and introducing himself as a member of the team, Dr. Brant interviewed Bryce about his difficulties achieving and maintaining an erection, as well as about his lifetime medical and sexual history. He also gave Bryce a standard physical exam and conducted some tests to assess the possible roles of neurological, endocrine, and vascular dysfunction, all of which are known physical factors in erectile difficulties.

Dr. Brant could find nothing physical to account for Bryce's difficulty, although he noted that an undetectable physical component could never be ruled out completely. He outlined for Bryce three main medical treatment options. One, a *penile implant,* was considered by the physician to be a far too radical solution in Bryce's case. The second was a *vacuum pump,* a device that draws blood mechanically into the penis, producing an erection; the erection is then maintained by the use of constricting rubber bands placed at the base of the penis. The third option was medication, specifically *sildenafil* (Viagra). Bryce had certainly heard of this drug. He had seen the commercials—happy geriatric men and women smiling in between commercials for the early morning news. Dr. Brant explained that a pill of sildenafil increases blood flow to the penis within 1 hour of taking it, enabling a man to attain an erection during sexual activity. Given that Bryce had no signs of coronary heart disease (a condition that would make sildenafil risky to take), the physician recommended this approach as a simple and safe way to solve his difficulties.

At the same time, the doctor suggested that after meeting with the others on the treatment team, Bryce might want to consider psychological therapy with or without sildenafil. After all, the patient was able to achieve satisfactory erections with masturbation, suggesting there was a situational component to his ability to have and maintain an erection. Psychological treatment, Dr. Brant explained, might assist him in expanding this existing capability to sexual situations with his wife.

> Sildenafil (Viagra) was discovered by accident. Testing it as a possible heart medication, researchers found that the drug increased blood flow to subjects' penises more effectively than to their hearts.

Bryce said he would have to think about it. He was very tempted by the sildenafil option. It seemed so simple and was likely to bring immediate improvement. On the other hand, he was hoping to avoid an artificial solution. He didn't want to take pills for the rest of his life to have sex. He later explained the various options to Mary. They both decided that before making a decision, it made sense to meet with the psychologist to learn more. Bryce returned with Mary to the Deer Creek Clinic to meet with Dr. Stella Cassidy, a psychologist who worked closely with Dr. Brant to help with a wide range of problems with sexual dysfunction.

A Spouse's Perspective "Concerned Yet Kind of Relieved"

When Bryce first told Mary that he had consulted a physician for his problem, she felt a strange combination of concern and relief. She was concerned because the doctor visit confirmed that her husband's problem was real and in need of solution rather than a difficulty that would pass on its own. She also felt relief because this was helping to put to rest a whole slew of suspicions and worries that had been building within her for months. Later that week, Mary called her older sister and unburdened herself:

At first I thought he was having an affair: It was the lowest I've ever felt in my entire life. "You're such an idiot," I would say to myself, "you should have seen it coming." He was always such a sex fiend. Well, maybe not a fiend but he was certainly always interested in sex. I loved him, but I could never keep up with him. And he always seemed to want more. So I thought that he'd eventually gotten tired of me.

I thought, "What am I doing wrong?" I tried to be sexier for him, but more often than not it seemed to backfire. I kept picturing him with some 20-year-old fact checker or hot young intern. I imagined the things they might do together, all the things he's tried to get me to do — things I would never do. I came to hate this perfect girl he was sleeping with — this girl who didn't exist.

I dressed up for him. I tried to say the things I thought he wanted me to say. But he just couldn't be excited about me. I would figure that he must be thinking about her. But then he would seem so genuinely upset when he couldn't have sex with me, that I couldn't be mad at him. I wanted to believe that he loved and wanted me but just had a problem. Much of the time, I did believe that. And of course I was concerned about him. So I told him to not worry about it.

Meanwhile, I myself had trouble thinking about anything else. I started going back to the gym, which I hadn't done in a few years. I bought a few new outfits, not that he noticed. But he just kept on being unable to perform. Other woman or no other woman, it really began to mess with my self-esteem, and I started to feel unattractive and uninteresting. I started to dread lying in bed at night, because he would so

Physicians wrote 120,000 prescriptions for *sildenafil* (Viagra) during its first month on the market in 1998, making it the fastest-selling new prescription drug in history (Adler, 1998). The current number of annual prescriptions for this and other erectile disorder drugs is more than 3 million (Marsh, 2017).

In one survey of heterosexual couples, women say they want an average of 19 minutes of sexual foreplay, and actually spend 11. Men say they want an average of 18 minutes of foreplay, and actually spend 13 (Castleman, 2017).

bravely start to be physical with me, and he would try so hard, but he would lose his arousal and I would know that neither of us were being satisfied.

It was so hard to face the idea that I was disappointing him or that he had found someone else who was more exciting, but I didn't let him know how upset I was. I also missed the feeling of being close to him, of having him make love to me. Maybe this sounds extreme, but I really thought I was going to lose Bryce. I tried to be as reassuring and understanding as I could, and all the while I was a wreck inside. I told him everything was fine and that it was normal, when I knew in my heart that everything wasn't fine, that something was dreadfully wrong. I told him that maybe all he needed was a little rest, maybe a vacation, maybe a doctor even.

And then Monday Bryce told me that he *had* gone to see a doctor. And I saw how scared he looked and I knew in an instant that there had never been another woman, that it had been ridiculous to even think such a thing. I felt relieved, but more than that I felt embarrassed for being so jealous, for distrusting my partner, and especially for not fully recognizing the fear and pain he must have been going through. Hopefully, this therapist—her name is Dr. Cassidy—will make a difference. To be sure, it's better than doing nothing or, worse, imagining things that aren't true.

Bryce and Mary in Sex Therapy Giving and Receiving Pleasure

A revolution in the treatment of sexual dysfunctions occurred in 1970 with the publication of William Masters and Virginia Johnson's book *Human Sexual Inadequacy*. The combination of cognitive, behavioral, couple, and family interventions that they used to treat sexual dysfunctions is the foundation for today's sex therapy programs.

Dr. Cassidy spent two sessions obtaining background information from Bryce and Mary. In the first session, she interviewed them together. In the second session, a week later, she met with Bryce and Mary separately for about half an hour each.

By the close of these sessions, Dr. Cassidy had determined that Bryce's sexual difficulty fit the DSM-5-TR criteria for erectile disorder, a type of sexual dysfunction. His difficulty had two key features: (1) a recurrent inability to attain or maintain an adequate erection until completion of sexual activity or decreased erectile rigidity that interfered with sexual activity and (2) significant distress or impairment over that inability.

Studies on erectile disorder had convinced Dr. Cassidy that in many cases psychological factors help produce the problem. Initially a man may have an instance of erectile failure due to stress, fatigue, mild physical impairment, alcohol intake, discomfort with his partner, or another such reason. Once such a failure occurs, he places extra demands on himself to perform in a productive manner. Given the recent failure, however, such demands tend to provoke negative expectancies. He may, for example, anticipate failure, disappointment, or ridicule. With such negative expectancies going through his mind, the individual focuses intensely on his performance during the sex act, searching for indications that he is not functioning adequately. This extra focus in turn produces an actual or perceived decrement in his erection. The continued concern and focus on performance eventually lead to an actual decrement in the erection, and the person becomes even more acutely focused on his performance. The cycle continues until the erection is lost entirely.

As a result of this episode of failure, the individual is primed for a similar result in the next encounter. Each encounter sets the stage for the next, causing negative expectancies, performance scrutiny, and erectile failure to become further and further entrenched. Dr. Cassidy believed that this psychological process must be reversed if an erectile problem was to be overcome. Sex therapy as she conducted it included a combination of cognitive and behavioral techniques, all of which were intended to accomplish a fundamental goal: shift the individual's focus from his performance to the sex act itself. As part of therapy, the psychologist also sought to reeducate clients about sexual matters and debunk any maladaptive attitudes about sex that they might have.

Sessions 1 and 2   The first two sessions were spent gathering both current and background information from Bryce and Mary. Toward the end of the second session, Dr. Cassidy explained the treatment plan to the couple. In practical terms, Bryce and Mary would undertake certain exercises at home that would minimize any anxiety about performance in sexual situations. At first the exercises would involve various types of massage and sexual touching, but later they would progress to more explicit sexual activities.

In the meantime, it was important, the sex therapist explained, that Bryce and Mary refrain from any "unauthorized" sexual activity. In fact, for the present, sexual contact should be limited to the specific exercises designed to further the treatment process. Both Bryce and Mary expressed a sense of relief. As matters now stood, all attempts at sexual relations had become a trial for them; indeed, the sense of obligation to keep trying to have sex, combined with the disappointing results, was turning into an unbearable burden. With Dr. Cassidy's recommendation that they stop making these attempts, the responsibility was off their shoulders. Bryce particularly seemed to welcome the idea of simply following instructions, especially as, from the sound of it, the types of things the psychologist would require of him were far less demanding than what he was requiring of himself.

Dr. Cassidy then explained what would be required of Bryce and Mary during the coming week. They would perform an exercise called *sensate focus*, in which the goal was to engage in pleasurable touching and caressing while undressed but to avoid any genital touching. The point of the exercise, the therapist explained, was for them to recapture a state of physical intimacy without any sense of demand. When conducting the exercise, they were just to immerse themselves in the sensations each received during the caresses and also to note the pleasure they were giving while administering caresses. Dr. Cassidy e-mailed Bryce and Mary each a copy of written guidelines, including a suggested sequence of body areas to caress,

People with *performance anxiety* during a sexual encounter worry that they will fail to perform adequately. In turn, they take a *spectator role* during the encounter; that is, they keep observing how they are performing, rather than relaxing and enjoying the sensations of sexual pleasure.

Sensate focus exercises are sometimes called *nondemand pleasuring*, or *petting exercises.*

as well as some pictorial supplements. The therapist recommended that the couple perform the exercise at least three times in the coming week.

Session 3   Bryce and Mary reported that as instructed, they had refrained from sexual activity. In addition, they had carried out the sensate focus exercise three times. Mary volunteered that she found the exercises enjoyable. Bryce echoed this but also observed that he had been tense during the first exercise, as it reminded him of his deficiencies. By the later two exercises, he had set aside his concerns and was giving himself up to the process; then he also found the exercises enjoyable.

Dr. Cassidy explained the next exercise, which involved a procedure similar to the sensate focus but with the inclusion of genital touching. Mary and Bryce were to take turns caressing one another as before but now were to include caressing each other's genitals as part of the sequence. The therapist noted that the inclusion of genital touching should not distract Mary and Bryce from the goal of the exercise, which was the same as before: just to enjoy the sensations.

The psychologist, as before, sent Bryce and Mary written guidelines for suggested approaches. For example, for Mary, part of the guidelines was as follows:

> Do as much of the general body caressing as you like initially. Then play with his penis. Play with the tip and the shaft and the testicles for a while. Then go to another part of his body. One that he likes. Caress his belly or his ears or his thighs, for example. Then go back to his penis. Use your fingers or lips as you and he please. (Adapted from Kaplan, 1987, p. 46)

For Bryce, the written guidelines included the following:

> Play with her whole body first. Then when you feel she is ready, or when she tells you, play with her breasts. Gently kiss and massage the nipples. Play with the area around her clitoris. Play around the vagina. Do not put your finger all the way into the vagina. Touch the clitoris lightly. Go somewhere else. Go back to the clitoris. Be as gentle and sensitive as you can. (Adapted from Kaplan, 1987, p. 49)

Dr. Cassidy emphasized once again that just as with the sensate focus exercise, the idea was simply to enjoy the sensations, no more and no less. Bryce and Mary said smilingly that they would "do their duty."

Session 4   Bryce and Mary seemed upset when they returned. Bryce told Dr. Cassidy that they had tried the new exercises, but they weren't working. The therapist asked Bryce for details, and the client indicated that they had conducted the exercises as instructed — including genital caressing — but that Bryce had failed to get an erection. "What was wrong?" he wanted to know.

Since both partners in a relationship share the sexual problem, regardless of who has the actual dysfunction, sex therapists believe that treatment is likely to be more successful when both are in therapy (Shifren, 2020).

Dr. Cassidy explained that there was nothing at all wrong. She had urged Bryce in the previous session not to focus on getting an erection. However, as often happens, these words can lose their meaning once a man is introduced to the sexual situation. The therapist went on to acknowledge that Bryce's situation in treatment was somewhat contradictory: He was being asked to avoid observing his erection during exercises, yet the whole point of the overall treatment was to promote erections.

Dr. Cassidy advised repeating the same exercises for the coming week, emphasizing that the question of erections should be set aside entirely. She recommended that Bryce and Mary just focus on giving and receiving pleasure, the same as they did with the nonsexual caresses. She also suggested that closing their eyes while receiving pleasure might help to keep it a purely touching experience. The therapist further suggested to Bryce that if he found he could not rid himself of the erection preoccupation, he should think of his goal as deliberately trying to avoid getting an erection during the exercise.

Session 5 Mary and Bryce returned in good spirits. Once again they reported a failure of sorts, only in this case, it was Bryce's failure to avoid an erection during the genital caressing exercise. Apparently, Dr. Cassidy's paradoxical instruction had its effect. Bryce found that the strategy of deliberately trying to avoid an erection allowed him to refocus his attention on the sensations of touching. By the second exercise, when adopting the same strategy, he found that he could not avoid the erection. During the third exercise, he was erect most of the time.

Clearly pleased with these results, Bryce said he was ready to "go for broke," meaning skip the intervening stages and proceed directly to intercourse. The therapist did not want to dampen Bryce's enthusiasm or rob him of his newfound sense of capability, but on the other hand, she knew from experience that jumping prematurely to later stages can be a problem if the results prove disappointing, as the patient's anxieties will then resurface. She explained, "I understand your desire to move things along. It's very possible that you and Mary could go ahead and have intercourse, and it would work out fine, but I'd prefer to stick to the original game plan. We only have a few weeks longer at the current rate, and jumping ahead, in case it doesn't work out, can sometimes make things take longer overall."

Dr. Cassidy then explained the next step in the sequence. In the coming week, Bryce and Mary would perform an exercise similar to the one they were already conducting, but one that would now include genital-to-genital contact. Specifically, first Bryce would give Mary the full body and genital caresses, and then Mary was to do the same for Bryce. This time, however, part of Mary's task would include sitting astride Bryce as he lay on his back and stimulating his penis by rubbing it against the exterior of her vagina. During this exercise, Bryce was to remain completely passive, as before, just thinking of himself as receiving a massage, paying no

Many sex therapists also provide *mindfulness* training in the sexual realm so that clients can develop a heightened awareness of the negative thoughts and feelings that travel through their minds during sex, learn to accept and disregard such thoughts, and better tune into erotic sensations (Graham & Bancroft, 2020).

attention to whether he got an erection or not. As before, the goal was simply to immerse himself in the sensations, and if trying to avoid getting an erection assisted him in this endeavor, he could use that device, too. The therapist emphasized that this exercise really differed from the previous week's only in that Mary would be using her genitals in addition to her hands. Mary and Bryce agreed to conduct the exercise at least three times in the coming week.

Session 6 Mary and Bryce reported that they had carried out the prescribed exercise four times. The first time, Bryce found that he became tense when Mary performed the genital-to-genital contact, and this seemed to prevent the involuntary erection that he had been getting from Mary's manual caresses. The second time that they tried the exercise, however, Bryce felt more relaxed, and Mary stimulating his penis with the exterior of her vagina did not evoke anxiety, nor did it prevent an erection. The third and fourth exercises similarly brought positive results. After each exercise, Bryce and Mary stimulated one another manually to orgasm, which was now permitted under the guidelines.

> **Common sexual myths:**
> **(a) A man is always interested in and ready for sex. (b) Sex is centered on a hard penis. (c) Sex equals intercourse.**

Dr. Cassidy: You two have been doing wonderfully with the exercises so far. The next step is only slightly different, in physical terms, from what you have been doing up to this point. Technically, it is sometimes called "vaginal containment." It means that you essentially do the same exercise as before, but now Mary is using the inside of her vagina to stimulate Bryce's penis, instead of just the outside. Once again, she sits astride, and she is in charge of the stimulation. She controls the insertion and moves her body just a little bit — without Bryce thrusting on his own — to maintain the stimulation. After a few minutes she then withdraws your penis and resumes manual stimulation.

Bryce: (pause) Well, I guess we've finally made it to the real thing.

Dr. Cassidy: Meaning?

Bryce: You know. We're finally doing it. I just hope it goes okay.

Dr. Cassidy: Okay in what sense?

Bryce: I mean, I hope I can keep the erection. I guess this will be the real test of all that we've been doing.

Dr. Cassidy: I understand your feeling. It's often hard not to look at this as a test of sorts, but in my view, it is no such thing. I'm looking at it as simply the next step in a progression. It's best if you can adopt the same frame of mind that you did with the other exercises. In other words, the idea is not to see if you are maintaining your erection but once again simply to immerse yourself in the sensations. The exercises should be considered a success if you can maintain that focus.

Bryce: I see what you mean. I guess I'm just anxious to get this over with, but I'll do my best.

After this exchange, the sex therapist was not entirely confident about Bryce's ability to approach the exercises in the proper frame of mind. However, there was little else to be said, and she felt it best just to wait and see how Bryce fared.

Session 7   Unfortunately, the intervening week bore out Dr. Cassidy's concerns. Bryce and Mary reported that they had abandoned the exercises out of frustration. They explained that they had begun the exercise as before, but that soon after Mary inserted Bryce's erect penis into her vagina, he started to grow soft; he then tried thrusting on his own to revive the erection, but to no avail. They then stopped the exercise. After experiencing a similar failure when trying the exercise the next day, they again stopped and did not attempt any more exercises for the remainder of the week. Once again, they were very upset, particularly Bryce. He was wondering if this was a sign that his problem would not respond to treatment after all. The therapist felt it important to normalize Bryce and Mary's experience.

Dr. Cassidy: What you experienced is very common at this stage of the treatment, and you shouldn't place too much importance on it. It's difficult not to think of the moment of insertion as a momentous event and to avoid examining how you're reacting, but that's what happened this time. As a result, your ability to immerse yourself in the sensations was probably undermined, your erection was reduced, and you became overly discouraged, causing you to end the exercise prematurely.

Mary: What should we have done?

Dr. Cassidy: In general, it's best to follow the exercise to its conclusion, regardless of what happens. As you may recall, I recommended that you resume manual caressing of Bryce's penis after vaginal insertion ended. In this case, even though the vaginal insertion ended sooner than expected—because Bryce became too soft to remain inside—you still could have resumed the manual caressing.

Mary: That's what I wanted to do, but Bryce was so discouraged. The idea just seemed to annoy him.

Bryce: Yes. I guess it wasn't the best reaction on my part. But as soon as I realized my erection was going down and I couldn't stay inside, I lost all interest in continuing.

The therapist felt that Bryce might benefit by increasing his psychological tolerance for the loss of an erection. The experience was becoming far too loaded for him, and unless he could get used to the idea that erections can come and go and then come back again, he would remain overly attentive to any decline in performance.

Dr. Cassidy: In the past, before this whole problem developed, how did you handle it when your erection went down during sex?

Bryce: I never had an erection go down before.

> Any physical problem that reduces blood flow into the penis can contribute to erectile difficulties. Common biological causes of such difficulties are heart disease, vascular problems (problems with the body's blood vessels), nervous system damage (resulting from such conditions as diabetes, spinal cord injuries, or kidney failure), the use of certain medications, and various forms of substance abuse (including cigarette smoking and alcohol abuse) (Rosen & Khera, 2021).

Mary:	(*Interrupting*) Actually, I beg to differ.
Bryce:	What? What do you mean?
Mary:	Well, I don't think you ever paid much attention to it before, but there have been plenty of times during foreplay when we've been taking turns on each other that you've gone soft for a time. I just stroked you for a little while, and you'd come back.
Bryce:	Really?
Mary:	Yes. It happened all the time. You just never seemed to notice or care about it, so it never became a problem.
Dr. Cassidy:	I think Mary has just made an important observation. It sounds like the critical aspect is not whether you lose an erection but how you interpret it once it happens. I gather in the past you never gave it any thought, so its very occurrence didn't trigger any alarms. I think it would be useful to do some exercises to promote that mindset again.

The sex therapy technique in which a man's partner stops caressing him whenever he gets an erection and does not resume caressing until the man loses the erection is sometimes called the *tease technique*.

The therapist explained a new set of exercises that she wanted the couple to try for the coming week. They would return to the earlier exercise, involving manual caressing and genital stroking. This time, however, there would be a new feature. During the time that Mary was stroking Bryce, if he was to achieve an erection, she was to stop stroking for a while, in a deliberate attempt to have him lose the erection. Then after Bryce lost the erection, he was to focus on stroking and caressing Mary for while; after that, Mary would resume stroking Bryce. Bryce's guideline, as usual, was to immerse himself in the sensations, giving no mind to the question of whether he got an erection at any given stage. The point of the exercise was for Bryce to learn to tolerate the loss of an erection and not see it as a signal to end the sexual episode, but rather as a typical part of the experience.

Session 8 The couple returned in a happy mood. They reported carrying out the exercise to the letter. During each of four attempts at the exercise, Bryce deliberately allowed himself to lose his erection after Mary stopped stroking him; he then turned his attention to caressing and stroking Mary. After that she returned to stroking him, and he found that his erection could gradually be regained. The exercise seemed to energize him. By the fourth exercise, he had developed a complete confidence in his ability to regain the erection and in fact he and Mary decided to resume the previous week's vaginal containment procedure. As before, Bryce began to go a little soft soon after insertion. He then withdrew and took his turn at caressing Mary. After that, Mary returned to stroking Bryce and, with his erection revived, she once again tried vaginal containment. This time, his erection remained hard as Mary continued moving on top of him. He ended up ejaculating inside her vagina. The following day, Mary and Bryce repeated this activity with similar results, and the next day they had regular intercourse without any difficulty.

The experiences were empowering. Now Bryce and Mary wanted to resume normal free-form intercourse. Feeling that the couple was ready, the therapist agreed to this plan. She requested, however, that Mary and Bryce stick to a few basic guidelines: (1) Intercourse should never be initiated as a test of sexual performance adequacy, but only out of a genuine desire for lovemaking. (2) If Bryce should lose an erection during lovemaking, he should not stop but switch to an alternative lovemaking activity, for example, manual stimulation instead of intercourse. (3) After switching to an alternative activity under such circumstances, intercourse could be started again, if desired, but only when a sense of comfort was restored. (4) If comfort was not restored, the couple should remain with alternative activities to complete the lovemaking.

Sessions 9 to 11   During the 9th session, Bryce and Mary reported making love twice in the previous week. Bryce had pressed for a third encounter, but Mary resisted, sensing that Bryce was doing it mainly to test his responsiveness. On the two lovemaking occasions, Bryce was able to complete intercourse both times, although the second time he appeared to become soft as he was trying to penetrate. In this case, switching back to foreplay for a while restored his comfort level, and in turn his erection, for another penetration.

At the 10th and 11th sessions, held 2 weeks apart, Bryce and Mary reported similar experiences: They completed intercourse four times, although there was one instance when Bryce did not attempt penetration again after first losing his erection, because, as he put it, "the desire did not return." On the whole, however, the couple felt that their sex life had been restored to a very satisfactory level and that by observing the guidelines, Bryce could avoid the type of performance anxiety that had been hurting him previously. They wanted to discontinue their visits to the sex therapist and just go it alone for the time being.

Dr. Cassidy agreed to the plan, with the strong suggestion that they call her if any difficulties arose and that either way Bryce was to text her in a month's time to provide an update on how they were doing.

> One survey has found that immediately after sex, 74% of couples cuddle, 50% watch TV, and 14% go on social media (Emery, 2018).

Epilogue

A text a month later confirmed that Bryce and Mary had maintained their progress. They were making love about twice a week and were completing intercourse almost every time. As before, there had been one occasion when Bryce's erection softened too much for penetration, and switching to an alternative lovemaking activity had created a satisfactory ending to the sexual encounter. The key point, they noted, was that Bryce did not get anxious or upset by the experience, so it had no carryover to the next encounter. Overall, they were both back in the pleasure business, as Bryce described their progress.

About 10 months after this conversation, Bryce left a message for Dr. Cassidy to say that he was planning to visit Dr. Brant at the Deer Creek Clinic because his problems in maintaining erections had become more pronounced in recent weeks. He was choosing a medical route because there didn't seem to be any anxiety component to his problem and also because he had noticed that maintaining an erection, even when masturbating, was proving difficult on occasion.

Dr. Brant reevaluated him with a complete battery of medical tests. They revealed that he had a mild venous leakage, which could account for his recent difficulty in maintaining erections. In this condition, which often occurs with age, blood flow to the penis is sufficient to produce an erection initially, but some of the blood then leaks out of the vessels and the erection softens. The physician noted that Bryce could continue dealing with the problem as he had been doing—that is, engaging in manual and oral stimulation with Mary rather than intercourse during some sexual encounters—or he could try one of the available medical remedies. Given that Bryce was still in excellent health, the physician recommended the use of sildenafil on occasion, as a kind of boost or insurance. This time Bryce agreed.

Over the following months, both Bryce and Mary were very pleased with the medication. It almost always helped Bryce to achieve an erection that was satisfactory for intercourse. At the same time, Bryce noted that he did not need the drug most of the time, and he preferred to do without it whenever possible. Overall, he felt that the combination of psychological and medical methods offered a perfectly reasonable solution for his periodic problem. Mary and he were once again back in the "pleasure business."

> Sildenafil and the other erectile dysfunction drugs help restore erections and enable sexual intercourse in 60 to 80% of men who use them, compared to a rate of 21% among men taking placebo drugs (Khera, 2021; Graham & Bancroft, 2020).

Assessment Questions

1. Define sexual dysfunction.

2. What contributed to the onset of Bryce's sexual dysfunction?

3. What factors may have led to Bryce's difficulty in completing sexual intercourse with Mary?

4. What percentage of men have erectile difficulties at least some of the time?

5. What may be some physical causes of erectile dysfunctions?

6. Why did Bryce initially decide that psychological therapy was a better option for him than sildenafil?

7. What were Mary's concerns regarding her husband's sexual dysfunction?

8. What types of therapy did Masters and Johnson use in treating sexual dysfunctions?

9. What are the two key features from the DSM-5-TR criteria for erectile disorder?

10. Why did Dr. Cassidy want Bryce and Mary to abstain from sexual intercourse at the onset of therapy?

11. Describe the purpose of sensate focus.

12. What are the factors that determine whether an erectile disorder is physical or psychological?

13. What were the basic guidelines requested by Dr. Cassidy once Mary and Bryce were able to resume successful sexual intercourse?

14. Why did Bryce eventually begin the occasional use of sildenafil?

CASE 12

Gender Dysphoria

Table 12-1

Dx Checklist

Gender Dysphoria in Adolescents and Adults

1. For 6 months or more, the individual's gender-related feelings and/or behaviors are contrary to those of their assigned gender, as indicated by 2 or more of the following symptoms:
   • Gender-related feelings and/or behaviors clearly contradict the individual's primary or secondary sex characteristics • Powerful wish to eliminate one's sex characteristics • Yearning for the sex characteristics of another gender • Powerful wish to be a member of another gender • Yearning to be treated as a member of another gender • Firm belief that one's feelings and reactions are those that characterize another gender.

2. The individual experiences significant distress or impairment.

(Information from APA, 2022, 2013.)

Nathan Living in the Wrong Body

Most people, called *cisgender* individuals, feel like and identify with their *assigned gender* (or *birth anatomy*), the gender to which they are born. In contrast, *transgender* individuals have a sense that their *gender identity* (one's personal experience of one's gender) is different from their assigned gender.

Nathan, a European American with Ukrainian and Polish heritage, was born in a suburb outside of Boston. Given his female birth anatomy, he was assigned female at birth and given the name Natalie. His parents, Julia and Paul, were both on their second marriage. Julia ran a successful online startup connecting people with rare medical conditions to health care providers around the world for second opinions. Paul worked full-time as a middle school teacher. Nathan was the youngest of four children, with two sisters and a half-brother from Paul's first marriage. Nathan had a carefree childhood, with lots of friends and a safe, family-friendly neighborhood. He was 4 years younger than his youngest sibling, but he always felt close and connected to his siblings, just as he did with his parents. In fact, growing up, Nathan believed he was the luckiest person alive to have the family he had.

His mother was his idol, brilliant and successful, changing the world by helping people access information from remote parts of the planet to understand how to diagnose and treat rare medical problems. His father was steady, reliable, a dependable presence to him and his siblings. This was especially true in the summer, when he was off from teaching. They would take trips together around the country, driving across the Midwest and plains to see the beauty and majesty of the Rocky Mountains. One year they went to Jackson, Wyoming. Another year they spent a month touring around Montana, counting the number of bears and elk they would encounter along the way. Once, he spotted an albino antelope darting across the highway into an arid field. He watched it until his eyes could no longer discern it from the horizon. He felt empathy for it and wished he could follow it, or protect it. He imagined what it would be like to be that antelope.

Nathan was never able to recall the moment he became aware that he felt different from girls his age. For as long as he could recall, he felt like he did not belong with other girls. As a toddler, he would play with more stereotypically masculine toys and would refuse to wear a dress or clothing that was highly feminine. He was highly imaginative as a child and always fantasized that he was a boy, playing with other boys, doing what they did, talking like they talked, and wearing what they wore.

Nathan didn't even like the words people would use to describe him when he was young. When other people called him "pretty" or a "little princess," he would become angry and loudly remind them that he was *not* a princess. His mother and other adults were generally amused by his initial resentment at these nicknames or compliments. However, when Nathan began to refuse to wear dresses or skirts, he and his mother engaged in a battle of wills for several years. His mother was a member of one of the local Christian church congregations and there was an unspoken dress code for Sunday mornings. Girls *always* wore dresses and boys *always* wore pants. Although Nathan's mother felt she could relent and let Nathan wear pants and shorts during the weekdays, the social embarrassment of allowing Nathan (who, at this point, was still "Natalie" to his mother and the church congregation) to wear pants to church was too much to tolerate. Beginning at age 3, Nathan and his mother would usually argue on Saturday nights about the outfit Nathan would wear the next morning. Occasionally, his mother would prevail by using a threat of punishment or promise of a reward. However, they often ended up skipping church when Nathan could not be coaxed into wearing something "appropriate." His mother felt that she would rather not attend services at all than face the judgment from others if Nathan were to show up wearing pants to church.

It was at this age when Nathan began to tell his parents that he wanted to be a boy. His parents were accepting, though confused. They wondered if this was a phase and assumed it was. They weren't familiar with what it meant for someone to be transgender, but they found they could think of Nathan as a boy in a girl's body, as he seemed in all other ways more like a boy than a girl. He even told them that he didn't just *wish* he were a boy, he truly felt that he *was* a boy and hated that other people didn't see him that way.

As a preschooler, Nathan continued to have a clear preference for toys and activities that were action-oriented. He received baby dolls and Barbie dolls for birthdays and Christmas until he was old enough to verbalize his own wish list. He asked for action figures, cars or trucks, play guns, and building sets. The dolls he owned became targets for battle reenactments, and he would create masculine

Most transgender people strongly prefer to use the name and pronouns that match their experienced gender identity rather than the gender assigned to them at birth, even when referring to events that occurred before they publicly transitioned. Correspondingly, this case presentation refers to the subject of the case as Nathan and uses male pronouns throughout.

outfits for the dolls and give them boys' names. He would play imaginary games with his action figures and call himself "Captain Nathan," fantasizing that he was a male soldier fighting in a war. His parents at first believed that his older brother's influence was to blame for Nathan's preference for boy's toys and activities. They redoubled their efforts to encourage Nathan to choose more feminine activities and toys, and they invited neighborhood girls over to play with Nathan whenever possible. These playdates did not typically go well as the girls preferred very different activities. Even at such a young age, Nathan remembered feeling like everyone wanted him to be someone that wasn't *right* for him.

As time went on, Julia and Paul began to accept their new reality. They had older children who had behaved more like the mainstream expectations for boys and girls. Their older daughters were very feminine, and their son was a "typical" boy, they thought, who acted like most other boys. As Nathan continued through elementary school, it became clear that he was different.

Nathan refused to let his mother style his hair with barrettes or bows or ribbons. He wore his hair in a ponytail and begged his mother for several years to cut it short. He loved and idolized his mother, but he also hated that she didn't seem to understand him. At age 8, his mother finally relented, telling Paul to take Nathan to get a haircut at the local barber and cancelling his appointment with Julia's hair stylist at the overpriced salon she had been going to for years. Paul, who was a bit more easy-going about Nathan's masculine traits, dropped what he was doing and took Nathan for the haircut. They walked in, and it was all men in the barbershop. Mario, the longtime barber Paul had seen since he was a kid, looked surprised when he saw Paul. "O my, what do we have here? Your little girl?" Nathan didn't skip a beat. "I want my hair to look like my dad's," he announced. Mario looked a bit puzzled but replied in a friendly manner. Nathan left the barber feeling relieved and comfortable, looking at himself in the mirror most of the way home. He got home and showed his mom and sisters, and they all said he looked great. Among themselves, they wondered whether "Natalie" was going to have difficulty in life as "she" got older, fearing that she would struggle to find herself and find others who accepted her as much as they did.

Throughout elementary school, Nathan excelled on the playground in all sports. He played basketball, dodgeball, and softball. He was one of the fastest kids in any race and would always be picked first for team games. Early on, the teams were composed of boys and girls but as the elementary years progressed, Nathan began to notice that fewer and fewer girls were participating. Soon, he was the only "girl" playing with the boys at recess. He was unconcerned with the gender separation, but his classmates continued to know him as "Natalie" and to think of him as a girl.

Nathan's best friend up to that point in life had been Raj, an Indian American boy from just down the street. They had grown up together, playing hide and seek

---

Sometimes transgender feelings emerge in children (Olson-Kennedy & Forcier, 2020). This childhood pattern may disappear by adolescence or adulthood, but in a number of cases the individuals become transgender adults (Elaut & Heylens, 2020).

Surveys of mothers indicate that about 1% of young boys wish to be a girl, and 4% of young girls wish to be a boy (Forcier & Olson-Kennedy, 2020a), yet only 0.6% of adults are transgender. This age shift is, in part, why many experts strongly recommend against any form of irreversible physical transgender procedures until the individual is at least 16 years of age, except in extraordinary instances (Endocrine Society, 2020, 2017).

in the neighborhood or chasing each other with soaker guns in the summer. However, by fifth grade, Raj was clearly distancing himself from Nathan in favor of playing with other boys. When Nathan asked why Raj had been avoiding him, his friend averted his gaze and replied, "I just like to play with the other boys, and my mom and dad don't think I should hang out with a girl so much." Nathan was crushed. It wasn't his fault he had been anatomically born a girl, and he felt it was so unfair to lose his friend because of something beyond his control.

At the same time, Nathan began to hear other girls making negative comments. They started to talk behind his back and to shy away from him in the lunchroom and on the bus. He stopped getting invited to the girls' birthday parties. He felt rejected and sad. The boys didn't want to play very often with a girl at that age, and the girls were excluding him. By the end of elementary school, Nathan felt increasingly lonely. Ostracized and ignored, he began to isolate at home, playing outside less, counting the days until the summer break, when he could once again go with his dad and siblings on another road trip out West.

The Teenage Years Terror Strikes

With horror, at age 12 Nathan's breasts began developing and started forming noticeable bumps in his shirts. He was terrified that his mother would notice and make him wear a bra, so he began wearing heavy, baggy sweatshirts at all times so no one would notice the changes in shape. As his breast development advanced, he became more and more desperate. He used his brother's sports bandages and began to wrap them tightly around his chest in an attempt to flatten the appearance of the breasts. He felt extreme disgust when menstrual cycling began at age 12. Nathan's mother told Paul that she was hopeful puberty would help reconcile "Natalie" to her gender, believing that when the "hormones kick in," their child would become interested in attracting boys and wearing cute clothes, makeup, and hairstyles. Though Paul and Julia were not opposed to Nathan dressing and living more as a boy, they were worried as parents that this would make the child's life exceedingly difficult. As Nathan's aversion to all things "girly" increased with puberty, both Julia and Paul became increasingly accepting of the reality that their child was experiencing emotional distress associated with being a female biologically while identifying as a male psychologically.

Nathan loved sports, and he continued to excel at softball as he got older. As a member of the girls' softball team, he was developing a strong arm and was accurate at hitting the strike zone. He had power and speed, and was extremely focused and competitive. He felt natural and free during games. His parents and family came and cheered loudly. He loved getting sweaty and dirty. His favorite moments came when he would slide into a base or dive into the grass to make a defensive play. On the other hand, he came to dread the 10 minutes in the locker

Some, but not all, transgender people experience extreme distress over their experience of incongruence and/ or find themselves impaired by it in their social relationships, at work, or at school. DSM-5-TR categorizes these individuals as having gender dysphoria. They often feel severe anxiety or depression, may display substance abuse, and may have thoughts of suicide (Guzman-Gonzalez et al., 2020; MHA, 2020).

Surveys reveal that 90% of transgender persons experience at least a moderate degree of distress or dysfunction at home, school, or work, or in social relationships, especially during adolescence (Lobato et al., 2019; Billard, 2018).

room before and after practice when the girls on the team would change into and out of their practice clothes. The locker room was a large open space with wooden locker doors that would swing open from the walls. Nathan chose the locker farthest into the room and tried to hide behind the door of his locker while changing. He hated the idea of the girls seeing his body or realizing how much effort he put into hiding his breasts. At that time, he wore two layers of heavy duty sports bras over tightly wrapped bandages. His breasts were not particularly large yet, so he was able to maintain the appearance of a flat chest as long as he wore baggy shirts. He also became increasingly uncomfortable with seeing the girls undressed. He was ashamed that he began to sneak furtive glances at the girls when they were changing. Although these teammates seemed foreign to him in so many ways, he also felt an increasing sexual interest in the girls' bodies. Nathan continued to excel on the field, but he struggled with the relationships off the field.

After high school graduation, Nathan desperately wanted to get out of his town. He thought that his lack of close friends was due to having grown up in such a judgmental place. He decided not to go to college, and instead took a job in a nearby blue-collar suburb at a manufacturing plant. His parents wished he would stay with them for the summer, and they had tried very hard to convince him to go to college, like their older children. They loved Nathan and supported his decision, but they were very worried for him. Nathan had saved some money from the part-time job he had during the last 2 years of high school at the local hardware store. He used that money to buy an old car and pay the first month's rent on a small apartment. He found himself hopeful for the first time he could ever remember.

It is estimated that 25 million people in the world are transgender—0.6% of the adult population (Elaut & Heylens, 2020; Tangpricha & Safer, 2021, 2020).

However, it soon became apparent that he had not left all of his troubles behind in his hometown. He found it just as difficult to make friends at work as he had in high school. Once again, he discovered that the world seemed to divide people based on gender, and he simply didn't fit into the right categories. The only difference between his new life and his old life was the fact that he now lived in a new suburb. He felt as alone as ever. Still, he kept at it, trying to make it all work, moving from the initial apartment to another nearby apartment, then to yet another on the other side of the city. He was an excellent worker and enjoyed the manual labor that came with working at the plant. He loved being around mostly guys at work. At the same time, they still saw him as a woman, and he hated when they tried to hit on him or made sexual jokes around him.

On his 21st birthday, he found himself alone without anything to do. His mother and father called to wish him a happy birthday. After the call, he found himself restlessly roaming his apartment until he finally grabbed his car keys and headed out the door. He had repeatedly passed by a bar near work over the past few years and had always wondered what it might look like on the inside. It had seemed like another one of those places full of people who "belonged," and he had felt envy and a small yearning each time he passed by. Today, on his "special" day, he decided to treat himself to a drink or two at that bar. He had drunk alcohol a handful of times over the years, and he knew that it calmed his anxiety. The idea of being able to drink something that would make him feel less anxious and alone was becoming more and more appealing. So, bemoaning the fact that he had, after all, never really had "normal" social experiences, he now decided that he could not tolerate letting his own 21st birthday pass without at least having one drink.

When he arrived at the bar, he gathered up all of his courage and walked inside. He almost walked back out when it felt like every person in the room turned to look at him. But he somehow made his way through the bar and ordered a beer, then another. He told the bartender it was his birthday. A patron overheard this and ordered him a shot. They talked briefly about birthdays and the Red Sox. Several hours later, Nathan felt relaxed and relieved. He had never felt so at ease in a public setting before. He came back the next week, and the next, eventually becoming sort of a regular. He knew the names of the other people who routinely came to the same bar. There was Frankie, Carl, and Ian. Sometimes the owners, Veronica and Kevin, would give him free shots of tequila or whiskey. Alcohol helped him feel more accepted and normal. He never developed any real friendships at the bar, but at least he was out meeting people, talking with the guys at the bar about the latest Celtics trade, questioning the decisions made by the Bruins upper management, and reminiscing about the days of Tom Brady and the Patriots dynasty. He also ventured further out of his comfort zone by visiting a bar known to be frequented by lesbians. He had known since high school that he was sexually attracted to women but he never used the term *lesbian* to describe himself because he didn't see himself as a woman in any way.

For several years, Nathan established a pattern of drinking regularly, engaging in one-night stands with women he met at bars, and keeping minimal contact with his family. His older brother was married now, living in their hometown and working as a firefighter after dropping out of college. His sister, Sophia, had graduated from the University of Massachusetts–Amherst and was working in Jamaica Plains at the Veterans Affairs Medical Center. His other sister, Maria, graduated from Boston University and worked in the city for a bank. Nathan was proud of his siblings even though he didn't feel like he really knew them.

One night, coming home from at an outing at a lesbian bar, Nathan was arrested for driving under the influence. It was then that he realized how dependent he had become on alcohol to provide him with the courage to interact with people in social settings. He also began to recognize that he was only able to have sexual encounters with women when he had been drinking and was disinhibited. Even so, he never felt truly like he was a lesbian, and he never was fulfilled by his sexual encounters. A few days later, as Nathan was surfing online, an advertisement caught his attention. It was for a clinic specializing in the treatment of gender dysphoria.

Sexual orientation is about whom one is sexually attracted to. *Gender identity* is about whether one considers oneself male, female, a mixture of the genders, or neither of the genders. Like Nathan, most transgender adults are sexually attracted to individuals whose gender is the opposite of their own gender experience (APA, 2022, 2013; Lawrence, 2010). However, transgender people may experience an array of different sexual orientations.

The clinic was in Boston, and the term *gender dysphoria* triggered his curiosity. He quickly did a Google search using that term and was astonished to find thousands of hits. He started clicking on the links, and, as he quickly read the information, his heart began to pound. He read about the symptoms of gender dysphoria, and his own life experiences flashed before his eyes. Given his mother's response to him as a child, he had been reluctant to ever discuss his internal feelings. He could not believe that his lifetime of distress and confusion was not something unique to him. The discovery that other people — lots of other people — experienced the exact same thoughts and feelings as he had was not only shocking, it was the biggest relief of his life. He stayed up the entire night reading Website after Website full of information and personal stories about gender dysphoria.

He even found an online support group for people with gender dysphoria. He read story after story and found tears running down his face uncontrollably. It was like waking up from a nightmare in which you thought you were completely alone in the world to find yourself surrounded by people who understood exactly what your life was like, who had in many ways lived the same life. For weeks, Nathan would rush home from work and search for more information online, paying particular attention to the support group. He slowly built up the courage to create an online profile on the support group's Website, and he wrote his first tentative post. He offered only a few brief sentences describing his situation and history. He waited anxiously to see if anyone would respond or if the responses would be judgmental or critical. To his amazement, the responses to the post came pouring in from all kinds of people. Everyone expressed support and understanding, and for the very first time in his life, Nathan felt totally welcome and accepted.

Nathan spent several more weeks posting and responding on the online support group. He learned about possible treatment options for his feelings of gender dysphoria. At first, he experienced a surge of hope that he might be able to find treatment and finally feel at peace in his life. However, it became clear that the treatments he read about were incredibly expensive and his minimal health insurance would probably not cover any of the costs. His initial hope was quickly shattered, and he tried to console himself with the fact that at least he had found a support group.

One day, however, one of his support group friends posted a link to a notice about a new research study at Massachusetts General Hospital on the treatment of gender dysphoria for transgender individuals. He excitedly clicked on the link. It led him to an advertisement seeking volunteers for the treatment study. Participants of either gender between the ages of 18 and 45 were eligible for the study, and there would be no cost associated with the treatment. Nathan sat back from the computer screen with his mind reeling. He felt as though he didn't breathe for over a minute, but eventually he was able to slowly reach into his pocket, pull out his cell phone, and call the number on the screen.

A positive development in recent years has been the increase in *support* programs for transgender people (Boskey, 2020; NCTE, 2020). Research indicates that such programs help prevent or reduce gender dysphoria among transgender individuals (Selkie et al., 2020; Johns et al., 2018).

Treatment Stage 1 (Psychotherapy)

Nathan sat in the waiting room at the counseling center with significant trepidation. It was full of children and their parents, a couple, and several individuals, and he felt as if every eye in the room was on him. To normalize his feelings, he tried to tell himself that everyone there was waiting to see a therapist, but the seconds ticked by slowly. He was surprised to be greeted by a woman who smiled warmly and said, "Hello, I'm Dr. Sloan." She led him to her office and said, "Make yourself comfortable—you can sit anywhere. Would you like a cup of coffee or decaf?"

Nathan introduced himself as Natalie. He chose a seat on the leather couch, noticing that the office was very nicely decorated—the perfect combination of homey and professional. He spent the next hour telling the therapist about his history. At first, he found it very difficult to discuss his childhood and the events leading him to the clinic, but Dr. Sloan was skilled at asking probing questions without being too intrusive. He found that the hour-long appointment was over quickly, and the therapist requested that they set up a follow-up appointment to discuss Nathan's eligibility for the treatment study and the likely course of treatment if he were to be accepted.

The next week crawled by as Nathan could think of nothing other than the treatment study. He alternated between feelings of extreme optimism and utter pessimism. He walked back into the clinic a week later having slept little and feeling as if his nerves were on end. At that point, he felt like he simply needed an answer regardless of the outcome. Dr. Sloan called his name and gave him a smile as they walked back to the office. Nathan sat down shakily and waited to hear the verdict. Dr. Sloan immediately put Nathan's mind at ease by simply stating: "The research team met and decided that you meet the diagnostic criteria for gender dysphoria and are an ideal candidate for the treatment study if you're interested in participating." After the anxiety of the past week, Nathan found himself flooded with relief.

The rest of the hour-long session was focused on discussing the course of the treatment protocol. Dr. Sloan described the treatment team as "multidisciplinary" and defined the term by stating that Nathan would work with physicians, psychologists, social workers, and nurses throughout the course of his treatment. The treatment included four stages and Nathan was informed that he could avail himself of any or all of the four. These stages included psychotherapy, hormone therapy, something called "real-life experience," and gender-affirming surgery. He would receive individual psychotherapy to address issues such as goal-setting, conflict resolution, and problematic emotions, beliefs, or behaviors. Nathan was able to set up a series of appointments to begin the psychotherapy stage immediately. He was informed that the length of psychotherapy before progressing to hormone treatments would likely be at least 3 months. That timeframe did nothing to discourage Nathan because he had already waited so long to reveal his

The DSM-5-TR categorization of gender dysphoria is controversial. Many argue that since a transgender pattern reflects an uncommon but healthy—not pathological—way of experiencing one's gender identity, it should never be considered a psychological disorder, even if it is accompanied by significant unhappiness.

true self. Indeed there were many issues to address during the psychotherapy stage, and his thoughts and feelings about hormone treatment were not fully developed yet.

For the next 4 months, Nathan met weekly with Dr. Sloan. These sessions focused on setting realistic goals for his future. They discussed Nathan's goals related to relationships, including those with his family and coworkers, and his future dating life. The therapist encouraged him to contact his mother and siblings and invite them to a therapy session. Nathan was terrified to disclose his transgender status and diagnosis of gender dysphoria to his family, but he was relieved to have the opportunity to do so with the help of his therapist. He could not bring himself to complete the call after 2 weeks of picking up the phone and then putting it back down. He finally chickened out and sent a group text to his parents asking if they'd be able to attend an important appointment with him the next week. His mother immediately called, terrified that Nathan had cancer or some other terminal illness. Nathan quickly clarified that he was fine but that he was seeing a therapist and really wanted his parents to come with him to the next appointment. His mother sounded hesitant and confused but promised that she and Paul would be there.

When his parents arrived the next week, Nathan was both relieved and slightly terrified. He had no idea how the session would progress or how his parents would ultimately react. He let Dr. Sloan start the session by explaining about the basics of transgender functioning and gender dysphoria to his parents. Then Dr. Sloan asked Nathan to describe his own experiences to them. He knew his face was red, and he began to sweat, but he was able to haltingly describe his early experiences of feeling like he was a male trapped inside a female body. He avoided eye contact completely until he finished speaking, then he looked up to see his mother's face smiling and tearful and his father's eyes beaming wide open and his head nodding. They said nothing at first, then Julia wiped her nose and face and said, "I love you so much, and I always knew."

> More and more studies are finding that when transgender individuals are supported in their identities by their family members and friends, they typically do not experience significant mental health problems (Herman, Brown, & Haas, 2019; Johns et al., 2018).

Dr. Sloan: I'm sure you can all agree that this has been very difficult for Nathan throughout his life, and it has also been very hard for him to talk about it with you in the past. Obviously, the whole family will need time to process the information, but I was hoping you could each give Nathan some initial feedback about how you're feeling after hearing his explanation of what's been going on for him.

Paul: Natalie, I love you dear. No matter what. Always. Like your mother, I've always really known all of this, but I just never realized how bad it was for you, and I hate that you've been so sad all your life. I just want you to be happy no matter what that means.

Dr. Sloan: Paul, I am very pleased to hear you and Julia voice your love and support for Nathan. One of the most difficult aspects of transgender functioning and gender dysphoria has been the sense of isolation that Nathan has felt most over the years. It's bound to give him some reassurance to hear a response that is both understanding and supportive. But I also realize that the rest of the family may not immediately feel so positive. I hope that the family can continue to explore all of your emotions and logistical concerns as we proceed in Nathan's treatment.

The session continued with Nathan's mother talking a lot about how she regretted not being a better mother when Nathan was younger. Paul consoled his wife but also explained that he too had always struggled with knowing what to do about Nathan's sense of himself. They ruminated shamefully about how they are accepting people and had tried to do everything they could to make things easier for him as a child. The session ended with a number of unresolved issues, but Nathan was generally relieved that the conversation had at least started.

Nathan and Dr. Sloan spent many sessions working through his concerns and hopes about the future. After discussing the pros and cons and spending countless hours considering both his past and his future, Nathan decided clearly and firmly that he did indeed want to live as a man. After that decision was finalized, he felt huge relief and excitement. In their sessions, Dr. Sloan was always quick to sort out and address Nathan's assumptions about the ways his life would improve if he were finally able to fully embrace his male gender. Moreover, to Nathan's great surprise, Dr. Sloan disclosed that she herself was transgender and had experienced gender dysphoria over the course of her teenage and young adult years. Assigned male at birth, Dr. Sloan was a transgender woman who had gone through the same treatment that Nathan was now embarking upon. Nathan was in awe. He had never suspected that Dr. Sloan might be transgender, and it gave him tremendous hope to identify with Dr. Sloan.

Over the course of therapy, Dr. Sloan also helped Nathan understand that all of his problems would not magically disappear with his self-acknowledgment and decisions. In fact, his alcohol use was a primary focus of treatment, and after 4 months of therapy without having a drop of alcohol Nathan was incredibly proud. Moreover, his family issues were not fully resolved. His brother was disapproving and couldn't understand why someone would "choose" to be a man after being a woman. He wrongfully believed that Nathan was simply making a choice, that it was more a whim than a deeply authentic sense of being. Indeed, he stopped talking to Nathan and the family. On the other hand, his sister Sophia's supportive reaction was a surprise, and their relationship slowly became closer. His sister Maria was verbally supportive, but she was preoccupied with her own life and seemed more distanced from Nathan as time went on. Nathan attributed this to Maria's demanding work schedule, but he also couldn't help but wonder if Maria felt uncomfortable or disapproving around him. His mother always wanted to talk

Transgender women (that is, people who identify as female but were assigned male at birth) outnumber transgender men (people who identify as male but were assigned female at birth) by around 2 to 1 (Nolan, Kuhner, & Dy, 2019).

to Nathan about his gender dysphoria, and whenever Nathan tried to change the topic, she would quickly ask more questions related to his gender identity and ongoing treatment. Dr. Sloan helped him focus on accepting the current state of his family relationships while continuing to make efforts to improve them.

Treatment Stage 2 (Hormone Therapy)

In hormone treatments, physicians administered the male sex hormone *testosterone* for transgender men and the female sex hormone *estrogen* for transgender females. Transgender females may also receive *antiandrogens*, drugs that suppress their bodies' production of testosterone (Elaut & Heylens, 2020; Ferrando, Zhao, & Nikolavsky, 2020).

After 5 months, Nathan and Dr. Sloan both agreed that he was ready to progress to the next stage of treatment. He met with an endocrinologist, Dr. Spratt, who discussed the process of hormone therapy. What seemed like an easy appointment turned out to be much more complicated than Nathan had imagined. He knew he wanted to take male hormones, but he had not realized all the issues involved with doing so. First of all, Dr. Spratt wanted to discuss fertility issues with him. One of the side effects of taking the male hormone testosterone, according to Dr. Spratt, was infertility. Nathan had never had any desire to conceive and carry a child, but Dr. Spratt presented an interesting alternative that he had never considered. He could have some eggs harvested and frozen in case he ever wanted children that were biologically related to him in the future. A part of Nathan wanted to avoid thinking about the issue entirely and move forward, but following the appointment, he found himself wondering if there would ever come a time that he would regret not acting now. Then again, the harvesting process was very expensive and wasn't covered by the treatment study. Furthermore, he would need to take female hormones for a month in order to maximize the number of eggs that could be harvested. After a few sleepless nights, he decided not to have any eggs harvested. He discovered that he was comfortable with the idea that if he later decided to have children, they would not be his biological offspring. He returned the next week to start the hormone therapy.

Nathan began taking testosterone that week. He had always had a fear of needles, so he was relieved to discover that he could use a transdermal testosterone patch instead of regular injections. Nathan was so eager for the testosterone to make an impact that he started scrutinizing his body immediately. After 2 weeks, he was disappointed to see that very little had changed. He went back to see Dr. Spratt who reassured him that it would take several months for the changes to manifest.

Over the next 3 months, Nathan began to notice that his voice became deeper. He was thrilled with this outcome because strangers on the phone began to refer to him as "sir" and "Mr." He also began to notice that his breasts were slightly smaller and less noticeable in his clothing. He continued to bind his breasts, however, and was still not entirely happy with their size. He also began to grow more hair on his body, including his chest and face. One day, he found himself in a pharmacy staring at the aisle carrying men's shaving supplies. Although the choices were a little overwhelming, he was excited to be doing something that felt inherently masculine. The appearance of hair on his face and chest was positive for Nathan, but, at the same time, he began to lose some of the hair on his head. He cut his hair even shorter, and saw that he was experiencing some male pattern baldness. He had a mixture of reactions to this discovery—on the one hand, he did not want to be bald, but on the other hand, he was relieved to be experiencing an issue that only affected men. To his relief, most of the side effects of the hormones were minimal for Nathan. He had read about problems with acne, emotional lability, and increased sexual desire, but his experiences with these issues were either absent or mild. After 6 months of hormone therapy, Dr. Spratt explained that Nathan had likely maximized the benefit from the hormones. He advised Nathan to continue on the same dosage and move forward with the next step of treatment.

Treatment Stage 3 (Real-Life Experience)

Of all the steps in treatment thus far, this stage was simultaneously the most nerve-wracking and exhilarating. During this stage, Nathan planned to officially and publicly change his gender identity. From this point on, he fully left behind the name "Natalie" and became Nathan, switched to using male pronouns, and began to live his public life as a man.

Nathan woke up the day after his therapy appointment and had to pinch himself to be sure that this was really happening. He got out of bed, took his shower, and opened his closet door. He had bought a new outfit for the occasion and was shaking a bit as he put on his new pants, shirt, and shoes. He decided not to shave that morning, feeling that the small amount of facial fuzz would help make him feel more masculine. He drove to work with great anxiety and almost turned around three different times. He sat in the parking lot for 15 minutes trying to find the courage to walk in. He had discussed his transition with his boss weeks ago. The look on his boss's face suggested shock and possibly disgust, but the boss's words were beyond reproach. He said he would support Nathan "as long as it doesn't interfere with your performance."

The manufacturing facility Nathan had worked in for years—with his generally female persona—had always been a place where he could simply blend into the surroundings. He had worked hard and been a model employee. However, he had only been promoted once while several other coworkers had been steadily climbing the ladder. He would not describe any of his coworkers as "friends" but they were generally cordial and comfortable around one another. When Nathan walked into work that day, he encountered a variety of reactions. Some of his coworkers didn't pay any attention to the change that seemed so monumental

> "Being told you are not who you know yourself to be is trauma."
> —Elijah C. Nealy, therapist

to Nathan himself. Others stared and left the break room soon upon his entering. He had requested a new name badge—with the name Nathan rather than Natalie on it—when he had met with his boss previously, and now he felt self-conscious wearing it.

Not a single employee addressed him as "Nathan" for the entire first week at work—they simply went out of their way not to say his name at all. He did overhear a conversation between two women at work who were known gossipers. One woman stated, "I'm not even sure what to call him/her. Should we now refer to him/her as 'it'?" The other woman burst out laughing before they realized that Nathan was standing behind them. His face was red, and he looked straight at the ground as they awkwardly walked out of the room. In some ways, Nathan was actually thankful that he had never established strong relationships at work in the past so that the contrast between "before" and "after" was now not too great in the social sphere. He found himself generally isolated and alone at work, much like he always had before. Dr. Sloan had certainly been right when she pointed out that changing his gender wouldn't necessarily solve all problems.

Nathan decided to meet with his sister Sophia as his first effort to come out to his family as a man. He felt that she would not be overly surprised by his appearance, given their recent discussions, and he felt like it would be a morale boost to start with the easiest family relationship and work his way up. He invited his sister to meet for lunch one day when she was in town for a conference. He sent her a quick text just prior to their meeting time that stated, "Didn't want to shock you but I'm now officially Nathan." His sister quickly responded with fist and smiley emojis, which immediately put his mind at ease. Sophia showed up on time, and they spent the entire meal rehashing the previous weeks and how hard it had been for Nathan to make the transition. She pointedly asked if he had told their parents, and he explained that everyone knew in the family. She tried to give him a pep talk about talking to their brother, but it was only half-hearted since Sophia was aware that the conversation would not likely be positive. She did come up with a recommendation that Nathan send him a text with an invitation to get together along with the rest of the family. Nathan loved the idea of meeting with his older brother, the lone person in the family who had been invalidating and unsupportive, as part of a group, and not alone. On the way home from meeting with Sophia, Nathan called his parents and they excitedly agreed to host a family meal the next weekend.

As the day to get together neared, Nathan became increasingly anxious about how his family would react when they actually saw him. The last time they saw him he looked very different. They were so used to knowing him as Natalie, but now he was 100% Nathan. He spent the night before the family get-together alone, drinking several beers in his apartment. It was his first drink in almost a year, but

According to surveys, 90% of transgender persons have been harassed or attacked in their schools, workplaces, or communities; 50% have been fired from a job, not hired, or not promoted; 20% have been denied a place to live; and 30% live in poverty (Rutherford-Morrison & Polish, 2020). Many have also been stigmatized, excluded from social groups, and denied access to appropriate health care (Forcier & Olson-Kennedy, 2020b; Seelman et al., 2018).

he felt like he had to escape his thoughts and feelings for one night. He texted Dr. Sloan the next morning; she responded that day, before he met with his family, helping him frame his drinking episode as a negative coping strategy and reminding him they would be meeting soon.

He went to the family home that day for dinner. His parents lovingly greeted him as he walked in. They cried together. His sister Sophia hugged and kissed him on the head, telling him how proud she was of him. Maria, too, was supportive and kind, telling him that she regretted not having the time to see more of him in the last year, and also telling him how much she loved him. Unfortunately, Nathan's brother cancelled that morning, saying he had to work. Nathan would need to wait until another time to see his brother. Nonetheless, his gender transition was now official to his family, and he felt like a major milestone had been achieved.

Despite various setbacks, some of Nathan's happiest times were during the first 6 months living as a man. He loved walking down the street and being clearly recognized as a man. It was like everyone could finally see who he really was. He enjoyed openly shopping in the men's department and using the men's restroom. He even found the courage to develop a profile on a dating app that promised a safe and inclusive space for transgender people. Although he had still not found the perfect match, he had been on a few dates and felt his confidence increasing each day.

Treatment Stage 4 (Surgery)

After a full year of living as Nathan, his treatment team began to discuss possible surgical options. Nathan was ambivalent about surgery for a number of reasons. For one, he worried about the financial costs associated with the surgeries. The treatment study would provide only partial funding for surgical treatments, anticipating that his insurance would cover the rest of the costs. However, he did not have fully adequate health insurance coverage, so he would be responsible for at least 50% of the medical costs of surgery, not to mention the cost of his missing work while recovering from the surgery.

He attended a few consultations with the surgeon and Dr. Sloan to discuss all of his surgical options. He was interested in having a mastectomy, but less optimistic about genital surgery. The long process of vaginectomy and penile reconstruction would likely take at least a year to complete. Thus, Nathan decided to focus on the mastectomy for now and reconsider the genital reconstruction later. He was able to use his savings to help offset the cost of the mastectomy. Despite his concerns about the surgery, he in fact had no complications. He was able to return to work after only 4 weeks, and he had saved up enough vacation time so that he did not lose any income.

Gender-affirming surgery—also called *gender reassignment surgery, gender confirmation surgery,* or *gender change surgery*—is usually preceded by 1 to 2 years of hormone administration (Ferrando & Thomas, 2020; Ferrando et al., 2020).

An analysis of 28 studies of transgender individuals who received hormone therapy and/or gender-affirming surgery found that 80% of participants subsequently experienced significant improvements in their symptoms of gender dysphoria (Tangpricha & Safer, 2021, 2020; Bränström & Pachankis, 2019).

Epilogue

Six months after the surgery, Nathan met with Dr. Sloan to check in on his progress. He was excited to report to her that he and his brother were working toward reconciliation. His brother had finally contacted him after a year of silence and agreed to meet him for dinner in the city. They had since seen each other twice and had been texting on occasion. Nathan felt like he had already grieved the loss of his brother's relationship, so any steps toward a positive relationship at this point were actually a bonus. His parents and sisters continued to be supportive. He maintained very limited alcohol use. Most important to Nathan, he had met a woman through the dating app he was using, and they had been in a relationship for the past 3 months. Overall, Nathan was very pleased with his progress during treatment and was very hopeful that his worst days were behind him.

Assessment Questions

1. What were the early signs that Nathan was experiencing a male identity?

2. How did Nathan's parents react to his transgender needs and functioning when he was a young child?

3. What effect did Nathan's gender dysphoria have on his social life as a child?

4. During puberty, what did Nathan do to try to hide his physical development?

5. What problems other than gender dysphoria did Nathan need to address in psychotherapy before proceeding to hormone therapy?

6. What were the effects of the hormone therapy for Nathan?

7. Why did Nathan choose not to have eggs frozen?

8. What were Nathan's biggest struggles during the "real-life experience" stage of treatment?

9. Why did Nathan decide not to undergo genital reconstruction surgery?

CASE 13

Schizophrenia

Table 13-1

Dx Checklist

Schizophrenia

1. For 1 month, the individual displays 2 or more of the following symptoms much of the time:
   (a) Delusions.
   (b) Hallucinations.
   (c) Disorganized speech.
   (d) Very abnormal motor activity, including catatonia.
   (e) Negative symptoms.
2. At least 1 of the individual's symptoms must be delusions, hallucinations, or disorganized speech.
3. The individual functions much more poorly in various life spheres than was the case prior to the symptoms.
4. Beyond this 1 month of intense symptomology, the individual continues to display some degree of impaired functioning for at least 5 additional months.

(Information from APA, 2022, 2013.)

Schizophrenia affects approximately 1 of every 100 people in the world during their lifetime (Fischer & Buchanan, 2020a; Hany et al., 2020).

Lucas's parents were born and raised in a small city in Brazil. They met when his father was 36 and his mother was 21 and decided to marry soon after his mother became pregnant. They then immigrated to the United States where they hoped to open a business. Their first few years on American soil were happy ones, but difficult financially. The couple went through several business failures before Lucas's father started a leather clothing manufacturing company that became successful.

After arriving in the United States, Lucas's mother, Maria, gave birth to three healthy baby boys in close succession. Lucas, born in 1973, was the third boy. Maria's oldest son became sick with a rare illness and died when Lucas was 2 years old. Devastated by the tragedy, Lucas's father, Antonio, soon stopped eating properly and began drinking heavily. His performance at work deteriorated over time, culminating in several situations where he lost his temper with employees. He eventually became so depressed that he could not function and had to be hospitalized briefly. The notion of being hospitalized for mental health reasons particularly concerned Antonio because his own mother and younger brother both had been repeatedly admitted to psychiatric facilities back in Brazil. During his hospitalization, Maria managed all of the affairs of the house. Despite her own unremitting grief, she managed to take care of the children and the home, all while spending as much time as she could at the hospital during visiting hours to see her husband. At nights, after everyone had gone to sleep, Maria would lock the door to her bedroom and weep for the loss of her child.

Two years after Antonio's hospitalization, Lucas's mother became pregnant again. This lifted Antonio out of his protracted depression, and he was able to stop drinking. By the time the new baby was born, he seemed restored to his former self. It was another boy. He later told family members that the birth of this child had been his "salvation." Maria was beyond herself with joy and excitement about the new baby.

Lucas Unfulfilled Promise

Throughout their childhoods, Lucas and his younger brother were the best students of the three boys and, as such, received most of the attention from their parents. Lucas was a prized pupil of his teachers, as well. He was enthusiastic and motivated, and he typically finished at the top of his class. As head of the debate club in high school, he led the school's debate team to victory in several tournaments. He was also among the top scorers on the state-wide scholastic achievement test. He was smart, analytical, and motivated to succeed. Everyone who knew him had high hopes for his future.

He was less socially skilled than he was academically gifted. He had a few friends, but mostly stayed home and did schoolwork or spent time with his brothers. There were many occasions when he would start talking rapidly about something he knew a lot about and could spend the next 20 minutes talking without a response from others. He was so smart that people usually chalked it up to him being a genius, but the truth is that most of the time he was misunderstood it was because he was not always making sense: Circumstantial and tangential thinking masqueraded as genius.

However, things began to change for Lucas toward the end of high school when Antonio suffered a serious heart attack. He was discharged after having surgery and given several medications known to prevent future cardiac problems after a heart attack. The incident was terrifying to Lucas. He became obsessively worried about his father, his mother, and the rest of the family. Thoughts swirled around his head throughout the day: What would happen to them all if his father died? How would they afford to live? Would they have to move? His schoolwork was suffering, as he wasn't able to concentrate or study as he used to. He coped as well as he could by using daily prayer and frequent attendance at church. Some weeks, he would pray throughout the day and go to church in the evening. His father did recover eventually, and Lucas became convinced that it was due to his prayers.

> If one identical twin develops schizophrenia, there is a 48% chance that the other twin will do the same (Hany et al., 2020; Gottesman, 1991). If the twins are fraternal, the second twin has a 17% chance of developing the disorder.

Despite poor grades in his final semester, Lucas graduated in the top quartile of his high school class; however, he seemed to have lost his sense of direction in life. He registered at a community college in the fall, but after a few weeks became lax about attending classes. He was bored with school and beginning to doubt the purpose of more education. Eventually, he stopped going to classes altogether and spent more and more time with some friends he had met in his community college classes. They would sit in their cars and spend time at local trails and parks drinking alcohol and smoking marijuana. Lucas had used marijuana in high school a few times but had never been in a group of friends that used it frequently. Now, with his new friends, smoking was common. It was illegal, but it was fairly easy to find at Lucas's age. Most people his age knew someone who could find marijuana for them if desired.

As the weeks and months went on, Lucas was using marijuana more and more, sometimes several times a week. On other days, he and his friends would eat psilocybin mushrooms. And, on other days, Lucas would spend practically the whole day watching TV in his bedroom. The extended time streaming and endlessly sifting through social media was not due to laziness, or lack of ambition, or lack of interest in people. Rather, Lucas was starting to believe that he had special powers. He would closely observe the movements of people on the screen, imagining he could communicate to them and trying to determine the extent of his influence. The more he watched, the more his suspicions were confirmed. He was seeing how his own thoughts were influencing what people would say or do. Sometimes, he noticed how people were wearing clothes or had tattoos with hidden messages intended for him. His effect on the characters was becoming too obvious to deny.

At first, this belief was just a suspicion, but eventually Lucas concluded that a specific change had occurred: He was acquiring the capacity to control other people's emotions and behavior. He explored this by going into movie theaters or to the mall and observing how people behaved when he thought about them. He noticed that if he looked at people long enough, he could cause them to rub their eyes, scratch their noses, or make other simple gestures. At first, he thought he had to be within a close range to have this effect. However, as time went on, he concluded that he could project this influence over great distances. He discovered this one day as he watched the morning news. While watching, Lucas observed that the reporter glanced down at her notes periodically. Lucas knew that he himself was directing these movements. From that moment on, he believed that he could guide characters on television to move in ways that they ordinarily would not. Gradually, he became convinced that not only people but objects, such as traffic signals and automobiles, were responding to his influence. If he stood on a street corner, for example, and observed the flow of traffic, he found he could direct the cars' movements.

> Delusions are strange, false beliefs that are firmly held despite evidence to the contrary. Delusions of persecution are the kind most commonly held by people with schizophrenia.

In the beginning, Lucas was not sure how he controlled people and things, but one day, while pondering his situation, he had a flash of insight. He concluded that he, like God, must have a "life force" in his breath. In effect, he influenced people and objects through his breathing.

This was a momentous revelation for him. It meant that his power was not just your garden-variety black magic or wizardry. Rather, he had been selected for some sort of holy mission. This suspicion seemed to be confirmed soon afterward when Lucas heard God's angels whispering that he had been chosen to be the Messiah.

With this discovery, Lucas also became increasingly convinced that people were talking about him in public. One day, for example, while picking up a pizza, he concluded that some of the customers in the restaurant were talking about him and that others were glancing at him and pointing. This, he presumed, meant they knew about his power. Another time, he saw a well-known movie star in a television advertisement for leather clothing, and he assumed the person was talking to him directly. In this instance, he felt confident and proud that he was being spoken to by the celebrity. He was certain that he was gaining a reputation with famous people for his newfound capabilities.

After having several experiences in which he walked into restaurants or other public settings and saw people talking about him, Lucas became extremely anxious. As confident as he was about the positive potential of his mind-influencing powers, he was afraid that other people, particularly those with evil intent, might somehow gain control of his power and use it for destructive purposes. The best solution, as he saw it, was to stay away from people as much as possible. He also began to use greater and greater amounts of marijuana because, he believed, "it reduces the oxygen in the breath and that reduces its effect."

As Lucas's discovery of his special powers evolved into the hearing of voices, then into his understanding that he would be the Messiah, and, finally, into his realization that others were talking about him, he became more and more confused. One day, as he emerged from his room after being alone for nearly 24 hours, his mother asked him how he was feeling, and he could only respond by babbling incoherently about "angels" and a "life force" in his breath. He was disheveled and growing long whiskers from his chin. He didn't smell very good either. His parents, who previously had seen their son as socially a bit awkward and withdrawn, now were alarmed, and they arranged for Lucas to see the family physician. At the clinic, the doctor was quick to notice Lucas seemed odd in his mannerisms and speech. She had in fact wondered in the past whether Lucas might be on the autism spectrum, but this time she was worried that his thinking and speech were strange and somewhat paranoid. He wasn't taking care of his basic needs, had little insight, and described hearing and seeing things that sounded delusional. She referred Lucas for the first of what turned out to be several psychiatric hospitalizations.

Hallucinations are sights, sounds, and other perceptions that are experienced in the absence of external stimuli. Auditory hallucinations—hearing sounds or voices—are the kind most commonly experienced by people with schizophrenia.

At the hospital, Lucas was given a diagnosis of schizophrenia, a label that initially meant nothing to his family but one they would eventually know all too well. At this hospital, Lucas was treated with thorazine, an antipsychotic medication. Within a week, his speech became coherent again and he stopped hearing voices. He continued to believe in his special powers, but he became less preoccupied with them. After a 4-week hospital stay, he had improved considerably and was discharged.

At home, Lucas continued to take the thorazine for a while and, as a result, was less troubled by symptoms. However, he lapsed into his previous lifestyle. Most of the time, he watched television or slept, emerging periodically for meals. He had no interest in returning to school or doing anything else constructive, in spite of his parents' urgings.

As the weeks passed, he decided to stop taking the medication because it made him tired and dizzy. Within a couple of weeks, his delusions, intense anxiety, and confusion returned. Once more he had to be hospitalized.

This pattern was, unfortunately, to be repeated again and again over the next decade. Lucas would be hospitalized periodically with a major flare-up of symptoms; he would be stabilized with antipsychotic medication; and, after a period of relief—sometimes just a few weeks, other times as long a year—he would either stop taking his medication or the medication would stop being effective. Even when his medication helped, only two of his symptoms disappeared: his hallucinations and incoherent speech. The delusion that he could control people and objects with his breath was only mildly lessened, and he remained isolated from normal events and activities.

At the age of 29, after 10 years of treatment disappointments, Lucas was still spending most of his time in his room at home, not having done any productive work for several years. He had one friend, someone he had known since grade school, whom he believed was immune to his breath's effect. Their interactions consisted largely of smoking marijuana together. Otherwise, Lucas socialized only with his immediate family.

Lucas's Mother Like Losing Another Child

Lucas's parents were at first devastated and then, over the years, exhausted by his schizophrenic condition. Particularly hard-hit was his mother, Maria. Having lived through difficult times at a young age, she found her son's deterioration to be a last straw, of sorts. Occasionally, she would attend a support group for members of the families of people with severe mental disorders. The people in the group were nice, and the discussions sometimes helped her cope with Lucas's condition. During one session, the focus was on her and she reflected on her reactions over the years to Lucas's disorder.

Psychosis is a loss of contact with reality. Various disorders or conditions (for example, substance misuse) can produce psychosis; schizophrenia is one of the most common causes.

At first, I just didn't want to let myself believe that his problem was serious. I'd been through so much, and I basically didn't want to think about anything. Lucas was one of the only things in my life that seemed truly fine. He was my hope that some day I would be able to look back on my life with a sense of pride and accomplishment.

Then, there was Antonio's heart attack. When Lucas kept talking about how he had saved his father's life, I indulged him. For one thing, I sort of believed it. We were all terribly upset and anxious, and I really did believe that Antonio survived through our love and our prayers to God. Even when Lucas started to insist that he and he alone had saved his father through prayer—a direct line of communication with God—I figured simply that he was being overly emotional about the situation. I thought that he had been overwhelmed by the horror of not knowing whether his father would die, and so he was now experiencing an unusual kind of relief and joy that Antonio had pulled through.

Soon after that, I became aware that Lucas had started using marijuana. But, again, I didn't think that was too bad. I'd tried it myself when I was young. I don't think I realized until later that he gradually was using more and more over time. And don't forget the problem with his room. He would spend increasing amounts of his time alone there. I guess I really didn't look into that closely enough. It just seemed normal for a teenage boy. His older brother was like that too, but not quite as bad. I just figured Lucas needed more alone time. I never tried to stop his withdrawal from others, and in hindsight, I never really saw how big his problems were.

But after this went on for a while, my shining honor student was starting to retreat into his own world. Of course, as a mother I had wanted him to become someone important, to do good for the world when he grows. It sounds silly, but I thought he could one day be a famous scientist or doctor. He was just so smart that it seemed inevitable. But then he seemed to start giving up, and nothing Antonio or I did seemed to help. At dinner, he would pull away from the conversation and stare at his food, mumbling when we asked questions, otherwise not talking or even acknowledging us. He was so moody, no longer the boy I had known. I didn't know what to think, but in our hearts we knew something might be terribly wrong. It wasn't just that he was ignoring us; that would have been hard enough. But he actually seemed to be paying attention to something else, something we could not sense.

Finally, one night he came out of his room muttering, like he was talking to someone in his room. He walked past me in the hallway as if I wasn't even there. Like he didn't even see me. When he passed by, I peeked into his room and saw that his TV was on and someone on it was talking. I went back down the hall to the living room and asked Lucas whom he was talking to. He cocked in head, paused, then said he was talking to the person on the TV. He said it in a mater-of-fact way, then started talking to me about something else. I asked him what he was talking to the person about on the TV. He told me he could make the people on the screen move and that he heard voices that confirmed this power. I froze. I had no idea what to

Approximately 10% of the first-degree relatives of people with schizophrenia (parents, siblings, and children) manifest the same disorder (Fischer & Buchanan, 2020b; Hany et al., 2020; Gottesman, 1991). Generally, the more closely related persons are to an individual with schizophrenia, the more likely they are to develop the disorder.

say. I was just petrified. I called Antonio home from work and we got Lucas to see our family doctor the next day, thinking she could fix whatever was wrong with him. But it wasn't that easy. Our doctor told us Lucas seemed to have symptoms of schizophrenia. We didn't know exactly what it meant, but we knew it wasn't good. She told me that my precious little boy may be seriously mentally ill and in need of antipsychotic medications. I hoped so much that this was wrong. I just couldn't face the idea that she might be right. At the same time, I couldn't think of any other explanation for what had been happening.

That was almost 10 years ago, and since then, our problems have been endless. For periods of time, Lucas will take his medicines, but even then he basically seems depressed and slow; and he is still, I am certain, focused somewhere else. And sometimes he has flare-ups; he gets really intense and has terrible psychotic episodes. He hears voices and may even scream back at them, which is terrifying for a mother to see.

We've had to spend so much money over the years, to put him in and out of hospitals, and to pay for his medications, that we've nearly gone into debt. We've never been able to move into the home we wanted, or to travel to the places that we've always wanted to see. We know now that it is unlikely that he, or our lives, will ever be normal again.

After the support group session, one of the members, a man Maria had not seen at past sessions, approached her. He said that he and his family had moved to the area around a year ago, and at that time he and his wife had sought a therapist for their 23-year-old daughter, whose severe problems sounded a lot like Lucas's. They made numerous calls — to their physician, to a referral service for people with severe mental disorders, to the leader of a support group, and to a university professor. The name Dr. Michael Hart kept coming up during these calls. Apparently, this psychiatrist had built a reputation for his successful treatment of people with schizophrenia — even individuals who had previously shown little improvement. Dr. Hart believed strongly that evidence-based psychological interventions must supplement antipsychotic medications if people with this disorder are to make successful and lasting recoveries.

The man said that his daughter had now been seeing Dr. Hart for the past 6 months and had been making real progress for the first time in years. When he heard Maria tell her story, it reminded him of his own situation, and he really believed that she should give Dr. Hart a try.

Maria had just about run out of hope, and so she was inclined to ignore the man's suggestion. But something about his enthusiasm, his joy — perhaps it was his hope — called to her. That night, she discussed everything with Antonio, and they decided to gear up for yet one more try. The next day, they had a long talk with Lucas, trying to persuade him to see Dr. Hart.

It was once theorized that people with schizophrenia typically had mothers who were cold, domineering, and impervious to their children's needs — so-called *schizophrenogenic mothers*. Research does not, however, support this theory.

Lucas was not interested in a new approach; he was certain it would be just another in a long list of disappointments. He objected, calmly saying "No thank you. I don't want anymore medications, or side effects, or another person trying to convince me that I don't know what I am talking about." Maria told him that she loved him, and asked him to please do her a favor and see this new psychiatrist. Lucas had always listened to his mother more than anyone else, and in the end he gave in. The disorder had worn him down quite a bit, and it was often easier, from his point of view, to go in whatever direction his parents pointed. He allowed his parents to make an appointment for him to see Dr. Hart.

Lucas in Treatment The Road to Return

As Dr. Hart directed his questions to his new patient, Lucas gave only minimal replies. Most of the time, he averted his eyes, looking miserable and frightened. Finally, however, he showed a spark of interest when the psychiatrist changed his approach and asked him what he considered to be the "real problem." In reply, Lucas stated that he had been seeing therapists since age 19, and this was the first time anyone had shown an interest in his view of the situation. "Usually, they only want to know about the voices," he said under his breath.

Lucas then told Dr. Hart, at length, about the special powers he possessed and the problems that this had created for him. He eventually explained that he didn't like secluding himself in his room at home, but he felt it wasn't safe in public and that he could use his unique abilities more easily when alone in his room. "It was like having the power of God," he explained. "At first it was fun," he went on, "but then it became a major burden—something I don't really want anymore." To cope with his predicament, he told Dr. Hart, he could emerge only for occasional meals, bathroom visits, and church services on Sunday mornings. By restricting his activities in this way, Lucas said he minimized the chance of doing anyone unintentional harm; also, it kept his power from falling into the hands of evil forces.

The patient admitted to Dr. Hart that he continued to hear the voices of angels; he also remained anxious that others were talking about him. Most recently, he said, he had been trying to understand his situation by immersing himself in Bible study, looking for scriptural evidence that he had been chosen for a special mission. He began to spend more and more time at this endeavor and, as his parents described it, his room was now strewn with biblical texts that he would study until the early hours of the morning.

Although at first skeptical about seeing yet another therapist, Lucas was grateful that Dr. Hart was interested in hearing him out on the subject of his religious concerns. Perhaps, he stated, the psychiatrist would help him explain to his parents why his recent biblical studies were his own business and not "craziness," as they believed.

"I shouldn't precisely have chosen madness if there had been any choice, but once such a thing has taken hold of you you can't very well get out of it."
—Vincent van Gogh, 1889

Research suggests that people with schizophrenia have excessive activity of the neurotransmitter dopamine, or abnormal interactions between dopamine and other neurotransmitters such as serotonin, glutamate, and GABA (Reid, 2021; Correll & Schooler, 2020).

After talking to Lucas and his parents at length and reviewing Lucas's history, Dr. Hart was certain that the young man's condition did indeed meet the DSM-5-TR criteria for a diagnosis of schizophrenia. He exhibited delusions, particularly the belief that he could control others with his breath; he experienced auditory hallucinations; and he suffered from avolition, the inability to initiate or persist in normal, goal-directed activities, such as work, education, or a social life. In addition, his social and occupational functioning were far below what might have been expected on the basis of his capabilities as a child and adolescent. Finally, Lucas's symptoms had lasted for a number of years and were causing significant impairment and distress in Lucas's life.

Like many clinicians and researchers, Dr. Hart believed that schizophrenia is best explained by a *diathesis–stress* model. That is, certain individuals may have a predisposing vulnerability (a diathesis) to schizophrenia, but the risk of actually developing the disorder is affected by the degree of stress in their lives. Theoretically, the diathesis must exist to some degree in order for a person to eventually develop the disorder; however, the diathesis can vary in severity. People who have a severe diathesis might develop schizophrenia even if placed in a mildly stressful environment. Those with a less severe diathesis, in contrast, might develop the disorder only in a very stressful environment. And those without the diathesis—the majority of the population—are unlikely to develop schizophrenia, no matter how severe their environmental stress.

Given this view of the disorder, Dr. Hart used an approach that integrated medication management with psychosocial interventions. This treatment approach included attending to *protective* factors available in Lucas's life—factors that could potentially lessen his vulnerability to schizophrenia or lessen the effects of stress on him. Medications could lessen his biological vulnerability; behavioral training in social and independent living skills could lower his behavioral vulnerability; and acceptance-based cognitive skills could help him learn to be less distressed by his delusional thinking or hallucinations. Similarly, the degree of stress in his life could be lowered by family counseling or supportive services, such as case management, special group housing, and a sheltered work setting.

Dr. Hart's treatment for schizophrenia followed a biobehavioral program that was initially developed in the late 1980s (Psychiatric Rehabilitation Consultants, 1991). This program includes 5 behavioral training modules designed to teach basic skills in areas where patients with the disorder are often lacking: medication and symptom management, grooming and self-care, recreation, job finding, and basic conversational skills. The approach also engages the patient as a collaborator in the treatment program.

Phase 1: Engaging Lucas as a Collaborator   Dr. Hart educated Lucas and his parents as thoroughly as possible about schizophrenia, including the diathesis–stress model. The psychiatrist also explained that symptoms would likely recur without continued medication and a combination of cognitive, behavioral, family, and case management interventions.

The most challenging part was in getting Lucas to try a medication treatment once again. Currently, the young man was not taking any medication, nor was he interested in returning to an approach that he felt had had no benefit for him in the past, only unpleasant side effects. Thus, Dr. Hart suggested that they work together to eliminate the burden of his "special powers," which Lucas was finding so troublesome.

Dr. Hart: I know these powers have been a huge problem for you for a long time, and I want to help make things better. You have a diagnosis of schizophrenia, and I believe that the power that you've noticed in your breath is a result of this illness. If we can treat your illness properly, I believe that this power will go away, or at least be weakened. Do you feel that this would be desirable?

Lucas: Yes. But I hate taking medications. They make me so tired, so tuned out from everything. I can't even think with them. You know I have taken so many different kinds of medications. Every time the doc tells me they will help. And you know what happens? Every time? They help at first, and then I hate how I feel and think. Or I forget to take them. Or I lose them. Or, and this also happens, I know that they are a way for the evil to take away the good in me. Doc, meds don't work. They don't get rid of any voices. The voices are much, much stronger than any pill ever made. You don't know. But here is one thing you should know: My power is as strong as ever.

Dr. Hart: I understand your reluctance to try medications again, but I'm going to take somewhat of a different approach. I think it is important that you feel that the medicine I prescribe is helping, otherwise I wouldn't blame you for not taking it. Therefore, I'm going to seek your guidance on this question, rather than just telling you what to take.

Lucas: What exactly do you want me to do?

Dr. Hart: I'm going to ask you to take some medicine, and then to keep track of the medicine's effect on specific symptoms, using a special record-keeping form. This way, we'll both be able to tell whether the medicine is producing any benefits.

Lucas: What if I don't think the medicine is working?

Dr. Hart: I'm going to take your opinion very seriously, and if you don't feel the medicine is working I'll accept that fact, and we'll have to consider our options. However, in return, I'm going to ask you to give the medicine a fair trial. It's going to take a little bit of trial and error. But I'd like you to bear with the process until we've had a chance to figure out how much benefit we can get from the medicine. This will mean living through a period when the medicine is not yet working to the maximum, or not working at all. I will tell you when I think I've got the best possible dose, and I'll seek your input about how much symptom reduction you've experienced each step of the way.

Lucas: It sounds okay. But I'm warning you, I'm not going to take it if I don't notice any change.

Antipsychotic drugs reduce or even eliminate the symptoms of schizophrenia in at least 70% of cases. Second-generation antipsychotics tend to be more effective than first-generation antipsychotics because they reduce both positive and negative symptoms of schizophrenia (Jibson, 2021; Stroup & Marder, 2020).

Dr. Hart: Okay. But we may need a month before we can tell whether the medicine has any benefit. How about bearing with this for a month, and then I'll accept your verdict?

Lucas: Okay. I'll give it a month.

Lucas's parents, who were present during this early discussion, were heartened that their son had agreed to take the medication, but his mother doubted that he could take it reliably. She asked if Lucas would let them monitor his medication use. After some discussion, Lucas grudgingly agreed to let his father watch him take the medication at bedtime.

Phase 2: Attacking Lucas's Symptoms This phase of treatment was devoted to finding a medication dose that would relieve Lucas's psychotic symptoms. There were three main kinds of symptoms that could be helped by the antipsychotic drugs: hallucinations (hearing angels talking), delusional thinking (Lucas's belief that his breath could control others), and suspiciousness (his concern that others were aware of his powers and were hostile toward him). To track Lucas's improvement, Dr. Hart and the patient would each regularly measure the severity of his symptoms on rating scales.

The medication that the psychiatrist had Lucas try was *risperidone* (Risperdol), one of the second-generation antipsychotic drugs. During the first 2 weeks, Dr. Hart slowly raised the dose of risperidone, while carefully monitoring symptoms and side effects in collaboration with Lucas. By the end of this period, the client complained that not only were his powers unaffected, but he was experiencing some unpleasant side effects: dizziness and fatigue. He said he was ready to stop taking the medicine. Dr. Hart reminded Lucas of their original plan to allow 4 weeks to decide whether the medication was producing any benefit. However, the psychiatrist also told Lucas that he respected his concern about side effects and would therefore slow the rate of drug increase, which should allow his body to get more accustomed to the drug.

By the fourth week, when Lucas had reached the full target dose, the side effects were minimal. On the other hand, he had noticed only a slight change in his target symptoms. Lucas pointed out that the 4-week mark had been reached, and he was leaning toward stopping the medicine.

Dr. Hart felt that the patient had not yet spent enough time at the target dose to determine whether that dose might eventually prove helpful. Still, he knew that he had, in effect, given his word to Lucas that he would respect the client's decision to stop the medication after 4 weeks. A critical juncture had been reached.

Dr. Hart: I know we had discussed using 4 weeks as the trial period for the medicine. However, it took a couple of weeks longer than I anticipated to help you get rid of the side effects. So I'm going to ask a favor, and

Risperidone and other so-called second-generation antipsychotic drugs operate on the brain's dopamine receptors and affect the dopamine activity of people with schizophrenia in ways that are different from first-generation antipsychotic drugs and so do not produce as many Parkinsonian symptom side effects (Liang & Tarsy, 2021; D'Souza & Hooten, 2020b).

request that you maintain this dose for another 2 weeks. Often it takes this long to determine a medicine's full potential once the maintenance dose is reached. I wish that the medicine had taken effect sooner, but I hate to abandon it at the point when we can finally find out if it's going to do any good.

Lucas considered Dr. Hart's request. The patient then said to the psychiatrist, "I can tell you're trying your best. And I know you are one of the good ones. You are not evil. I know this. I will go another 2 weeks. But if I find out that you are being controlled by any evil forces or I get word that I am following the wrong path, you won't see me again."

Lucas maintained the target dose for 2 more weeks, and by the second week, he noted a significant decrease in the symptoms on his rating scale. Correspondingly, he stated that although he believed he still had some power in his breath, it now seemed weaker, so he didn't have to think about it all the time. He also noted that the angels had stopped talking, and other people seemed to be talking less about him. Thus, he was willing to continue taking the medicine.

During this same period, Dr. Hart asked Lucas to enroll in the psychosocial skills training program at a nearby mental health center. In particular, Lucas was assigned to the medication self-management group and the symptom self-management group. In these groups, each of which met twice a week over a 3-month period, he learned (1) the importance of continuous medication regimens (that is, that medicine does not work from dose to dose but as a result of cumulative doses), (2) how to work out medication problems with a psychiatrist, (3) how to identify the warning signs of relapse, (4) how to intervene early to prevent relapse once these signs appear, (5) how to cope with psychotic symptoms that continue despite medication, and (6) how to avoid alcohol and drugs, which exacerbate the symptoms of the illness.

With Maria and Antonio's nudging, Lucas was attending these groups regularly, providing the first change in his weekly structure in years. More important, in the groups he learned skills that were directly relevant to his situation. For example, he had always believed that smoking marijuana was beneficial, both because it had a place in his delusions and because he believed that it lowered anxiety. He learned in his training that drugs and alcohol usually increase the symptoms of schizophrenia, and also lower motivation and interest in normal activities.

Over the course of 3 months of group meetings, Lucas increasingly seemed to recognize the purpose and benefits of antipsychotic medication and became more responsible about his adherence; eventually, his family no longer needed to keep a careful watch over his taking of the medication. Lucas also stopped using marijuana.

Phase 3: Stabilization After 3 months of taking risperidone, Lucas's symptoms persisted, but at a much lower level. His delusion about having a power in

A growing number of therapists now act as *case managers* when treating people with schizophrenia. They not only treat the patients but also try to coordinate available community services, guide patients through the complexities of community services, and protect patients' legal rights (NIMH, 2020e; Bustillo & Weil, 2019; Schneeberger et al., 2017).

his breath remained, but he was much less focused on it and such beliefs occurred less often. As a result, he had stopped looking through religious texts for a sign that he was the Messiah, although he continued reading the Bible for a large portion of the day. Perhaps most important, he had successfully avoided hospitalization during this period. His life was beginning to stabilize.

The next aim was to help him set some longer-term goals and teach him the skills to achieve them. Potential goals included employment, financial security, adequate housing, friendships, dating, finding healthy and enjoyable hobbies, and family support. When discussing these matters with Dr. Hart, Lucas identified two priorities: improving his relationships with his family and developing an ability to function independently. It was agreed that the psychiatrist would conduct behavioral family management sessions with Lucas and his family, and that Lucas would attend a separate individual behavioral skills training group.

Behavioral Family Management

During the early sessions devoted to *behavioral family management*—a set of procedures designed to improve family functioning—Dr. Hart had Lucas and his parents discuss the problems they had been having. The parents started to discuss the problem of their son's remaining in his room continually, and things soon broke down into a shouting match. Lucas explained that the time he spent in his room was necessary for his Bible reading, but Antonio was soon arguing that the main problem was his son's laziness. Maria interrupted, saying that Antonio had no idea what went on most of the time because he was usually away at work. Antonio in turn replied that he was able to see enough to figure out that his son had become a "good-for-nothing" and that his wife was enabling him. Lucas listened to most of this conversation with his eyes turned upward in the "Oh, brother!" mode. Other times, he looked down and stared at the carpet. Eventually, however, he joined the conversation, saying that a major reason he stayed in his room was so he didn't have to listen to "this kind of crap." Antonio yelled that "this crap" was due to their utter frustration in dealing with their son's problems. In no time, all of the family members were yelling.

Dr. Hart could see that family interactions were characterized by high levels of *expressed emotion*. Research has shown that individuals whose families display high levels of expressed emotion—frequent critical, hostile, or intrusive remarks during family communication—are more likely to experience a relapse of schizophrenia than those whose families have lower levels.

Dr. Hart: I can see that you all have been experiencing a lot of frustration in connection with Lucas's problems, which has led to a lot of arguing. Having a family member with an illness such as Lucas's is stressful for most families. It would benefit everyone if we could reduce the general

According to research, interventions that also address the social and personal difficulties of people with schizophrenia significantly improve their recovery rates and reduce their relapse rates (Jones et al., 2020; NIMH, 2020e). Such approaches offer practical advice; teach problem solving, decision making, and social skills; make sure patients are taking their medications properly; and help them find work, financial assistance, and proper housing.

tension and bad feeling. In particular, it will be helpful for Lucas and for you all if there is a focused effort to reduce the criticism and hostility expressed in the house. One thing we have learned through studies is that these kinds of communications in the family may make it more difficult to recover from schizophrenia. I would like to hold several sessions devoted to showing you how to reduce the arguing and improve communications.

The family agreed, and the next 12 sessions with the psychiatrist were devoted to behavioral family management.

Several of the first of these sessions concentrated on education: simply sharing some of the latest scientific information with the family about schizophrenia. Dr. Hart gave the entire family some written material on the disorder, including descriptions of the problems produced by it. The psychiatrist also had the family watch a video that explained that most people with schizophrenia have difficulty performing routine activities. In the video, a series of examples were given of patients who had stopped being able to work, go to school, or attend to even the most basic needs, such as eating or taking showers on a regular basis.

Lucas's mother and father acknowledged the resemblance between Lucas and the cases shown in the video. They had previously believed that Lucas's limitations were largely due to his not trying hard enough or to his downright refusal to face up to his responsibilities. Now they were feeling regret at having criticized him constantly for his failures. Dr. Hart cautioned the couple not to blame themselves unfairly for their reactions or for Lucas's illness. He reminded them of something else shown on the video, that families typically react with a certain degree of distress over the limitations of the disturbed family member, finding it difficult to understand how someone who once seemed so capable and full of promise had fallen to such a level. The task now, he said, was to put their new knowledge to good use, beginning with the next phase of family therapy, which would be devoted to communication skills training.

Among the communication skills that Dr. Hart attempted to teach the family members were acknowledging positive actions in others, making positive requests of others, and expressing negative feelings constructively. They also learned how to communicate with Lucas in a way that better respected his boundaries and need for autonomy. Lucas's parents were open to these suggestions.

The psychiatrist explained that in many troubled families the simple art of praising one another for positive actions is lost. Criticism of a person's shortcomings or mistakes becomes the sole form of providing feedback, while the person's positive efforts are taken for granted or ignored. Lucas's parents, for example, found it easy to point out whenever Lucas failed to pick up his clothes, forgot to take out the trash, or spent an entire day holed up in his room. But they had given up praising any positive efforts by Lucas, such as his mowing the lawn or sticking to his

Brain scans indicate that people with schizophrenia have a dysfunction of the brain circuit that includes the prefrontal cortex, hippocampus, amygdala, thalamus, striatum, and substantia nigra (He et al., 2021; Bristow et al., 2020).

medications. Similarly, for his part, Lucas had gotten into the habit of noting only what his parents failed to do for him, while ignoring their positive efforts.

Thus, Dr. Hart had the family members perform an exercise. Each of them had to identify something positive that one of the others had done in the past few days. Each member was then to practice stating their appreciation in Dr. Hart's presence. Lucas, in particular, was coached to make better eye contact and to make his statement of appreciation with more vocal emphasis: "Mom, when you made my favorite meal the other night, I really felt good. Thanks a lot." To keep up with this task on a daily basis, the family had to record, over the next 2 weeks, all occasions when this skill was successfully practiced. With time, this kind of communication increased in frequency and became more natural.

To learn another skill, how to make positive requests, the family was asked to cite examples of things that irked them, and how they had specifically communicated that annoyance to one another. Lucas's mother volunteered that just that morning she had gotten fed up with the pile of laundry in Lucas's room. When asked what she had told her son, she replied that she had said, "The laundry in your room is a disgusting mess. You simply must start shaping up." Dr. Hart then used this example to explain to the family how to rephrase concerns or requests in positive and specific terms rather than negative and global terms. "Positive" statements indicate what the person should do under the circumstances, as opposed to what the person should not do or should stop doing. "Specific" statements clarify what should be done; they are not just some vague demand for better performance. Maria was asked to restate her concern in line with these guidelines. Her new statement was: "Lucas, please bring the laundry from your room down to the basement at the end of the week." Again, the family members were told to record each successful practice of this skill over the next few weeks.

Similar training was carried out for expressing negative feelings constructively, that is, effectively letting persons know how their actions upset you. Often, family members neglect this piece of the communication process, keeping feelings of dissatisfaction or disappointment to themselves and then moving directly to criticism and insults. Expressing a feeling is a way of telling a person that there is a problem but without making incorrect assumptions or accusations. Thus, for example, Lucas's father was guided to say to his son, "When you look away while I'm talking, it makes me feel that you don't care what I'm saying," instead of, "You don't care about anything you're told."

Over the course of six sessions, the family members became more able to use the new communication skills, and the skills became a more natural part of their interactions.

Now the family was in a position to learn the final set of skills in behavioral family management: problem solving. To introduce these skills, Dr. Hart had Lucas and his parents choose a concrete problem to solve. They decided to work on

According to some studies, family therapy—particularly when combined with drug therapy—helps reduce tensions within the families of people with schizophrenia and therefore helps relapse rates go down (Worthington et al., 2020).

the problem of Lucas's staying in his room continually. He acknowledged that it was not just his religious concerns that kept him there all day; he was also trying to avoid his parents' arguments and criticisms of him. If he left his room, he would usually hear them arguing with each other, or they would criticize something he was not doing enough of, or maybe something he was doing too much of. His parents agreed that there were many arguments in the home, but too often they blamed Lucas's withdrawn behavior as the cause. If he could bring his activities more into line with those of the household in general, they felt that some of the arguing would be reduced.

Dr. Hart explained the principles of problem solving. All members would have a few minutes to reflect on solutions to the problem; then they would propose their specific ideas, with each member withholding judgment on any stated idea until all alternatives had been listed. Maria suggested that Lucas come down for meals three times a day. Antonio had the same suggestion, but also added that Lucas might be allowed to leave the table if he felt anxious or uncomfortable. Lucas proposed that he join the family for a dinner out once a week—he felt that his parents would be less likely to argue in public—and that he have some of his new friends (from his self-management groups at the mental health center) over for dinner on another night of the week. Several other possibilities were spun, and then the family members discussed the advantages and disadvantages of each alternative. Dr. Hart urged them to reach a solution by consensus. It was eventually decided that Lucas would join the family every night for dinner, provided that the family would eat out on one night a week, and that Lucas would have a friend come to the house for dinner on another night.

The family put this plan in action, and it did eventually reduce the usual arguments about Lucas's participation in household activities. Other sessions were devoted to similar problem-solving exercises following the same format. With time, the family members developed some skill at finding solutions to problems on their own.

Individual Behavioral Skills Training

As some of the stress in Lucas's life became relieved through medication and behavioral family management, he expressed his growing desire to function independently, inspired in part by the example of other patients he had met in his self-management classes. One friend there, John, had improved to the point where he got a paying job as a clerical assistant at a small social services agency called Helping Hands, which housed people experiencing homelessness. Lucas visited John at his job and was impressed to see that he had his own desk and was given respect and responsibility. Lucas thought about developing his own work skills, with the hope that he could ultimately live independently. He raised this hope with

"I feel cheated by having this illness."—Individual with schizophrenia, 1996

Dr. Hart, who encouraged him and had him enroll in the mental health center's training group on personal effectiveness for successful living.

This group was set up along the same lines as the medication- and symptom-management groups that Lucas had already attended, but this group was geared toward individual problems. Led by a social worker, the group used traditional behavioral techniques, such as modeling, role playing, corrective feedback, and behavioral practice exercises, to train members in various skills needed for managing in the world. The group also applied newer evidence-based *acceptance* interventions designed to help group members learn ways to tolerate unpleasant thoughts with a distanced perspective.

After a few sessions, Lucas told Ms. Candace, the social worker, and the other group members that his immediate goal was to go on interviews for jobs advertised online, something he had never done before and had no idea how to approach. The group broke the process down into separate skills: (1) researching online for appropriate ads, (2) telephoning or e-mailing for further information and requesting an interview, (3) arriving at the appropriate time and place, and (4) being interviewed. First, the group focused on telephoning or e-mailing for an interview. One member, who had a fair amount of interview experience, played the prospective employer, while Lucas acted out his own role as the applicant. The pair went over the process repeatedly, while Ms. Candace and group members gave Lucas corrective feedback on his telephone conversation. Lucas also wrote several sample e-mail requests for an interview and brought these to the group where the e-mails were edited and revised.

Lucas's homework assignment was to make five telephone calls in response to ads and to report the results at the next group meeting. The point of the homework exercise was not for him to obtain actual interviews, just to practice his telephone behavior. In fact, to reduce pressure, it was understood that he would not be going on any of the interviews he might actually obtain. He would simply cancel them for now.

At the next session, Lucas was excited to report that he had made the five phone calls. On three of them, he was told that the positions had been filled. On two others he was told he could complete an online application. He felt he had become much more comfortable with the process by the fifth call, and he decided to make five calls each week.

During this time, Dr. Hart had been continuing to work with Lucas in individual therapy to find a medication level that would make a further dent in the young man's belief that he had power over others. Although Lucas had certainly improved while taking risperidone, he felt that his breath still had some power to affect people. Dr. Hart tried increases and then decreases in the level of risperidone and added and subtracted some additional drugs as well. Perhaps it was the medication changes or perhaps it was the impact of the personal effectiveness group, or perhaps it was both—but at one point, psychiatrist and patient hit on a medication combination that made a large difference. Lucas began to notice a significant drop in the intensity and frequency of his main symptom. He told Dr. Hart that the medicine seemed to have "neutralized" his capacity to influence other people through his breath. The patient also noticed that other people had stopped talking about him when he went out in public.

In addition to the medication, Dr. Hart helped Lucas practice *acceptance-based* techniques. He taught Lucas to be able to notice when his thoughts were odd or even delusional. Once he noticed such thoughts, he learned to recognize that they may not be literally true but rather experiences produced by his brain that he could observe and describe. This didn't make his thoughts less distressing, but he learned that even if his thoughts were distressing, he did not have to believe they were true, thus allowing him to gain a helpful perspective, and, in turn, enabling him to make choices about what to best do with regard to his actions and decisions.

Stabilization Phase   This change produced a sense of confidence and optimism that Lucas had not felt in years. For the first time, he believed he was ready to seek paid employment. He discussed this with the members of his group, and he eventually decided to try a volunteer position as a stepping-stone. He chose to pursue a lead given to him by John, his friend who worked at Helping Hands. John told him about another agency that delivered hot meals to homebound elderly people. Despite all his years of disability, Lucas was able to drive and had in fact maintained his driver's license in good standing.

Once again, the various components of obtaining the job—the initial call, the interview, the first day on the job—were practiced in the group setting, with group members playing the roles of phone screener, interviewer, and fellow employees.

Lucas made the initial call and several days later was accepted for an interview. At the interview itself, he was well-prepared to ask and answer questions. The interviewer was impressed with his sincerity and motivation, and told him that they would be glad to accept him on a trial basis as a volunteer assistant to one of the paid drivers. He could begin the following Monday, working 3 half-days a week.

The following Monday, at noon, Lucas arrived at the agency to meet the driver for his assigned route. He was extremely nervous at first, but once he began working and saw how readily he took to the job, his confidence rose. Over the course of the next several weeks, he worked hard and, eventually, was offered a job as a paid driver.

The *acceptance-based intervention* for psychosis is largely derived from the cognitive-behavioral approach *Acceptance and Commitment Therapy*. The intervention tends to be most helpful in reducing positive symptoms such as hallucinations (Yildiz, 2020).

Epilogue

Over the following years, Lucas continued both to take medications and to attend his group meetings on a weekly basis. It would not be accurate to say that he made it all the way back to a fully functioning and productive lifestyle. In fact, he experienced several periods in which his notion of having power over others and his belief that others were talking about him returned to some degree. On the other hand, those ideas never again took over his life as they had in the past, and they were always temporary. Adjustments to his medications eliminated the ideas within days or, at most, weeks, and in the meantime, Lucas was able to use the acceptance-based techniques he had learned to keep these ideas from derailing his life.

As much as he wanted his independence, Lucas was not able to make it out of his parents' house and into his own apartment. He tried moving out several times, but found life on his own too stressful. He had great difficulty keeping up with making his own meals, cleaning his clothes, and keeping things straight, and so he eventually concluded that he did indeed need the help of his parents. Furthermore, his job, although a huge improvement over years of unemployment, did not represent the level of work or responsibility that he had seemed destined for when he was young. Although he hadn't made it all the way to a full recovery, his progress was clear. A decade of repeated hospitalizations, full-blown delusions, isolation, and confusion had come to an end. He was now leading a much more normal life—and Lucas and his parents were relieved and grateful.

> Occupational training and job opportunities are important features of recovery from schizophrenia (Wang et al., 2020). Fewer than 20% of people with schizophrenia have jobs in the competitive job market (Holm et al., 2021; Bustillo & Weil, 2019).

Assessment Questions

1. What are the statistics for development of schizophrenia among identical twins?

2. What were three of Lucas's initial symptoms that signaled a mental disorder?

3. What was the diagnosis Lucas received after he was hospitalized?

4. Why did he stop taking his medication and what symptoms returned when he stopped taking his medication?

5. Explain Dr. Hart's theory of the diathesis–stress model of schizophrenia.

6. Describe the combination of biomedical and behavioral therapy used by Dr. Hart.

7. What are some abnormalities in the brains of individuals with schizophrenia?

8. How do antipsychotic drugs work to reduce the symptoms of schizophrenia? What are some of the downsides of using these medications?

9. Why are the newer second-generation antipsychotic drugs usually preferred over the earlier first-generation antipsychotic drugs?

10. What six factors were a part of the psychosocial skills training program for Lucas in conjunction with his medication program?

11. What were the two long-term priorities for Lucas once his medication stabilized some of his symptoms?

12. Why was it important to involve Lucas's family in his rehabilitation?

13. What particular communication skills were important for Lucas's family to learn?

14. What were some individual behavioral skills Lucas learned in order to become more independent?

15. Why did Lucas eventually decide to continue to live with his parents rather than on his own?

CASE 14

Antisocial Personality Disorder

Table 14-1

Dx Checklist

Antisocial Personality Disorder

1. Persons repeatedly disregard and violate the rights of other people in three or more of the following ways:

   (a) Little or no adherence to social and legal norms.

   (b) Deceitfulness.

   (c) Impulsivity or poor planning.

   (d) Irritability and hostility, marked by repeated fights.

   (e) Careless disregard for safety of self or others.

   (f) Failure to behave responsibly in the spheres of work or finances.

   (g) No regret for hurting or mistreating others.

2. Persons are at least 18 years old, but showed signs of conduct disorder before they were 15 years old.

(Information from APA, 2022, 2013.)

Around 3.6% of adults in the United States meet the criteria for antisocial personality disorder (Fisher & Hany, 2021; Alarcon & Palmer, 2020). The disorder is as much as four times more common among men than women.

Dee was a 24-year-old single, biracial, cisgender, bisexual woman recently admitted to the psychiatric unit of an academic medical center in Minneapolis. She had expressed suicidal ideation and threatened to take action the night before in an argument with her girlfriend. What started off as a joke Dee made about her girlfriend's flat chest turned to physical violence after the girlfriend called Dee cruel and lacking empathy and then accused Dee of stealing a large sum of money from her (the girlfriend's) mother. Dee, fearing she would be caught for this crime she knew she had committed, yelled and screamed in denial, claiming falsely that she had not taken the money. When her girlfriend yelled back, Dee pushed her down and stood over her, pointing her finger and telling her never to do that again.

The neighbors in the adjacent apartment heard the commotion and called the police. When the police arrived, Dee's girlfriend was furious and agitated. Dee was calm. She lied to the police, telling them that her girlfriend had smoked some weed and become paranoid, making "crazy" accusations, and physically threatening her. Her girlfriend angrily denied these allegations. When the police saw bruises on her arms and challenged Dee, she became enraged and defensive, saying that she "may as well kill herself." The police officer asked her if she was thinking of harming herself, and she fabricated another lie, explaining that she had been thinking of killing herself for a long time, and that she just might do it after this altercation with her girlfriend. The police officer, unsure of the truth but now more concerned that

Dee might harm herself, asked her if she needed to be taken to the emergency room. Dee, believing that she might otherwise go to jail for assault or theft, told the officer she was worried for her safety and wanted to go to the hospital.

At the emergency room, Dee told the psychiatric nurse practitioner that she could not bear life any longer and was thinking of ending it all. Dee said she had spent the past month writing out a plan and gathering means to kill herself. She disclosed tearfully that she had been sexually abused as a child by an uncle, and she had endured years of physical abuse from her father before he abandoned Dee and her mother. She went on to explain that she had attempted suicide before and had cut her wrists numerous times when she didn't know what else to do to take the edge off of her emotions. The nurse practitioner listened intently and took notes. Dee was new to this hospital, and there were no electronic medical records to corroborate this information. Trained to take great efforts to rapidly build rapport and trust in emergency room settings, the nurse practitioner took Dee's words at face value. Why wouldn't she?

Dee reported that she had been actively thinking about and planning to die by suicide since she was 21. She had overdosed at 18 with the intent to die, she explained. She had been hospitalized in Minneapolis when she was 22 for self-injurious behavior, that time for cutting her wrists and legs. The nurse practitioner eventually had to leave to attend to other patients, and a licensed clinical social worker later came to the emergency holding room Dee was placed in. The social worker was a young Dominican woman who appeared to be roughly the same age as Dee. Her name was Teresa, and she disclosed that she had recently finished her degree and licensure.

Teresa had an earnest way about her, and she passionately asked about Dee's personal history. She took fastidious notes and asked a lot of questions related to the risk for self-harm. To Teresa, Dee seemed deeply upset. Occasionally she would stop speaking and bury her face in her hands. When the social worker asked her which psychiatric disorder she had been diagnosed with in the past, Dee replied, "You name it, I've got it." She said that she had recently lost both her job and now her girlfriend, and currently her mother was gravely ill, among other things. She feared that unless she got some help, she was going to "go off the deep end and do who knows what to myself."

Teresa and the psychiatric nurse practitioner huddled at the nurses' station and decided it would probably be best to keep Dee in the psychiatric emergency unit holding room. This way she could be safe while the medical team conferred about the next steps. Because she was not a patient known to this medical system, the team decided later that night to play it safe and admit her to the psychiatric unit at the hospital. Luckily, there was a female bed available. Dee was transported safely to the unit, where she was checked in, given a room, and oriented to the unit rules and schedule.

In one classic study, clinical psychologists viewed videos of statements made by individuals and evaluated their truth or falsehood. The clinicians were only able to identify 62% of the lies, a performance similar to that of federal judges (Ekman et al., 1999).

People with antisocial personality disorder are often impulsive, taking action without thinking of the possible consequences (Lykken, 2019).

Dee Playing Her Hand

Soon after arriving on the inpatient unit, Dee was interviewed by a different licensed clinical social worker. This social worker asked her about her family and social history, current and past medical conditions, and a host of other questions about what kinds of things stressed her out and how she coped with stress. The attending psychiatrist and psychiatry resident on the unit knocked on the door and interrupted. A medical student stood quietly behind as the two doctors began talking to Dee. The social worker stayed and listened, hoping to learn important information that could assist with a discharge plan and smooth transition back into Dee's community. After introducing herself, the attending psychiatrist observed as the resident, Dr. Krishnan, led the conversation. It was clear to Dee that the two psychiatrists were concerned that Dee would consider suicide again. This wasn't surprising to her, given her earlier statements about being unable to restrain herself from self-harm. But Dee wasn't, in truth, considering suicide. She also had no plans to harm herself. She had impulsively made up this story as a way to evade the police officer's questions about the crime she had committed, stealing from her girlfriend's mother. Dee was saying what she needed to say, and she figured she could outsmart the doctors.

Later, a unit staff member brought Dee to the nurses' station, a large semi-circular area enclosed in safety glass, where a half-dozen staff were busily typing patients' notes into the computers. Upon seeing Dee, a nurse exited the station, introduced herself, and took Dee to the dining area, down a long, bare corridor adjacent to the main TV room in front of the nurses' station. In the dining area, a nurse showed Dee how to acquire food and drinks, and where to throw her garbage away. Dee ate quietly next to another woman. The food was bland and soft, "like prison food," said yet another woman across from Dee.

After eating, Dee flopped down on her bed and buried her face in her pillow. An hour later, the resident psychiatrist, Dr. Krishnan, came by to give Dee a routine physical examination, which seemed to perk her up a little. Dee greeted the physician with a friendly, "Hi, Doc," and the doctor examined her heart, lungs, blood pressure, and other vital signs. To make conversation, he remarked on an "interesting" tattoo that Dee had on her arm, an obscure Celtic symbol. With obvious pride, the patient explained, "Yeah, I got it in honor of my mom." After the physician left, Dee donned her hospital pajamas, got into bed, and slept soundly through the night.

The next morning, she joined the other patients in the dining area, where breakfast was being served. As she took her place at the table, she announced that she was "hungry as a mule," and began eating demonstratively. After she finished her own food, she glanced over at a patient across the table and noticed that the man, a patient with schizophrenia, had only nibbled at his eggs and toast. "Hey, old-timer," Dee called out, "you don't mind if I take some of your feast, do you?"

The man just stared, glassy-eyed, while Dee, without waiting for a response, took his plate and started scraping its contents onto her own dish.

Another patient sitting at the table reprimanded Dee for taking the older patient's food. "We're not supposed to share food. It's against regulations. Besides, that guy is pretty sick. He has been throwing up and hasn't eaten for days. You wouldn't want to eat anything he's touched."

Dee was unimpressed by that patient's disapproval. "You the unit police?" she asked. "I guess you want all the food for yourself. Well, sorry my guy, I beat you to it." The other patients watched the confrontation with curiosity. A few walked away fearfully. Several others stayed and kept their eyes on Dee. She was a sight to behold to them. Younger than them all, brash and full of personality, Dee commanded attention. And then there were those eyes. She had piercing blue eyes which moved quickly against light brown skin. Her mother was Scottish, also with blue eyes, and her father was biracial, his own mother from France and his father from Senegal. As a result, Dee and her older brother had caramel skin and wavy black hair, long limbs, and a tall thin physique. She was an imposing person to be around, and the other patients quickly found themselves in two camps: those who were afraid of her, and those who were compelled by her.

Dee in Treatment Using Therapy to Her Advantage

Later that morning, Dr. Krishnan arrived to meet with Dee. Dr. Krishnan found the young woman standing on the ottoman in the television area, holding court to several patients about how she could help them get their rights back. They felt trapped, stuck, stripped of their civil liberties by being held involuntarily. She picked up on this as a primary complaint from many of the patients that morning. As a way to ingratiate herself with them, she highlighted how they really had no choices, no rights, and how this was illegal and unethical. As soon as Dr. Krishnan approached, Dee looked up and smiled. She had an appealing, cheerful quality, and at first Dr. Krishnan wasn't sure who she was. She stood tall on the ottoman and spoke clearly and passionately. It reminded Dr. Krishnan of a time he was in Hyde Park in London, back in his medical school days, listening to the soliloquies of the Sunday morning Londoners on their soap boxes. Looking at Dee, he instinctively stopped and listened. Despite being admitted for suicidal ideation and threats, this patient was seeming more like a religious leader, full of emotion and energy. Dee turned around and saw him, then stopped her preaching and stepped down, extending the warmest, happiest greeting he had seen as a new psychiatrist.

"Hey, Doc. Good to see ya," she said. "I'm just shooting a little straight talk here." Dr. Krishnan explained that as Dee's doctor while she was hospitalized, he was hoping to meet with her each day. They walked back to her room together. Once inside, he asked Dee to take a seat and told her that he wanted to know all about

> Antisocial personality disorder was called "moral insanity" during the nineteenth century.

the troubles she had been having and why she had been contemplating suicide. Dee confirmed that she was "real depressed" and didn't know if life was worth living. When the psychiatrist asked what she was depressed about, the patient replied, "Everything and anything." She went on to explain that it was mainly her girlfriend but, basically, she "just felt like giving up." She said, "Frankly, Doc, it's too painful to talk about." Dee didn't look particularly pained, however.

Dr. Krishnan told her that they would have to discuss these matters eventually, if she was to get any help. At this, Dee said she didn't think that talking would do any good. "Don't they have meds for depression?" she asked. "What's there to talk about when all I need is to take a pill to feel better? How about giving me some Prozac? Or Paxil?"

"Did you ever take Prozac?" Dr. Krishnan asked.

"Me? Oh, no."

"Did you ever take any psychiatric drugs?" he asked.

"No," Dee insisted, "This is my first time in the loony bin, or even talking to a shrink."

"How about street drugs? Did you ever try those?" the psychiatrist asked.

"To be perfectly honest with you, I have tried marijuana—but who hasn't? I stay away from the harder stuff, though."

Because Dee would not discuss her feelings, Dr. Krishnan tried a different tack, asking the young woman about her living situation, work, and family. Dee replied simply that she had been living with her girlfriend, but "I suspect that is over after what happened." She explained that she had recently lost her job as a bartender in Willard-Hay after another employee had stolen money and blamed the theft on Dee. Dr. Krishnan tried to inquire more about that matter, but Dee said she was too upset to talk about it and was getting tired. She wanted to lie down and nap.

Before he departed, the psychiatrist asked her whether she was still having thoughts of suicide. Dee replied that she was feeling more secure now that she was in the hospital, and she was hopeful that Dr. Krishnan could help her. The psychiatrist explained that, in order to help her, she would have to talk more about her feelings. The patient promised that, in time, she would. She just had to develop "more rapport" with Dr. Krishnan first. She covered her face and started to cry, then turned away.

Dee lay down and put her head on a pillow, but then sat up as if having second thoughts. She said she really appreciated the time that the psychiatrist had given her, and hoped that they could talk more. As she spoke, Dr. Krishnan observed that Dee did not have any tears on her face and did not look sad. For a moment, he considered confronting Dee with what he had just seen, but he decided to wait until another time.

The next morning, Dr. Krishnan sought Dee for another visit. This time he found her seated in the dining area. She apparently was enjoying herself immensely,

> Most individuals with antisocial personality disorder are not interested in receiving treatment. Those who do receive treatment typically have been forced to participate by an employer, their school, or the law (Fisher & Hany, 2021; Black, 2020).

laughing loudly with another patient, while the other patients stared glumly at their food or into space. As he approached, the young woman looked up and greeted him with a cheery, "Hey, Doc! I'll be ready in a minute, as soon as I am done eating." The psychiatrist walked away and waited for Dee in his office behind the glass in a secure area, completing notes from his rounding.

A few minutes later Dee walked up and asked the nurse at the desk if the doc was around. He came out, and they walked back to her room. Dee told Dr. Krishnan that he had upset her, that he had hurt her feelings by leaving her in the dining area, and that she didn't trust him. Going even further, she told him that she had thought he was a better doctor than that, but that he was probably just like all the other doctors—too busy in the electronic medical record writing notes to spend time with his patients. "You chose to treat the chart, but good doctors treat their patients," she mused. The psychiatrist was momentarily dumb-struck. Dee was accusing him of dehumanizing her, when he was simply doing his job. "What were you thinking walking away from me?" she asked.

Dee explained that she didn't like it when people walked away from her. "Speaking of which," she added, "I can't take being cooped up in here all day and night. I know I was suicidal before, but I think I'm coming out of it. Can I have leave soon?" Then she went on, "Look, I'm sorry about being mean to you. It was stupid of me. I had a rough childhood, remember, I'm sure you've seen what I told them in the emergency room. So sometimes I get pissed when people walk away from me. I just want to be loved, you know, and …" She trailed off. "And, what?" Dr. Krishnan asked. Dee closed her eyes and stayed quiet for a long time. "And, nothing. Just that. I've got no one, OK, a shitty, lonely, miserable life. But I promise not to kill myself, and that I am not thinking about suicide anymore."

Dr. Krishnan explained that in order to be discharged, she would have to dis-cuss her situation more openly. Dee's attitude then changed, and she said she was ready to speak frankly. First, she apologized profusely for any trouble she had caused. She said that if she was sometimes disrespectful, it was a front she had developed out of fear that others might take advantage of her if she didn't act like she could take care of herself. She admitted to Dr. Krishnan that she had spent time in prison for a "stupid petty theft"; while in prison, she was bullied constantly because of her appearance. The Black inmates made fun of her for having white facial features and wavy hair. The white inmates taunted her with racist language. That experience had hardened her, she said, and now she sometimes lashed out at others, even among people who had her best interests at heart.

Dee went on to admit that she hadn't really been considering suicide; she had simply claimed that to gain admission to the hospital. In her opinion, however, it was no exaggeration to say that she was at the end of her rope. She said that since being paroled, she had had tremendous difficulty finding and keeping a job. She had tried everything, from bartending to retail and restaurants, but in each

People with antisocial personality disorder tend to respond to warnings or expectations of stress with low brain and bodily arousal, such as slow autonomic nervous system arousal and slow electroencephalogram waves (Fariba et al., 2021). This may help explain the inability of many such individuals to experience constructive levels of fear or to learn from negative experiences.

case she was fired within a few weeks because of her temper and difficulty with people.

In addition, she explained, falsely, that her mother's heart condition had worsened considerably, forcing her to be hospitalized. Because neither one of them was now working, they lost their apartment. Moreover, her girlfriend, with whom she sometimes lived, had gotten fed up with her losing jobs and her inability to contribute to the rent and had demanded that she leave. After being kicked out by her girlfriend, she had gone to a homeless shelter—until being hounded out of there by "ruthless thugs" who stole what money she had left. Feeling that she was losing this daily struggle for survival, she had maintained she was having thoughts about suicide.

Dee said she was sorry if she had offended anyone with her charade for getting admitted, but she felt she was suffering as much as any patient, and her false claim of suicidal thoughts showed just how desperate she was. She said he felt she was experiencing a "crisis of confidence" and needed some intensive therapy to help her through this period. "Look," she concluded, "I could tell you that I still want to end my life, but I'm trying to be honest with you now in the hope that I'll get the right kind of help."

Dr. Krishnan listened to Dee's story with an open mind. Although skeptical about her claims, he decided against recommending immediate discharge. Instead, he decided to proceed with a personality disorder consultation from a psychologist. This would include a mental status exam, including testing with the Minnesota Multiphasic Personality Inventory-3 (MMPI-3) and the Structured Clinical Interview for DSM-5 Personality Disorders (SCID-5), two research-based personality tests that are commonly used in diagnosing personality disorders. Dee's case conference would be held in two days, at which point the treatment team would decide whether to discharge her or proceed with a higher level of treatment at the state psychiatric hospital.

Dee was upset that she would not be discharged right away, but even more so that she had to meet with a psychologist for testing. Knowing she needed to stay on Dr. Krishnan's good side, Dee said she would cooperate with the testing procedures and promised not to be difficult. During the following days, the patient was true to her word. She was well-behaved and cooperated fully with all the testing procedures. The psychologist used the MMPI-3 to conclude that there was a high probability that this patient was being untruthful, trying to present herself in a particular way that was inconsistent, and was high on the personality trait of *psychopathy*. Additionally, the results from the SCID-5 indicated that Dee likely met criteria for *antisocial personality disorder*. This diagnosis was obtained after Dee further admitted that she had been truant, started many fights, and been arrested for stealing twice before the age of 15. Since the age of 18, she reported behaviors that showed a clear disregard for the rights and well-being of others. She admitted

> A mental status exam is a structured interview in which the clinician asks about specific symptoms, such as anxiety or hallucinations; observes other symptoms, such as emotional expression or motor activity; and tests certain cognitive capacities, such as memory or abstract reasoning.

that she had continued to break the law (but would not disclose details about how), was prone to impulsive aggressive outbursts, and didn't care much for how the people she harmed may have felt. She denied symptoms of schizophrenia, and, upon probing questions, stated that she had been depressed before but had never had a manic episode.

The case conference that followed included Dr. Krishnan, the social worker, and the psychologist. They reviewed her history, the results from psychological testing, and observations of her behaviors. It was unanimous—Dee appeared to meet criteria for antisocial personality disorder and was characterized by psychopathy (meaning that Dee showed a lack of empathy for others) and affective instability (meaning that she showed dramatic changes in mood). Her affective instability was believed to be part of her personality disorder symptoms rather than part of a bipolar disorder or the like. The team concluded that she was not a risk to herself and could be discharged and referred for outpatient treatment.

Dee was discharged from the hospital the next day. She went back to her girlfriend's apartment, but her girlfriend wasn't home and the door was locked. Unsure of where to go next, she went out onto the streets of St. Paul and walked around. She quickly got bored and got onto a bus. When the bus driver insisted she pay, Dee stormed off the bus and kept walking. She had her phone and called a friend. No answer. She called her brother. No answer. She texted a former girlfriend, asking if she wanted to get together. While walking and waiting without hearing back from anyone, Dee decided to go back to a place she knew well.

After walking a couple of miles, Dee knocked on the door of her mother's home. It was her childhood home, and as much as she needed a place to stay, she hated everything about her home. It reminded her of all the trouble she got into as a child, all the times she was caught and punished. Dee's mother answered the door, smiled politely, and let her in. "You can stay here for a few days, but no more than that, you understand?" Dee hugged her mother warmly, feeling nothing, but knowing this was what her mother would want, and hoping it might help her stay longer than a few days. Her mother, having seen this behavior before, was aware of Dee's intentions. She had come to understand what to expect from her daughter. She showed her to a small spartan guest bedroom. "You can stay in here," she said, without any feeling. Dee closed the door. Her mother stood silently in the hallway, holding back tears.

A Parent's Tale Watching Antisocial Behavior Unfold

The next day, Dee's mother Emily told her friend, Marlena, that Dee had returned. She recounted her experiences raising Dee. Even when she was a toddler it seemed like there was something wrong. "Her brother had been such a sweet boy,

---

Research participants with antisocial personality disorder display deficient functioning in their prefrontal cortex, anterior cingulate cortex, amygdala, hippocampus, and temporal cortex—brain structures that, collectively, help people follow rules; plan and execute realistic strategies; and display sympathy, judgment, and empathy (Kolla et al., 2021; Kaya, Yildirim, & Atmaca, 2020; Blair et al., 2019).

DSM-5-TR requires that there be evidence of *conduct disorder* prior to the age of 15 in order to meet the diagnostic criteria for antisocial personality disorder.

and we expected the same from Dee. But it never happened. She had a temper, was selfish, and didn't seem to care about others. Things got much worse when she was old enough to go to school. That's when the real trouble started."

At about the time that Dee entered first grade, she seemed to develop a "thing" for jewelry or, more accurately, for stealing it. For example, she would take items from Emily's jewelry case and sell them one by one to classmates or to older boys in the neighborhood, often for no more than pocket change, which she would spend on candy. Emily and her husband learned what Dee was doing after she tried to sell a pair of heirloom pearl earrings to her second-grade teacher for $50.00. Emily scolded her harshly. Her father spanked her with a belt. He beat her when she was caught stealing each time thereafter. He also beat her when she was disrespectful to him. Dee grew indifferent to her beatings. Emily was at a loss. She refused to lay a hand on her daughter, but at the same time she knew she had no control and hoped her husband's discipline would have an effect. Eventually, they decided that the only way to deal with the situation was to keep their valuables—credit cards, jewelry, cash—under lock and key in a safe.

Emily explained to her friend how they had provided Dee with a generous weekly allowance in an effort to reduce her desire for stealing. Unfortunately, it turned out that her desire could not be satisfied so easily. By the age of 10, Dee began breaking into neighbors' houses and cars to steal items to sell. In many ways, she became quite ingenious in these break-ins. She learned from a neighbor's older brother how to pick locks, disable alarms, and slip into small openings. At the same time, however, the way in which she would dispose of the stolen items often seemed remarkably careless and thoughtless, according to her mother. She tried to sell stolen goods to people in the neighborhood, sometimes the very people whose homes and cars she had broken into. It was obvious to them she was the thief. She thought it was funny that she could steal in daylight, walking into homes when people would be away at work or church. But the daylight also brought witnesses, and she would get caught. In addition, Dee had a big mouth, and was prone to boasting about her latest thefts.

Her first arrest happened at age 11, but she was remanded to the custody of her mother, her father no longer in the picture after having left for another woman. Her mother told the judge that she would figure out a way to control Dee. She did indeed try to control her antisocial ways by keeping a more careful eye on her. When Dee went to school, for example, Emily would actually escort her into the building to make sure that she was attending classes. But the girl would smile, wave her hand, wait a few minutes, and then cavalierly walk back outside, inevitably to get into some kind of trouble.

Dee's stealing eventually took a more serious turn. She joined up with a group of teenagers who made a profession of shoplifting. They saw in Dee an opportunity to acquire stolen goods with a reduced risk of detection, since Dee was much

Twin research has found that 67% of the identical twins of people with antisocial personality disorder also display the disorder themselves, in contrast to 31% of the fraternal twins of people with the disorder (Poore & Waldman, 2020; Waldman et al., 2019).

younger and less likely to be suspected. Typically, the teenagers would case a store, locate items of interest, and then send Dee inside to remove the items according to their instructions. They would then sell the items in return for cash, marijuana, and alcohol.

Associating with these older boys led Dee to develop more varied and sophisticated interests and a precocious sexual awareness. The turning point in her antisocial childhood came when, at age 15, she lured a 12-year-old neighborhood girl into an alley behind her house, undressed her, and tried to force her to perform oral sex on her. When the young victim started screaming, a woman came running outside and discovered them up against a fence. Dee at first claimed that the girl had tried to steal from her. When that didn't work, she offered the woman $20.00 "to keep her mouth shut." The woman refused and walked toward them. Dee threatened her, telling the neighbor she had better take the money or else "shit could go down!"

With this incident, Dee entered the world of serious legal trouble and was sentenced to a year in reform school (now called juvenile training centers). There, sadly, she learned more advanced methods of taking advantage of others. As soon as she was released, she began experimenting with auto theft. She learned how to hot-wire a car and would do so whenever she needed cash or transportation. Why take the bus, she reasoned, when there were cars all around? Dee's mother estimated that she hot-wired 50 cars before finally getting caught in the act, leading to another term in reform school, this time for 2 years.

When Dee was released, at almost 18 years old, Emily explained how she tried to persuade her to return to school and pay enough attention to her studies to get a high school diploma. The teenager agreed to attend school and promised she was a changed person. Her mother had accepted that her daughter likely could have ongoing legal problems the rest of her life. She blamed herself for not doing more and for marrying a man who beat her daughter. Emily tried to get Dee help from mental health professionals, but Dee always found a reason to not stay in therapy. The therapist was a "dumb shrink," a "bitch from the suburbs," "an old clueless dude," and so on.

Emily was crying. Her friend Marlena gave her a tissue and kept listening. Dee barely graduated from high school and never found regular employment. At age 21, she was living from home to home, sleeping on couches or staying with a boyfriend or girlfriend. She knew how to be charming, especially to people she just met, and she would use this as a tool to gain access to a place to live, food to eat, and, of course, things to steal. It all came to a head when she was caught stealing a sports car one night outside a hockey arena. During the game, she wandered through the parking lot looking for the perfect car. She wanted to be challenged, felt bored, and knew there was a rush of excitement that came with each new vehicle she stole. An Audi S7 appeared before her. The closest source of light was

One study found that middle school children who were attracted to antisocial peers went on to themselves engage in antisocial behavior in order to gain acceptance (Juvonen & Ho, 2008).

According to research, the parents and close relatives of people with antisocial personality disorder have a higher rate of this disorder than do people whose relatives do not have this disorder (Alvarez-Garcia et al., 2019).

several cars away, and she slipped into the darkness between vehicles, dropping low and using her gadgets to swiftly slide down the base of the window, disarming the alarm system, then opening the door. It was a hack she learned a year before, and this was the most expensive ride she had used it on. The door opened, and she went inside, removing the panel to use her well-honed skills to jump the ignition. She backed the car out and drove slowly down the aisle. Turning left, moving through the arena lot, she felt the rush she was seeking. In her mind, she was already counting the dollars that this car would yield. However, due to a combination of bad luck and carelessness, Dee was pulled over for speeding within blocks of the arena. At first, she attempted to flirt her way out of trouble as she had done before, but the officer didn't bite, and it eventually became apparent that she was driving a stolen vehicle when she was unable to produce a license or registration.

After awaiting trial in jail for several months, at age 22, Dee was sentenced to 3 years in a state penitentiary. Not being the violent sort, she was paroled after 18 months for good behavior. Upon her release, she went back home to see her mother. She knocked on the door, but no one answered. Dee made her way down to a local bar, where she would meet up with some old friends from the neighborhood. For the next few years, before ending up in the hospital by threatening suicide, Dee lived with various partners. Things didn't last long with any of them. She was fun at first, but would soon show her antisocial tendencies, selling drugs, robbing, or trying to con until she got caught. She had learned how to get what she wanted, but she couldn't trick people for long. Just as she always had since childhood, Dee seemed to repeatedly make mistakes and get caught. Emily concluded by shaking her head. "Marlena, my daughter is a criminal, but not a particularly smart one."

> It is estimated that at least 35% of people in prison meet the criteria for antisocial personality disorder (Azevedo et al., 2020; Douglas, Vincent, & Edens, 2019).

Dee After Her Hospital Discharge

Once back home, Dee tried to reunite with her girlfriend. They exchanged texts until finally her partner agreed to talk on the phone. Dee didn't love her, but she profusely apologized and professed her love. This was her pattern with partners. Dee showed no concern about the age, appearance, or character of the partner. Rather, her interest in them seemed largely a matter of housing, money, and, to a lesser extent, sex. No feelings of love or attachment were ever involved.

At the time that Dee had been admitted to the psychiatric unit, she was, her mother believed, in truly desperate straits. Emily suspected that in seeking hospital admission, her daughter had simply been looking for a place to stay, or had been running from something else. Now that Dee had landed in Emily's home following the hospitalization, the mother insisted that her daughter share the contact information for the therapist recommended by the psychiatric team. Dee gave it to her, knowing full well that her mother had no control over her and that by allowing her mother to believe she was able to control her, Dee could maintain the upper hand. She was trying to buy more time in the house while she tried to reunite with her girlfriend. Sure, her mother had said she could only stay a few days. But Dee was certain she would be able to find a way to stay as long as she wanted.

Emily demanded that Dee go to therapy. She threatened to kick her out and never let her return unless Dee contacted the therapist she was referred to by Dr. Krishnan and his team. Dee agreed to go. The therapist was a portly man with an expressionless face and a double chin. Dee thought he looked like a cartoon character. She couldn't take him seriously. He told her that he was interested in getting to know her, that they could take as long as needed, and that he wanted to know anything about her that she was willing to share. Dee obliged, treating the session like a game. She lied about everything she could, trying to use the things she saw in his office as cues to make up stories. It was a trick she saw on a movie once. It was her favorite movie — *The Usual Suspects* — and she had always wanted to try it out. At some point, the therapist caught on, but, hoping to gain Dee's trust, he decided to not confront her and played along, answering sympathetically as she tearfully improvised imaginary traumas.

Dee never returned to therapy. "Mom, he was a dull fat man who didn't say anything. I don't think he had any idea what to say." Emily gave her a week to find another place to live. Dee left willingly when she was able to cajole a previous girlfriend into giving her a place to crash. This failure of treatment certainly did not surprise Emily, although it did cause her disappointment. After the psychiatric hospitalization and Dr. Krishnan's referral for therapy, Emily had briefly allowed herself to feel a glimmer of hope.

After Dee moved out, Emily saw her own therapist for a follow-up booster session. She shared her disappointment over this latest episode with her daughter. They had discussed Dee's behavior before, and her therapist was unsurprised to learn that Dee had been diagnosed with antisocial personality disorder—it fit with the pattern of criminal behavior, lying, impulsive and reckless behavior, and callous disregard for others Emily had previously described. The therapist explained to Emily that although many people with this personality disorder exhibit criminal behavior, their brand of criminality is, like Dee's, often marked by idiosyncratic qualities. For one, their criminal acts often seem to be inadequately motivated. The individual may, for example, commit a major crime for very small stakes. In this regard, Dee's mother recalled that Dee tried to sell her pearl earrings for far less than they were worth when she was younger. Also, the criminal acts of these individuals often seem to be committed without much sense of self-preservation. They may fail, for example, to take obvious precautions against detection when carrying out their crimes. Here, again, Emily recalled Dee's attempts to sell items to the very source from which they were stolen.

In short, Dee showed the disorder's classic overall pattern of long-standing antisocial behavior, dating from childhood, aimed largely at the immediate gratification

Research finds that treatments for people with antisocial personality disorder are typically ineffective (Fisher & Hany, 2021; Black, 2020).

of transient desires. Her behavior did not seem to be deterred by any sense of shame, remorse, or even plain self-interest.

Sympathizing with Emily's disappointment, her therapist told her that, unfortunately, today's clinicians have generally despaired of devising an effective treatment for antisocial personality disorder. There is a treatment known as *moral reconation therapy*, a cognitive-behavioral technique that aims to teach patients to apply moral reasoning to their decision making. However, this technique is normally used in prison settings, and the prognosis for outpatient therapy is not good. Perhaps the main reason for this limited success is that people with the disorder, by definition, have no recognition that their behavioral pattern is problematic. They usually reject the value of or need for psychological treatment, and so they are unlikely to initiate it or adhere to it for very long.

Unfortunately, many clinicians have concluded that currently the single greatest hope for improvement in this realm may lie either with treatment during incarceration or with the simple passage of time. It appears that a number of adults with this pattern, who often begin a criminal career as teenagers, significantly reduce their level of criminal activity after age 40. That is, they experience fewer convictions and serve less time in prison as they grow older. The reason for this shift remains unclear, but, as Emily's therapist described, it may be that antisocial behavior "burns out" somewhat over time. Emily was grateful to see her therapist again, and she drove home feeling some hope. Dee was off into the world again, likely repeating the same kinds of behaviors as she had since childhood, but maybe in time Emily's daughter would make some improvements—and find some peace.

> Studies have not typically found that efforts to improve a person's moral thinking in daily decision making, as practiced by some cognitive-behavioral therapists, are particularly successful in the outpatient treatment of antisocial personality disorder (Black, 2020).

Assessment Questions

1. What is one of the most common reasons individuals with antisocial personality disorder end up in therapy?

2. Throughout this case study, what behaviors did Dee manifest that fit a diagnosis of antisocial personality disorder?

3. What did Dee do that is consistent with antisocial personality disorder during her time in the emergency room?

4. What are the statistics regarding the gender of people with antisocial personality disorder?

5. How did the clinical interviews in the inpatient admission unit help inform Dee's diagnosis?

6. Give three examples from Dee's mother's story to her friend Marlena that suggested Dee met the criteria for antisocial personality disorder.

7. What are some possible biological explanations for antisocial personality disorder?

8. Why is treatment usually ineffective for this personality disorder?

9. Which of Dee's behaviors is consistent with the personality trait of *psychopathy*?

10. What is the eventual outcome for many individuals who display antisocial personality disorder?

CASE 15

Borderline Personality Disorder

Table 15-1

Dx Checklist

Borderline Personality Disorder

1. Individuals display pronounced, wide-ranging, unstable, and impulsive patterns in their relationships, sense of self, and emotions. Such patterns begin by the time they reach their mid-20s.

2. The individuals specifically exhibit at least five of the following symptoms:

   (a) Desperate efforts to avoid perceived abandonment.

   (b) Fluctuations between idealizing and denigrating family members, friends, and coworkers.

   (c) Highly changeable self-concept.

   (d) Self-damaging displays of impulsivity.

   (e) Repeated self-mutilating or suicidal acts or gestures.

   (f) Significant fluctuations in moods and emotions.

   (g) Long-term sense of emptiness.

   (h) Experiences of extreme and often uncontrollable anger.

   (i) Periodic, short-term paranoid ideas or dissociation during times of stress.

(Information from APA, 2022, 2013.)

Kareem, a 28-year-old cisgender, homosexual, single, and unemployed Black man, was admitted to University Hospital after deliberately taking an overdose of benzodiazepines and alcohol, with the stated intention of dying by suicide. He made this suicide attempt when the man he had been dating for 2 months told him he was moving to another city and wanted to end their relationship. Kareem lost consciousness from the overdose, and after his roommate found him unresponsive in his bed, he was taken by ambulance to the hospital, where he would spend the next 2 days in the intensive care unit.

Because doctors at the hospital were reluctant to discharge him until they were certain that he would receive follow-up counseling, Kareem called his therapist and asked him to tell the hospital staff that he was indeed in counseling. The therapist, however, did not respond as Kareem expected. He pointed out that this was his third suicide attempt in the past 2 years, and, as a result, he was unsure that their therapy was effective. In fact, the therapist did not think that he should continue to treat Kareem. He described the suicide attempts to the social worker

People with a personality disorder display an enduring, rigid pattern of inner experience and outward behavior that impairs their sense of self, emotional experiences, goals, capacity for empathy, and/or capacity for normal relationships and intimacy.

on the intensive care unit as another example of Kareem being "manipulative," and said that he was using the suicide attempts and other forms of self-harm to draw attention to himself and to avoid confronting his underlying feelings about his childhood traumatic experiences.

Kareem had been deliberately physically harming himself since his teenage years by cutting his arms and legs. He inflicted the injuries in a slow, deliberate fashion, typically when alone and feeling ashamed, rejected, or abandoned. He would sit down with a razor blade in hand and watch closely as he dragged the blade across his flesh. The cuts were relatively superficial, but deep enough to draw a thin line of blood that he observed with fascination. For a brief moment, he felt less intense negative emotions and was distracted from the self-judgmental thoughts and worries about the future that had held a tight grip on him. The pain was physical, real, and, in his mind, deserved. Indeed, he had a deep and long-standing sense that he was a fundamentally bad and broken person, someone who should endure suffering and misery, someone who deserved to experience physical pain and carry visible wounds as a reminder to him—and to others—of his irreparably damaged being.

The frequency of Kareem's cutting, and his use of drugs and alcohol to deaden emotional pain, varied according to his relationships with men. When he had a steady boyfriend, he generally felt more positive, as though life had meaning and focus. On the other hand, the slightest hint of problems in the relationship could trigger deep emotional distress and panic.

Kareem A Typical Relationship

Kareem's relationship with Ervin, a 29-year-old who worked at the airport as a baggage handler, was in many ways typical. They met in a gay bar and immediately had sex that evening. They met up the next weekend at the bar and went back to Ervin's apartment, where they would spend the weekend together, drinking alcohol and smoking marijuana between periods of intense and enjoyable sexual intercourse. For the next 2 weeks they were together almost every night. Kareem felt safe with Ervin, like he found someone who might love him. He had been with other partners, many in fact, but this time he believed he may have found a partner that would last. After only a week, he started to fantasize about their life together. They lived in a very gay-friendly city in California, and both were open about their sexuality. They could move in together, take walks together by the beach, spend time with each other's friends and family, maybe get a pet together. When he was with Ervin, Kareem stopped drinking alone in the evenings and was able to refrain from cutting himself or thinking about suicide.

As time passed, they stopped seeing each other every day, but Kareem's focus on Ervin remained. In fact, it was obsessive. While at work, he would check his phone and social media several times an hour to see if Ervin had left any messages or posted anything. If he was home in the evening and he hadn't heard from Ervin, Kareem would frantically text him.

With time, Kareem grew more and more sensitive to signs that Ervin might be pulling away. He would keep asking him about his feelings for him, and he became irritated if Ervin seemed evasive. At first, Ervin had said he was "so into you" and "let's do this thing!" But, as had happened with Kareem's previous partners, after a while Ervin said he didn't understand why they had to spend so much time together. He began texting Kareem less and less, responding to Kareem's texts with longer and longer delays. Kareem had figured this would happen. It was a familiar pattern. He felt unwanted and rejected. He imagined he was defective, like a present a child might receive Christmas morning: something that would be the center of attention at first, but in a short time would break and be relegated to a pile of other broken, cheaply made pieces of plastic in the corner of a room, eventually thrown unceremoniously into the trash and hauled away to decay in a giant heap of rotting and worthless garbage somewhere outside the city.

On nights when he had no contact with Ervin, Kareem would sit alone in a darkened room just holding his phone in his lap. He would frenetically scan his various social media apps to see if he could determine where Ervin was and whom he was with. Often, when his anxiety was especially high, he would text Ervin. Sometimes Ervin would text back, but his responses were usually short and could be hard to interpret. When Kareem would try to pin him down as to when they could get together, he would just reply, "Not sure." And on those few occasions in which Ervin texted him first, he rarely asked Kareem to get together. In fact, such Ervin-initiated texts tended to be a bit incoherent, occurring late at night after drinks or smoking marijuana.

One night, Kareem and Ervin went to a restaurant together, and just as they were taking their seats, Ervin said he wanted to say hello to someone whom he recognized. Kareem immediately became jealous and worried, as he recalled seeing a muscular and very attractive man waiting on a table when they walked in. The good-looking man was tall, with broad shoulders and an angular jawline—just what Ervin was most attracted to. Kareem demanded that Ervin stay with him. Ervin left his seat anyway, explaining that he would be right back. Kareem then reached out, grabbed his arm, and yanked him back in his seat with surprising force. Ervin was momentarily shaken, but after collecting himself, he rose again and stalked out of the restaurant. Kareem followed him out to the sidewalk; by the time he reached the curb, Ervin was already across the street and moving briskly. Kareem stood on the side of the street screaming, "Ervin! Where are you going? Come back! Please! Don't leave, I'm sorry." Ervin kept walking, never turning his back, but picking up his phone from his side pocket and making a phone call. "No! Who are you calling! Come back," Kareem wailed, now crying uncontrollably.

Studies have found that people with borderline personality disorder typically have poor skill at *mentalization*—the ability to recognize and understand their own mental states (needs, desires, feelings, beliefs, goals) and those of others (Cyrkot et al., 2021; Jorgensen et al., 2021).

Kareem returned home, devastated. He tried to call Ervin over and over again but only got voice mail. He took a shot of vodka, pulled out a new cartridge, and took several puffs of an indica strain he thought would settle him. After about 10 minutes, he started to feel buzzed, but instead of feeling calm, his mind began to race with paranoia. He ruminated over whether he would ever see Ervin again, whether he would ever find happiness with a partner, and whether he would ever be truly loved. The bottle of vodka by his side, he took several more shots, and after another 30 minutes drank two more. His mind continued to race, but at this point it was less linear and more jumbled, with worries and shameful speculations about being alone interspersed with moments of anger, even rage. How could Ervin just get up and walk away without responding to any of his calls or texts? How could he? Unable to find any sense of peace, and now well into the early hours of the morning, Kareem found himself shifting into a familiar pattern of resolve. He began mentally berating himself, went into the bathroom, and pulled out his razor blades. Upon looking at them, he immediately felt more focused and calm. His breathing slowed down, he stopped thinking about Ervin, and he cut himself several times superficially on his right thigh. It didn't hurt very much, but it shifted his focus to the sensations in his thigh. He felt a bit calmer, and he sensed that this was the endcap of the series of events that evening. He saw that there were red marks forming in lines where he had cut, but there was no blood. He felt exhausted and went to sleep.

When Kareem finally was able to reach Ervin the following day, he tried apologizing, but Ervin told him he didn't want to see him anymore. Kareem pleaded with him, declaring that he loved him and couldn't live without him. He promised to be more considerate, less reactive, and less jealous. Ervin said that he just didn't think it was working out and that he wished him the best. At this, Kareem became furious, hung up, and threw his phone across the room. He found a bottle of wine to ease his misery, but even after drinking it all, he still couldn't bear the pain of separation. He began obsessively checking his social media, and sure enough, Ervin had posted something cryptic about ending relationships and beginning a new chapter in his life. There was an accompanying meme with a picture of a cat walking away from a collapsing building, unharmed and relieved, with the word "intuition" in block letters at the top of the image. Kareem was furious and felt humiliated. He posted a response to Ervin's meme with vomit and anger emojis. Immediately after doing so, Ervin responded publicly to his emojis, calling Kareem out for his difficulties with anger, drug use, alcohol, and self-harm. Kareem was stunned that Ervin would do this. He stared at the screen and soon saw that some of their friends were empathically responding to Ervin, ignoring Kareem's response.

A wave of shame washed over him. Then came a sense of foreboding terror and alienation, then numbness. He reached for a bottle of vodka, poured a glass, and took several gulps, then several more. Within minutes, his emotional shock

According to many theorists, self-mutilation by people with borderline personality disorder serves to produce physical pain that competes with—and, hence, partially reduces—the much more painful experience of negative emotions (Harned, Fitzpatrick, & Schmidt, 2020).

Approximately 70% of people with borderline personality disorder attempt suicide at least once in their lives. Of the people who attempt suicide, as many as 10% will actually die of suicide (Salters-Pedneault, 2020).

had given way to an overwhelming desire to flee from everything. He thought about how poorly his relationship had ended with Ervin. He thought about all of the previous relationships that had ended similarly. His memories went back further, and he sat, now sipping his vodka, vividly recalling the times when he was physically abused and emotionally neglected by his father as a child. And then it hit him. He knew what to do. It was time to end his life. Now extremely inebriated, Kareem went to the bathroom, reached for a bottle of benzodiazepines, poured them into his hand, and swallowed about 10 pills.

When Kareem's roommate, Donna Jean, came home, she found Kareem unconscious on the floor of her bedroom. Donna Jean phoned for an ambulance, and Kareem was rushed to the emergency room.

In some ways, Kareem's intense relationship with Ervin had been better than many of his relationships. Ervin, for example, did not physically assault or sexually take advantage of him, as some of his past boyfriends had done. Kareem was so desperate for the sense of worth he received from being in a relationship—any relationship—that he would tolerate more than most people would. When a relationship did end, it was almost always his partner who wanted to break up. Each time, Kareem felt a profound sense of emptiness, abandonment, and despair.

Unrewarding though his relationships typically were, he considered almost all of them preferable to being alone. When not in a relationship, he practically felt as if he didn't exist. Indeed, he never developed lasting personal interests or career ambitions, and, like a lost sailor who had been too long at sea, he had an uncertain sense of direction in his life. Thus he would drift from one relationship to another, feeling anchored by newfound purpose with each boyfriend, only to later feel dejected and untethered when the relationship ended.

A Roommate's Perspective "Six Months of Hell"

After finding Kareem near death and finally getting him to the hospital, his room-mate, Donna Jean, was shaken and drained. At first, she thought she would get over it within a few days, but a week later she took stock and realized that she was feeling, if anything, worse. Her family persuaded her to make an appointment with a therapist to discuss what had happened. During her session, Donna Jean declared that finding Kareem on the bedroom floor was, in fact, the culmination of "six months of hell."

Donna Jean explained to her therapist that she had met Kareem after post-ing an ad on Craigslist for a new roommate. At the time, Kareem did not really confide in Donna Jean about his emotional problems. He did say that he was "in therapy" and described himself as "really crazy, totally neurotic." However, since Donna Jean herself had been in therapy, she thought little of it, and even believed that their common neurotic tendencies might be a way to bond. As it turned out, the 6 months that followed were far from a bonding experience.

As Donna Jean told the therapist:

At first Kareem was a lot of fun, but then he would become really depressed and easily agitated. For the first month, I thought we were having fun living together, discovering that we liked a lot of the same movies and music and things. Then one night, about 2 months after he moved in, I was getting ready to go out with a friend, and Kareem demanded to know where I was going. I told him I was going out. That wasn't good enough for him. Where was I going? Who was I seeing? What was I doing?

Then he tried to make me feel guilty for going. "Fine, just leave," he pouted. He complained that we were no longer spending any time together, which was ridiculous because we had just spent a whole day shopping together. When I pointed that out to him, he got hysterical, yelling at me, telling me that I only cared about myself and that I was leaving him with nothing to do. By then, I was mad, and I told him in no uncertain terms that I did not plan to spend every waking moment of my life with him just because we were roommates. I stormed out.

When I came home that night, it was really scary. There was a little blood on the floor, and it made a trail that led to his bedroom door. When I banged on the door to see if he was all right, he said that he'd accidentally cut himself making a sandwich and everything was fine. I wasn't sure I believed him, but I preferred to go along with that, rather than consider the possibility that he might be seriously disturbed.

After that evening, he was distant from me for a while. He seemed very angry, and I must admit that I was really put off. The last thing I needed was to be living with someone who wanted all my attention, who was so high maintenance. I wasn't so much scared as annoyed. Dealing with him was starting to take a lot out of me. Eventually, he got over being angry with me and went back to his old ways: constantly draining my attention and making me feel guilty about not spending more time with him. No matter how much time I did give him, it was never enough.

Then he started dating this guy, Keith, and I thought that things were getting better. I didn't know much about Keith, but Kareem was spending almost no time at home, and that was just fine with me. When I did see him, he would gush about how incredibly happy he was—I mean, this was just weeks after he had met Keith—how deep their relationship was and how perfect everything was. He was sure this was "the one." Of course, by now I knew how unbalanced Kareem was, and I suspected he was probably being crazy like always, but I didn't want to look a gift horse in the mouth. He was no longer my problem for the moment.

I should have seen what was coming next but, like an idiot, I didn't. Keith left him, and Kareem was totally my problem again. He stayed home and cried for days at a time. He made me take care of him, telling me he was too depressed to do anything for himself. He even fantasized about the violent things he would do to Keith when he eventually felt up to it. And that's pretty much how it's been ever since.

According to surveys, 6% of the adult population may display borderline personality disorder (Chapman, Jamil, & Fleisher, 2021; Skodol, 2021).

After Keith, there was Brent, then Vincent, then Bruce. Always the same story, always the same ending. And always with me in the middle—having to smile while he gushed endlessly about the latest relationship and having to pick up the pieces when the relationship would end.

Kareem The Early Years

Kareem grew up in a working-class family that seemed stable and loving to those who didn't know any better. His father was a manager at a local drug store and active in the church. His mother worked at the neighborhood health clinic and volunteered at the school. Kareem also had two older brothers who were excellent students.

In private, however, the family was violent and chaotic. Even as a toddler, Kareem was frequently beaten with a belt by both parents. Some of the beatings were inspired by misbehavior. Others were carried out on general principle, to "keep the devil out of him," in his father's words.

His parents were extremely unpredictable. His father might hold him on his lap and tell him he was a "good little boy" and how much he loved him, but minutes later he would once again be "beating the devil out of him." Nor was the abuse Kareem suffered at the hands of his family the only trauma in his young life. Beginning at about age 6, his parents left him and his brothers with a neighbor when they were at work and needed child care. The neighbor was a lovely older woman, but she often left Kareem alone with her teenage son and his friends. Oblivious to their antisocial tendencies, she would leave Kareem with them while she went to the store for groceries. While away, her son and his friends would abuse Kareem sexually by forcing him to perform oral sex on each of them while the others watched. This occurred about a dozen times and continued until Kareem reached the age of 11. After molesting Kareem, the boys would call him a "little bitch" who was "worth shit."

Years later, when Kareem graduated from high school, he left his family and moved to a small apartment in the adjacent neighborhood. He found work at a local diner, started dating a man he met there, and moved in with him just a few weeks later. His new boyfriend, Jorge, an emergency medical technician who was older, began dominating Kareem in short order. In many respects, their life together was a replay of Kareem's upbringing.

Jorge suspected, without basis, that Kareem was flirting with other men and carrying on affairs behind his back. He made him quit his job and kept him a prisoner in their apartment. He demanded that Kareem leave the house only with him or to do necessary food shopping. On one occasion, Kareem visited his former coworkers at the diner despite Jorge's house rules. When Jorge found out, he confronted him as being "deceitful" and beat him when he defended himself.

Studies have often found instances of great trauma in the early lives of people who develop borderline personality disorder (Chapman et al., 2021; Marchetti et al., 2021; Walker & Kulkarni, 2020).

When not in a jealous mood, Jorge could be very nice to Kareem. Often, he would take him out for dinner or dancing, tell him he was "the hottest dude he ever met," and apologize for any of the hurtful things he had done. He would describe his hopes of making "a pile of money" someday and his desire to then treat Kareem "like a king." Such affection was typically short-lived, however. The next day Jorge might very well return home from work and yell at Kareem for allegedly flirting with other men online.

Kareem's family background made it extremely difficult for him to accurately assess his life with Jorge. Of course, he hated being physically intimidated and abused, but he could not judge whether this treatment was undeserved or whether he might be able to find better treatment elsewhere. As it happened, he never had to leave, because Jorge was killed in a car accident not long after their tumultuous relationship began.

After Jorge's death, Kareem went through a period of utter confusion, in which feelings of both devastation and relief rose to the surface. He was now free from Jorge's cruelty, but Kareem had nevertheless become completely dependent on him. Kareem felt lost and alone, hopeless and helpless, leading to his first psychiatric hospitalization at the age of 19.

Kareem underwent 10 more psychiatric hospitalizations over the next 13 years. He received a wide range of diagnoses during this period, and many different medications were prescribed for him, without much benefit. For example, he had been prescribed antidepressants such as sertraline, fluoxetine, and duloxetine for depressive symptoms. For anxiety, he had tried buspirone, clonazepam, and diazepam. To help manage his anger and emerging paranoia, the doctors had given him mirtazapine, quetiapine, and olanzepine. Worse, it was in the psychiatric hospital where he first learned about cutting and self-injury as a way to cope with intense negative emotions. He saw people come in with cuts on their arms or legs and the nurses and doctors talking to them about why they cut, what triggered cutting, what happened afterwards, and so on. It was here that he realized cutting was something that could lead to intensified focused attention and care from medical staff.

When not hospitalized, Kareem would support himself with work at restaurants or warehouses. Work was of little importance to him, however. It was relationships with men that filled his thoughts and his dreams, as he moved from one intense and unrealistic attachment to another.

Kareem feared abandonment more than anything else in life. He had attempted suicide three times, and indeed, all three of the attempts were direct responses to being left by men to whom he had formed passionate attachments.

During those 13 years, in addition to his hospitalizations, he saw at least 10 different outpatient mental health providers—psychiatrists, psychologists, licensed professional counselors, and social workers—each for no more than a year, with

As many as 85% of people with borderline personality disorder also experience another psychological disorder at some point in their lives (Tong et al., 2021; Beeney et al., 2020). Common ones are depressive disorders, substance use disorders, bulimia nervosa, posttraumatic stress disorder, and other personality disorders.

half of them seen only one time for an intake evaluation. Most of these providers described themselves as "compassionate," "flexible," "person-centered," and "focused on the healing relationship." A few of them said they practiced "eclectic" therapy, mixing and matching techniques from various therapy modalities. A few branded themselves as psychodynamic, interested in talking about Kareem's childhood traumatic experiences and letting him express his thoughts freely and loosely during therapy sessions. Most seemed like nice people. All had been referred by one hospital social worker or another after a discharge. However, none seemed to be very helpful, despite being kind and seemingly well-intentioned.

Kareem in Treatment "Like Learning a New Language"

After Kareem's third suicide attempt and his therapist's refusal to continue working with him, the hospital discharged him to the county social services system, where he received once-a-month medication management and weekly group therapy. After a while, he concluded that his treatment there was not helpful, and he was about to stop when, without warning, his life took a very positive turn. In what he would later describe as "the break of a lifetime," a staff member at the mental health center recognized Kareem's broad pattern for what it was and referred him to Ms. Melvinna Seals, a clinical social worker specializing in *dialectical behavior therapy*, called DBT for short.

During a lengthy initial session, in which Kareem described his problems and history, Ms. Seals grew confident that his condition met the DSM-5-TR criteria for a diagnosis of *borderline personality disorder*. That is, Kareem repeatedly engaged in frantic efforts to avoid abandonment; he exhibited a pattern of unstable and intense interpersonal relationships; he had a markedly unstable self-image, or sense of himself; he engaged in recurrent suicidal behavior and self-mutilation; his moods were unstable; he had chronic feelings of emptiness; he frequently displayed inappropriate anger; and he became paranoid when acutely emotionally distressed.

Using the *biosocial model* of dialectical behavior therapy, Ms. Seals hypothesized that Kareem's symptoms of borderline personality disorder were the consequence of difficulties with *emotional dysregulation*—an inability to regulate one's emotions, particularly negative emotions such as sadness, anger, and anxiety. According to the biosocial model, emotional dysregulation is linked to multiple factors, including biological vulnerability, social skill deficits, and an oppressive childhood environment in which an individual's emotions were frequently disregarded or invalidated. Biological vulnerability to emotional dysregulation features such inborn characteristics as a high sensitivity to emotional stimuli, intense reactivity to such stimuli, and a slow rate of recovery from emotional arousal. When such characteristics combine with significant skill deficits, individuals will have difficulty inhibiting inappropriate behaviors or exhibiting appropriate behaviors if they experience strong

Borderline personality disorder has been linked to abnormal activity within and between certain brain structures, including the amygdala, hippocampus, prefrontal cortex, and other parts of the frontal lobes—structures that help us plan well, form accurate judgments, make good decisions, exercise self-control, and express emotions properly (Chapman et al., 2021; Khoury et al., 2019).

emotions, particularly in social situations. Moreover, according to the biosocial model, these difficulties will be even more pronounced if the individuals have been subjected to family and relationship environments throughout childhood in which their thoughts or feelings were not taken seriously or supported, particularly environments marked by chronic physical, emotional, verbal, and/or sexual abuse and victimization. Children who grow up in such environments may learn to not trust their own feelings or thoughts—and they may develop little sense of who they are. They must depend on other people for direction, support, and meaning. They are prime candidates for borderline personality disorder.

Like other dialectical behavior therapists, Ms. Seals would typically address such problems in stages throughout treatment. During a pretreatment stage, she would explain the principles of dialectical behavior therapy and ask clients with borderline personality disorder to commit themselves to the treatment program for a minimum period. Then she would move on to three treatment stages. In the first stage, she would address issues fundamental to survival and functioning, such as decreasing suicidal behaviors, decreasing therapy-interfering behaviors, decreasing behaviors that interfered with the quality of a client's life, and increasing behavioral skills. In the second stage, the clinician would work to reduce distress due to past trauma, such as sexual abuse. And in the final stage, she would address longer-term issues, such as increasing self-respect and achieving career, social, and interpersonal goals.

Also, like other dialectical behavior therapists, Ms. Seals would typically conduct treatment on two fronts. She would have clients participate in behavioral skills training groups, where they would develop needed behavioral skills. At the same time, she would conduct individual psychotherapy sessions with her clients, focusing on what was happening at the moment. The goal of individual therapy was to develop a trusting and safe relationship and motivate clients to make changes using new cognitive and behavioral skills, and to help them through crises. As with any therapy, the relationship between client and therapist was a key part of treatment; Ms. Seals would strive to create a validating environment that had been, according to the dialectical behavior therapy model, missing in the client's past.

In addition, Ms. Seals would encourage clients with borderline personality disorder to contact her by telephone between clinic visits. This telephone consultation was not therapy. Instead, it was an opportunity to provide immediate support to manage emotional dysregulation or crises, giving clients a chance to generalize the skills they were learning in therapy to real-life situations. Whereas other therapy approaches might view between-session contacts from clients with borderline personality disorder as attention-seeking, manipulative, or problematic, Ms. Seals would encourage her clients to use calls to help implement skills to regulate emotions, tolerate emotional distress effectively, use mindfulness techniques, or improve interpersonal effectiveness. These calls would be short, structured, and

Although termed *behavioral*, the techniques of dialectical behavior therapy also draw from cognitive, psychodynamic, humanistic, and sociocultural approaches.

focused, more like coaching than therapy. Ironically, because there was so much structure to them, Ms. Seals was usually glad to hear from her clients when they called. It meant they were trying to use the skills they were learning in therapy to create a life worth living.

Pretreatment Stage   Ms. Seals's primary goal during the pretreatment sessions was to obtain a commitment from Kareem to stay with therapy for a minimum period. She considered such a commitment essential in cases of borderline personality disorder, in light of most such clients' disappointing past experiences in therapy and their explosive reactions, which could lead to impulsive, premature terminations of therapy.

At the same time, Ms. Seals recognized that, prior to obtaining any sort of commitment, it was important first to discuss Kareem's history fully and gain a proper appreciation of his experiences, both in therapy and out. Only then could Kareem feel that the therapist's recommendations were well considered. Accordingly, Ms. Seals spent three full sessions with Kareem before asking for a commitment to treatment. During these sessions, she empathized with how much fear and mistrust of the treatment process Kareem must have developed because of his unsuccessful past therapies. She also expressed empathy for Kareem's own attempts to handle his feelings through the use of self-harm, dependent relationships, and alcohol. Finally, the social worker expressed admiration for Kareem's persistence in trying to improve his situation despite a long history of invalidation and abuse.

Kareem expressed surprise at the clinician's recognition of his strengths, noting that more typically therapists would shake their heads over how "messed up" he was. Ms. Seals replied that she recognized Kareem indeed had problems, but that she also recognized Kareem was probably coping with them in the best way he knew how. "You are doing your best, and you need to do better," she said. "Both things can be true at the same," she went on, "and that is an example of a dialectical way of thinking. When two things seem like they contradict each other, sometimes there is a middle path where both are true."

The term *dialectical* is meant to suggest that the goals and methods in dialectical behavior therapy often involve achieving a balance between two opposing forces, especially a balance between self-acceptance and making changes for the better.

To help her client decide whether to commit himself to this therapy, Ms. Seals described the principles and techniques of dialectical behavior therapy. To begin, she explained that Kareem's problems fit a pattern known as borderline personality disorder, a term that Kareem said he recognized from some of his previous treatments. The therapist explained that the term *borderline* was an old term from the middle of the 1950s that was used by clinicians to characterize the condition as "on the border" between neurosis and psychosis. She said that current thinking on this disorder was that it primarily involved difficulty in managing strong emotional feelings; many of the behavior problems—self-harm, impulsive behavior, interpersonal difficulties—were now seen as stemming from the individual's understandable need to manage these emotions. The treatment, Ms. Seals explained, would involve learning more effective ways of regulating emotions so as to be more skillful and effective in a wide variety of life situations. She then described the various stages of treatment and two of the primary modes of treatment Kareem would be doing, namely, weekly group skills training and individual psychotherapy.

Kareem said he was impressed with the organization and structure of the treatment approach. In all his previous therapies, a systematic plan had never been laid out for him. He said the approach made sense to him, but he was wary of his ability to succeed. Ms. Seals expressed empathy for his ambivalence, and also tried to shift some of the burden of success, explaining that success was dependent not only on Kareem's efforts but on her ability to apply the treatment appropriately. They agreed to work together for at least 6 months. Ms. Seals estimated that the total treatment time might be 1 to 2 years.

First-Stage Treatment: Addressing Issues of Survival and Basic Functioning   In the first stage of treatment, Ms. Seals focused on issues critical to survival and functioning: increasing behavioral skills, decreasing suicidal behaviors, decreasing behaviors that interfered with therapy, and decreasing behaviors that reduced the quality of one's life.

> Research indicates that individuals with borderline personality disorder often improve markedly during treatment with dialectical behavior therapy (Chapman & Dixon-Gordon, 2020; Linehan, 2020; Zeifman et al., 2020).

Increasing skills (group therapy)   Kareem began attending a weekly dialectical behavior therapy skills training group, designed to teach cognitive and behavioral skills in a systematic fashion, using a combination of didactic teaching, group practice exercises, and weekly homework assignments. Four skills modules would be taught over 6 months: (1) mindfulness, (2) interpersonal effectiveness, (3) emotion regulation, and (4) distress tolerance.

Mindfulness skills refer to the ability to step back from and look at one's emotions while at the same time not being judgmental about them. Interpersonal effectiveness skills involve being able to make and decline requests, while at the same time maintaining self-respect and sound interpersonal relationships. Emotion regulation skills involve being aware of intense emotional arousal and behaving effectively in spite of emotional dysregulation. Distress tolerance skills refer to the ability to cope with negative emotional arousal, by employing such techniques as distracting oneself during a crisis, soothing oneself, or considering various responses.

At first, Kareem was reluctant to participate in the skills training group, asking why he couldn't just see Ms. Seals for the individual sessions and forget about the "group thing." The social worker, however, explained the importance of learning the skills; she also pointed out that if the individual sessions were spent entirely on skills training, there would be no time to deal with Kareem's day-to-day concerns. The client agreed to attend as part of his commitment and, after a few weeks, began to feel that the group training was worthwhile. In addition to gaining mastery in certain skill areas, he came to feel comfort in the emotional support supplied by the group and a sense of gratification in providing support to others. He continued to attend the group for one year, rotating through the four skills modules two times, feeling a greater sense of self-efficacy in the second cycle learning the skills than during the first six months, when it was all new information to him. "Like learning a new language," he told Ms. Seals, "it all made more sense the second time through the skills."

Decreasing suicidal behaviors In the first individual therapy session, Ms. Seals explained that she would like to focus on Kareem's tendency to harm himself. She shared an electronic file full of various forms and handouts she liked to use and adapt to each client. Ms. Seals began by having Kareem keep a daily record detailing his level of suicidal ideation; overall misery level; self-harm urges; self-harm actions; urges to use illegal drugs, alcohol, or benzodiazepines; whether he used these substances; what he did to cope with any self-harm urges; and his use of new skills learned from group. The self-monitoring tool was called *a diary card*, and it would be used to set an agenda and structure each individual therapy session.

In the second session, the diary card revealed that the client had cut his upper arms or inner thighs with a razor blade two times the past week. The injuries, which he bandaged himself, were visible to others only if he wore shorts or a tank top. Unlike Kareem's previous therapists, Ms. Seals was careful not to criticize him for creating these injuries, label them as "manipulation," or threaten to stop treatment if the behavior continued. Instead, she responded to each instance with a *behavioral analysis*, trying to get Kareem to see how the cutting was serving a function. The behavioral analysis worked by looking at each link in the chain of events immediately before, during, and after self-harm. Ms. Seals even called it a "chain analysis." In one chain analysis, a man whom Kareem had met at a party took his phone number, then failed to text him the next day. Kareem's misery level rose as the hours passed without a text, and, after drinking a vodka and club soda and smoking a bowl of marijuana, he eventually made two superficial cuts on his upper thigh, which briefly reduced his emotional pain. At that point in time, Kareem had called Ms. Seals to tell her what he had done and to receive support.

During the next session, when reviewing the incident and Kareem's reactions, Ms. Seals validated his disappointment and worry, and also recommended that he start coping differently with urges to cut. She explained that she wanted Kareem to begin managing his emotions using the skills he would learn in group, and that he could contact her for skills coaching *prior* to self-harm. In fact, she explained that in this treatment there is a "24-hour rule" prohibiting Kareem from contacting the therapist for skills coaching for at least 24 hours following any deliberate self-injurious behavior. The rationale was twofold. First, calls or texts to the therapist immediately after self-harm have no problem-solving value because the

Because people with borderline personality disorder are more emotional than analytic, dialectical behavior therapists teach clients how to make a *behavioral analysis* of problems. The therapists help them to see a larger context: that their problems—emotional, behavioral, or interpersonal—are usually just one element in a chain of events.

behavior has already happened. Second, the rule against speaking with Ms. Seals until 24 hours after any self-harm would create an incentive to use skills and skills coaching before self-harming behavior, thereby decreasing its probability.

In the early morning following this session, at about 3:00 A.M., Kareem called Ms. Seals. Breathing heavily and almost sobbing, the client said that he had not yet cut himself but desperately wanted to do so. He was afraid, on one hand, that the therapist would reject him if he carried out the cutting and, on the other, that Ms. Seals would be angered by him calling so late at night.

Though groggy and startled, Ms. Seals made it clear to Kareem that it was "absolutely wonderful" that he had taken this step, and she was glad he had taken the risk of calling rather than cutting. These words alone had a very calming effect on the client. She reminded Kareem of some of the distraction, self-soothing, and distress tolerance strategies he had learned in the recent skills group. The client, in turn, decided to make himself a cup of hot cocoa, take a hot shower, and scroll through TikTok to decrease his emotional arousal and urges to self-harm.

Kareem made a similar call 2 days later, and the day after that. In both cases, Ms. Seals encouraged him to use distress tolerance strategies, and Kareem was able to resist the urge to cut, instead soothing himself and distracting himself with emotions and activities that would disrupt his learned pattern of using self-harm to regulate emotions.

At the next session, Kareem's diary card revealed no instances of self-harm for the week. Ms. Seals devoted most of the session to analyzing this achievement, noting how Kareem had successfully replaced cutting with more constructive coping strategies. Still, Kareem's misery level had remained high during the week: a 10 on a scale of 10 on most days. On top of this, he had drunk more alcohol and used more marijuana this week than in the past several weeks.

Over the next 3 months, Kareem contacted the therapist an average of three times a week and succeeded in avoiding all self-harm during this period. Correspondingly, his misery level began to improve. Then he started seeing a man to whom he was strongly attracted. As had happened with previous men, they had sex on their first night out together. At his therapy session the next day, Kareem announced that he had found the perfect man and felt certain he was in love. He was brimming with enthusiasm—more than Ms. Seals had ever seen in him. The psychologist supported his feelings, noting how wonderful it was to be in love.

Unfortunately, the man didn't share Kareem's enthusiasm and failed to text the following day as promised. When Kareem finally reached him and suggested they get together, he said he really didn't feel like "getting involved." Kareem was devastated and, over the next several days, cut himself multiple times before calling Ms. Seals. When he did call to tell the therapist what had happened, he felt certain that Ms. Seals would reject him for having self-harmed. He begged her not to end the treatment.

The theory and techniques followed by Ms. Seals and other dialectical behavior therapists are based largely on the work of psychologist Marsha Linehan.

Around 35% of the identical twins of people with borderline personality disorder also display the disorder themselves, in contrast to 19% of the fraternal twins of people with the personality disorder (Chapman et al., 2021; Skodol, 2021).

Ms. Seals:	In the past, when you have cut yourself, have previous therapists talked about ending treatment with you?
Kareem:	Yes! The last two therapists said they didn't think they could help me when this happened. They referred me to other therapists and said that I was too complicated. That I needed a specialist. It was humiliating and only made things worse.
Ms. Seals:	I see. Well, it makes a lot of sense based on this past learning why you are worried the same thing could happen with me. You're thinking if it happened before it could happen again, right?
Kareem:	Exactly. Please, please don't fire me…
Ms. Seals:	Kareem, even if that happened to you in the past, I want you to see if you can come up with any ways in which this treatment is different from your previous ones.
Kareem:	This treatment? This treatment is different in so many ways! That's why I don't want to lose it.
Ms. Seals:	Exactly. It is different in many ways! Now, let me ask you something. Why would I, using *this* treatment, want to stop working with you for doing the very thing that you need help with, and that brought you to therapy in the first place?
Kareem:	I started cutting again, and I didn't even try to call you to get help.
Ms. Seals:	What kept you from calling?
Kareem:	I just felt so alone, and like a piece of shit.
Ms. Seals:	But you're calling now, and that's great! I understand your reluctance to call. It's perfectly natural. No one likes to bring bad news. But try not to think of this as such bad news. You were under a lot of stress for the first time since our therapy began; it's understandable that you might not be able to manage it perfectly. But, look at what you did do. You did stop the cutting eventually, and you did call me. I think it's best to look at this as a temporary slip, as opposed to a complete relapse. I think you'll find that you can get back on track again and avoid the cutting once the distress from this experience subsides.
Kareem:	I think I can stop cutting now. Just hearing you tell me that it was natural to get upset helps. But I feel so miserable.
Ms. Seals:	I know. Let's discuss some concrete things you can do now to cope with that feeling.

Ms. Seals then reviewed some concrete problem-solving strategies. Kareem agreed to make out a schedule of things to do for the rest of the day, including three errands and one recreational activity, to reduce his thoughts about being rejected. In the evening, he would go to the gym to work out rather than staying in his apartment, where the probability of self-harm was higher.

At the next session, Kareem said he had carried out the scheduled activities the day before, and this had helped turn his mind away from being lonely. However, now he was feeling "completely hopeless" about the progress of therapy itself. He said there was no point in continuing with something that just didn't work. He demanded that the social worker admit that he was a hopeless case who could never live a normal life and only deserved pain and suffering.

Ms. Seals was momentarily at a loss for words. But before she could speak, Kareem himself came to her assistance. "Don't be upset," the client said, smiling. "Sometimes I say these things. If you don't overreact, if you believe in me, it's easier for me to believe in myself, and not in the hopeless part." She told him that she certainly did believe in Kareem, and then offered the client a parable. She said that the way out of misery is like finding your way out of the desert; you walk and walk, and often things look just the same: dirt, sagebrush, rocks, no water, no shade, no relief. However, if you follow a fairly straight path for a long time, even though things look and feel the same, you're in a very different place, much closer to getting out of the desert.

A number of times after this exchange, Kareem expressed the same kind of hopelessness and claimed to be giving up. However, such claims were typically followed by him working even harder and achieving new goals the next day or week. He gradually came to appreciate that he had a tendency to experience hopelessness, and that he should not believe such frequent and intrusive thoughts were literally true.

Over the next year, Kareem had only two episodes of self-injury, which he described as mainly due to habit. He then remained free from self-harm for the remainder of treatment.

Decreasing therapy-interfering behaviors Kareem frequently displayed two kinds of therapy-interfering behavior. He would repeatedly express extreme hopelessness and insist that he could not follow the treatment plan any longer, and he would experience extreme anger toward the therapist.

Although Kareem seemed, overall, to have warm feelings toward Ms. Seals, there were many occasions when feelings of fear, hopelessness, shame, or depression caused him to lash out. He would turn bright red and criticize her or call her names. For example, on one occasion, he said, "Thanks for your brilliant suggestion. You know, other therapists I've had were stupid, too, but at least they cared about me."

Although at first taken aback by comments such as this, Ms. Seals recognized that they were signs that she had unwittingly invalidated some aspect of Kareem's experience. She knew that it was important not to respond defensively to an attack or an insulting remark from him. Indeed, the most therapeutic reaction, for

Because therapists are frequently confronted with the emotional crises, self-destructive acts, and intense anger of, and even insults from, clients with borderline personality disorder, treatment is emotionally demanding for the practitioners. Thus, dialectical behavior therapists often consult with other therapists to help them remain professional and stay on track with the principles of dialectical behavior therapy.

Kareem's sake, was for Ms. Seals to admit right away that she might indeed have said something unwise or hurtful, or that *something* legitimately triggered Kareem's ineffective interpersonal behavior. During the initial stages of therapy, for example, she would respond to Kareem's outbursts by saying something like, "I must have really messed up for you to be this angry. What am I missing? I really want to know what's going on." As therapy progressed, Kareem was able to exercise more and more self-restraint in his angry reactions. Instead of criticizing or attacking Ms. Seals, he would say something like, "Hey, I don't think you're understanding me."

Other times, the anger that Kareem expressed toward Ms. Seals actually had more to do with people he had encountered and had been upset by outside of therapy. With time, he was able to distinguish between these reactions and the feelings produced by Ms. Seals's words. At later points in therapy, he was able to simply tell her, "I'm in a bad mood. It has nothing to do with you. It's okay. I'll get over it." Ultimately, through identifying and using skills to change therapy-interfering interpersonal patterns with Ms. Seals, Kareem was able to generalize learned skillful responses from the therapy setting to his interactions with people in his daily life.

Decreasing behaviors interfering with quality of life
When Kareem began therapy with Ms. Seals, he was abusing alcohol, marijuana, and benzodiazepines. These target behaviors were addressed most directly as what Ms. Seals called "quality-of-life behaviors." As therapy progressed and Kareem no longer was self-harming and began to develop greater control over his emotions and actions, they began more actively addressing quality-of-life targets, starting with substance use. Ms. Seals taught Kareem some additional distress-tolerance skills that were specifically applicable to substance use. These skills would help him tolerate urges to use; communicate more effectively to his friends, coworkers, and family about his substance use; and change his social habits to reduce the probability of using. Kareem also asked his primary care doctor to stop prescribing benzodiazepines, disclosing his problems with substance abuse.

Second-Stage Treatment: Reducing Distress Due to Past Traumas
The focus of the second treatment stage was to help Kareem overcome lingering feelings of distress due to past traumas, such as his sexual abuse. In fact, his abuse history had been addressed to some degree from the beginning of treatment. Indeed, in the first stage of therapy, Kareem had developed skills that could help him better tolerate his abuse memories. He had learned, for example, to soothe himself—to do especially nice things for himself, such as eat favorite foods, dress in favorite clothes, or go for a walk in his favorite park; and to distract himself, by finding constructive and engaging projects to work on, such as working with reclaimed wood to make picture frames and doing photography.

Psychotropic medications, particularly antidepressant, mood stabilizing, antianxiety, and antipsychotic drugs, have helped calm the emotional and aggressive reactions of some people with borderline personality disorder (Chapman et al., 2021; Newton-Howes & Mulder, 2020). However, given the heightened risk of suicide by these individuals, the use of medication on an outpatient basis can sometimes be risky.

In the second stage of treatment, however, the goal was not only to manage the emotional distress that resulted from abuse memories but to reduce the capacity of the memories to produce distress. Ms. Seals used *exposure techniques* similar to those used in the treatment of posttraumatic stress disorder, in which clients undergo repeated, controlled exposures to stimuli—external or internal—that have been linked to past traumas.

Initially, the therapist asked Kareem to describe his past abuse experiences in general terms only. As the client described the same experiences over and over again as a regular exercise, the exposure seemed to result in reductions in his distress levels. Thus, after repeatedly describing how he was sexually abused by the neighbor and his friends in general terms—three times per session for three sessions—Kareem's distress level was relatively mild by the ninth description. The procedure was then repeated using greater and greater levels of detail, until even the most detailed descriptions of his traumatic experiences produced only moderate distress. The same procedure was applied to Kareem's other traumatic memories, with similar results.

Third-Stage Treatment: Addressing Longer-Term Issues   The focus of the third stage of treatment was to help Kareem gain greater self-respect and achieve career, social, and interpersonal goals. In fact, in his case, the achievement of these goals had been occurring naturally over the course of therapy, as a result of the gains he had been making during the first and second stages of treatment. As Kareem had stopped injuring himself, developed stable behavior patterns, increased his interpersonal effectiveness, and stopped using substances, he was in fact valuing himself increasingly and providing a more dignified existence for himself—a "life worth living," as Ms. Seals had called it during their first therapy appointment.

Epilogue

Kareem remained in individual therapy once a week for a total of 2 years, and now continues with periodic follow-up sessions or phone calls every month or two. Overall, his life has improved greatly, especially compared with what it was prior to beginning dialectical behavior therapy with Ms. Seals.

Above all, he no longer hurts himself, even when extremely upset. He also rarely uses alcohol to deal with feelings of distress, and he has not been hospitalized since his last suicide attempt, a month before therapy began. He works part-time at the airport and part-time as an assistant in the medical records department of a local hospital, and he takes courses at a nearby community college, with the goal of becoming an IT technician. He sells his wood frames and photography on Etsy, and though he doesn't make much money from this, it gives him a great sense of

Close to 75% of the people who receive a diagnosis of borderline personality disorder are women (Salters-Pednault, 2020).

meaning to create and inspire others, and he feels like it is something he has to offer to the world that adds value.

Most important, Kareem has regained control over his life. As he puts it, "I get to have my feelings, and nobody has the right to control me anymore." In addition, he feels that a major achievement of therapy has been "my recognition, deep down inside, that, like other people, I am an acceptable human being and that life can be safe. My life is my own now." Still single but no longer getting involved in dysfunctional relationships, Kareem is confident that he will one day, when it happens naturally, find the partner that is best for him.

Assessment Questions

1. What led to Kareem's admission to the University Hospital?

2. Why did Kareem's previous therapist decide to discontinue treatment with him at the time of his admission to the hospital for an overdose?

3. How many individuals with borderline personality disorder attempt suicide?

4. Describe Kareem's typical intimate relationships before he began treatment with Ms. Seals.

5. What was Kareem's "greatest fear" that led to his frequent suicide attempts?

6. How did Kareem's behavior meet the DSM-5-TR criteria for borderline personality disorder?

7. Describe the concept of dialectical behavior therapy. Be sure to describe the main points of this type of treatment.

8. What is Ms. Seals's primary goal during the pretreatment stage? How did she relate this to Kareem in their initial therapy sessions?

9. What were the primary modes Ms. Seals told Kareem would be part of his treatment program?

10. List the four specific skill areas covered in the first stage of treatment with Kareem.

11. Why is it common for certain individuals to use self-destructive behaviors when they are disappointed by life events?

12. How did Ms. Seals handle Kareem's cutting behaviors, not only to help him prevent the behaviors but also to support him when he relapsed?

13. What were two therapy-interfering behaviors frequently displayed by Kareem?

14. What was the focus of the second treatment stage? What types of therapeutic interventions did Ms. Seals use with Kareem during this time?

15. Describe some other disorders that individuals with borderline personality disorder may also develop.

16. What is the ultimate achievement Kareem feels he has realized from his treatment?

CASE 16

Attention-Deficit/Hyperactivity Disorder

Table 16-1

Dx Checklist

Attention-Deficit/Hyperactivity Disorder

1. The individual presents one or both of the following patterns:

   (a) For 6 months or more, the individual frequently displays at least 6 of the following symptoms of inattention, to a degree that is maladaptive and beyond that shown by most similarly aged persons: • Unable to properly attend to details, or frequently makes careless errors • Finds it hard to maintain attention • Fails to listen when spoken to by others • Fails to carry out instructions and finish work • Disorganized • Dislikes or avoids mentally effortful work • Loses items that are needed for successful work • Easily distracted by irrelevant stimuli • Forgets to do many everyday activities.

   (b) For 6 months or more, the individual frequently displays at least 6 of the following symptoms of *hyperactivity* and *impulsivity*, to a degree that is maladaptive and beyond that shown by most similarly aged persons: • Fidgets, taps hands or feet, or squirms • Inappropriately wanders from seat • Inappropriately runs or climbs • Unable to play quietly • In constant motion • Talks excessively • Interrupts questioners during discussions • Unable to wait for turn • Barges in on others' activities or conversations

2. The individual displayed some of the symptoms before 12 years of age.

3. The individual shows symptoms in more than one setting.

4. The individual experiences impaired functioning.

(Information from APA, 2022, 2013.)

Christopher was the first of three children. He was born after a normal, uncomplicated pregnancy, a healthy baby who grew rapidly and reached the standard developmental milestones—sitting, standing, walking, talking, and so forth—either at or before the expected ages. His parents marveled at his exuberance and his drive to be independent at an early age. He was sitting by the age of 5 months and walking at 11 months. Once mobile, he was a veritable dynamo (in fact, they called him "the Dynamo") who raced around the house, filled with a curiosity that led him to grab, examine, and frequently destroy almost anything that wasn't nailed down.

Christopher From "Dynamo" to "Dynamite"

During his toddler period, Christopher's parents had no inkling that his activity level was at all unusual and, in truth, in many ways it was just an exaggeration of tendencies that most toddlers exhibit. Still, his parents found it exhausting to cope with his behavior. Just watching over him was a full-time job. Christopher's mother, Shelley, had contemplated doing some freelance accounting at home to earn extra money. However, with her very first project she realized that this was completely unrealistic. Shelley had hoped she could contain Christopher by keeping him in a playpen while she worked, but she found that he wouldn't tolerate such confinement for more than 2 minutes before he was yelling to get out. Once out, he was likely to get into trouble by bumping into or knocking things over, becoming easily distracted and leaving a mess of toys, or even injuring himself accidentally. Within minutes, Shelley would hear a crash or some other noise that demanded her attention, making it difficult for her to get anything else done.

When Christopher's mother became pregnant with his sister, Christopher was well into the "terrible twos," and his mother and his father, Greg, were beginning to doubt their suitability as parents. Of course, other new parents often remarked on how demanding children were, but Shelley and Greg could tell that the other parents felt nowhere near the same sense of desperation.

When Christopher was two, his sister Emma was born. When he was four, his brother Tommy arrived. In raising Christopher's sister and younger brother, it became crystal clear to Shelley and Greg that their problems in handling Christopher were not simply due to their inadequacy as parents, as they had previously worried. As an infant Emma—unlike Christopher—did not try to squirm and break free every time she was held. Later, there were other differences. As a toddler, she was content to sit quietly for long periods just playing with her toys, and she listened until the end of the entire story when Shelley read to her, whereas Christopher routinely would get restless and run off within a couple of minutes. During his preschool years, Christopher had been put on probation from the school for biting another child in the line for the bathroom. At the same time, his brother Tommy, now 12 months old, was easygoing, calm, and receptive to his parents, showing none of the same behaviors that Christopher had at that age. Something was different about Christopher, and his parents were starting to realize it.

When Christopher reached school age and Shelley and Greg received more objective feedback from teachers about his difficulties, they began to understand with greater clarity what was going on. After his first month of school, his kindergarten teacher described him as "a nice boy, but he needs to exercise better self-control." At their first ever parent–teacher conference, the teacher told Christopher's parents that his activity level was well above that of the other children. In the first and second grades, as the academic component of the curriculum increased and the demands on the children for behavioral control increased

> Between 7% and 10% of all children may have ADHD at any given time (Krull, 2021a; Polanczyk, 2020).

correspondingly, Shelley and Greg started to receive stronger complaints from his teachers. In addition, Christopher's academic progress was slowed because of his problems with attention. Although he eventually learned to read, he didn't really begin to master the skill until the second grade. Now in the third grade, Christopher was falling behind the other children in a wide range of academic tasks. With encouragement—actually, insistence—from his teacher, Ms. Freedman, his parents decided to seek help for him at the Ripple Center, a local clinic affiliated with a larger hospital enterprise throughout the state.

Christopher at Home A Parent's Perspective

By age 8, Christopher rarely carried out his parents' requests or instructions, or he carried them out only partially before becoming caught up in some other activity. He could be easily distracted. Trouble seemed to follow him everywhere. Making matters worse, since the first grade he had become increasingly anxious. There were times when his anxiety was about ordinary things kids his age get worried about—lightning, thunder, darkness, and the like. But typically his anxiety was about other things. He worried about his health, the safety of his family, what other kids thought about him, and, more generally, his future. Like a game of whack-a-mole, when he felt less anxious about one thing, up popped another worry. The endless parade of worries, on top of his difficulty paying attention, staying focused, and being thoughtful with his actions, was more than his parents could handle on most days.

> Many children with ADHD also have great difficulty controlling their emotions, and some have anxiety or mood problems (Shapero et al., 2021).

One evening shortly after his eighth birthday was illustrative: Christopher's father had just finished preparing dinner when he went to his son's room and asked him to stop playing his video game, wash his hands, and take his place at the dining room table. "Okay, Dad," Christopher answered.

"Thank you, Christopher," Greg said as he went back down to the kitchen to do some final preparations. However, only 5 minutes later he realized he still had not seen Christopher. He went back up to his room and found Christopher playing on his gaming device. He had never turned off the game, and didn't even pretend to notice or worry about his father when Greg stepped into the room.

"Christopher, I mean it. Stop playing now!" he told him.

"OK. In just a minute Dad," he said, and turned away.

"No! I asked you 5 minutes ago and you ignored me. Let's go Chrissy!" That was the name Greg called his son whenever he wanted to get his attention. He tried it years before, and it worked, snapping Christopher's attention into place momentarily. It kept working, so it stuck.

Although this was Greg's second effort, Christopher was now coming without too much of a struggle, so his father was relieved. "Go wash your hands," he reminded him.

"Okay, Dad," Christopher replied, "but do you think I am going to get sick if I don't wash my hands? Am I gonna die if I don't wash my hands, Dad?" Greg stood in the hallway, unsure of what to say before telling him not to worry, and to please just wash up and head downstairs. As he headed down the hall toward the bathroom, Christopher caught a glimpse of his younger sister already seated at the dining room table, holding a new doll. His younger brother Tommy was away visiting his grandparents. At the table, Emma was talking to the doll, giggling. The doll cocked its head and blinked, then moved its head up and down, like it was saying yes to Emma. Shelley walked into the room and smiled, touching Emma on the shoulder lightly and quietly speaking to the doll. Christopher stood and watched all of this, puzzled.

"Hey, cool!" Christopher exclaimed. "Let me try." He immediately ran downstairs, clumsily grabbed the doll from Emma's hands, and tried to find buttons to make it move or talk. The doll was still, and Emma whined to their mother that she wanted her toy back. "Does the doll do anything else?" Christopher asked, ignoring Emma. He started to walk away with the doll, unfazed by Emma's protestations and tears.

"How does it work?" Christopher wondered aloud.

"Mommy!" Emma cried.

"Chrissy!" Greg's voice boomed as he thundered down the stairs.

"Christopher," Shelley said as she calmly looked him in the eyes. "Hand it to me." He looked at her, and after she repeated herself, he gave his mother the doll, without any awareness of his sister, or his father for that matter. Emma wiped tears from her cheeks. Greg shook his head, and Shelley shrugged her shoulders.

Later, as they ate dinner together, Greg and Shelley were talking about what was happening in the world news. Emma ate quietly, eyes down at her food, her fork sweeping across the plate with purpose. Christopher had oscillated between eating his food vigorously and ignoring it altogether, occasionally staring off into space before suddenly returning his attention back to his plate. Shelley shared with Greg her convictions about how the president of the United States was leading the country down a dangerous path in the management of tensions with China. Greg agreed with her, but because he enjoyed intellectual conversation, he took the opposing side of the argument, just for the sake of stimulating more conversation. He knew she would like it, gentle debate as a temporary reprieve from the stress of parenting, perhaps even a reminder of what their conversations used to be like when they were dating many years ago. As they verbally sparred about foreign relations, both Emma and Christopher now were watching. The conversation was playful but serious, with Greg laughing at Shelley's criticisms of his viewpoints, and Shelley steadfastly sticking to hers.

Confused, Christopher interrupted his parents. "Mom, Dad—Are we all going to die when China takes over the world? Because I don't wanna die, and I don't want you to either."

> More than twice as many boys as girls have ADHD (Krull, 2021a; Polanczyk, 2020).

"Oh no, sweetie, no no no," Shelley said leaning toward her son and shaking her head. "China isn't going to take over the world. You don't need to worry about that. China is a large country with a long history, and I was telling your father that I don't like the way our president in talking to the leaders of China. I don't agree with how he is handling things. That's all. No one is taking over the world, and you don't need to worry about dying because of what I was talking about."

"Okay, but," Christopher nervously kept going, "one of the kids at school was talking about how his parents were talking about people dying, or getting sick. Will I get sick too?"

Greg reached out to his son and touched him on the top of his head. "Christopher, you are not sick, and neither are we or your sister or brother. Let's enjoy the food and be grateful for everything we have. Let's not worry so much about all of these other things, okay bud?" Christopher nodded. The conversation ended, and they ate the rest of the meal in silence, Greg and Shelley casting furtive glances when the kids were not looking, connecting with each on their shared frustration and hopelessness about how to handle these kinds of situations.

What had begun as a simple attempt to get Christopher to wash his hands and come to the dinner table had become an emotionally distressing situation. His anxiety during dinner had further compounded the level of stress and tension. It was not the first time this kind of thing had happened.

Unless Christopher was escorted through every task of the day, he'd get sidetracked, and it often ended with an argument, something getting broken, or another problem. Consequently, his parents often found it easier just to do things for Christopher—wash his hands, clean his room, get him dressed—because getting him to do the tasks himself was the greater effort. When he became anxious, they would tell him not to worry, to let go of whatever it was that was bothering him.

When left to his own devices, Christopher's behavior was disruptive in other ways. He jumped on the beds, ran through the house, or played shrill games of hide-and-seek under the dinner table with his unwilling parents or siblings. If his mother was on the phone, he would think nothing of yelling out demands for a drink, a snack, or help in finding some lost toy, despite Shelley's numerous warnings not to interrupt her.

Even playing out in the yard was not a solution, because if Christopher wasn't watched closely, in a flash he might run out into the street after a ball without any regard for traffic. When playing indoors with neighborhood children, Christopher was bossy, continually grabbing their toys or refusing to share his own. His play dates had to be closely supervised by his parents to avoid squabbles. Because of these problems, Christopher had few friends. Instead, most of his leisure time was spent watching television or playing video games, activities that Shelley and Greg were reluctant to encourage, but which they felt forced to accept since he could

In the past, ADHD was known officially as *hyperkinetic reaction of childhood,* and it was commonly referred to simply as *hyperactivity* or *hyperkinesis* (the latter term from the Greek for *over* and *motion*).

do little else without supervision. All of these restrictions and layers of challenges contributed to Christopher's anxiety. He worried about whether he might get injured playing. He worried about having to go the hospital. At least weekly, he self-consciously asked his parents why no one wanted to be his friend.

Christopher at School A Teacher's Perspective

Christopher's third-grade teacher, Ms. Freedman, found his behavior extremely disruptive in school. She was also concerned that Christopher's behavior problems were interfering with his ability to learn. She believed he was a bright child, but his inattention, anxiety, and associated behavioral problems were causing him to fail to complete his lessons and hampering the other children's ability to complete theirs.

One day at school in mid-April Ms. Freedman had called the class to attention to begin an oral exercise: reciting a multiplication table on the digital whiteboard. The first child had just begun her recitation when, suddenly, Christopher exclaimed, "Look!" The class turned to see Christopher running to the window.

"Look," he exclaimed again, "a cool airplane!"

A couple of children ran to the window with Christopher to see the airplane, but Ms. Freedman called them back, and they returned to their seats. Christopher, however, remained at the window, pointing at the sky. Ms. Freedman called him back, too.

"Christopher, please return to your desk," Ms. Freedman said firmly. But Christopher acted as though he hadn't heard her.

"Look, Ms. Freedman," he exclaimed, "the airplane is flying so low!" A couple of other children started from their desks.

"Christopher," Ms. Freedman tried once more, "if you don't return to your desk this instant, I'm going to send you to Miss Warren's office." Christopher seemed oblivious to her threats and remained at the window, staring excitedly up at the sky.

Ms. Freedman, her patience wearing thin, addressed Christopher through gritted teeth. "Christopher, come with me back to your seat." She took him by the hand and led him there. She also considered making good on her threat to send him to Miss Warren, the principal, but she glanced at the clock and realized Miss Warren would not be in her office now. Finding someone else to supervise Christopher would probably be more disruptive than disciplining him within the class, so she settled for getting him back in his seat, then took her place once more in front of the class. By now she was almost 10 minutes into the lesson period and still had not finished a single multiplication table.

Ms. Freedman tried to resume the lesson. "Who can tell me the answer to 3 times 6?" she asked. Fifteen children raised their hands, but before she could call on anyone, Christopher blurted out the incorrect answer. "Thank you, Christopher,"

Half of children with ADHD also have learning or communication problems, many perform poorly in school, a number have social difficulties, and about 80% misbehave, many quite seriously (Retz et al., 2021; Tenenbaum et al., 2019).

she said, barely able to contain her exasperation, "but that is not correct, and I would like you to please raise your hand like the others."

Ms. Freedman tried again. "Who knows 3 times 7?" This time Christopher raised his hand, but he still couldn't resist creating a disruption.

"I know, I know!" Christopher pleaded, jumping up and down in his seat with his hand raised high.

"That will do, Christopher," Ms. Freedman admonished him. She deliberately called on another child. The child responded with the correct answer.

"I knew that!" Christopher exclaimed.

"Christopher," Ms. Freedman told him, "I don't want you to say one more word for the rest of this class period."

Christopher looked down at his desk, feeling ashamed, ignoring the rest of the lesson. He began to fiddle with a couple of rubber bands, trying to see how far they would stretch before they broke. He looped the rubber bands around his index fingers and pulled his hands farther and farther apart. This kept him quiet for a while; by this point, Ms. Freedman didn't care what he did, as long as he was quiet. She continued conducting the multiplication lesson while Christopher stretched the rubber bands until finally they snapped, flying off and nearly hitting two children. Two of the children watching the whole episode gasped out loud when the rubber bands went flying, then started laughing. The class turned toward them.

"That's it, Christopher," Ms. Freedman told him. "You're going to sit outside the classroom until the period is over."

"No!" Christopher protested. "I'm not going. I didn't do anything!"

"Really? Where did these two rubber bands come from? I don't think they dropped from the sky. You shot those rubber bands across the room," Ms. Freedman said.

"But it was an accident."

"I don't care. Let's go!"

Christopher stalked out of the classroom to sit on a chair in the hall. Some of the kids giggled as he walked toward the door. He noticed, looking at them and seeing their smiles. He smiled back, turning his head away as he moved from the classroom to the hallway. After sitting alone in the hallway, Christopher started to get anxious. What if there was a fire alarm? What if a tornado hit the school? Where would he go? What would he do? He nervously fidgeted in his chair, contemplating going back into the classroom—or maybe the principal's office. He could go there and say he felt sick. The school nurse would take care of him. He even thought about leaving the school to try to find his way home. It would be safer at home.

Soon, the school bell rang, signaling the end of the period and the beginning of recess. Ms. Freedman was thankful to get some relief from the obligation of controlling Christopher, but she was frustrated that almost the entire math period had been wasted due to his disruptions.

Children who are hyperactive may be viewed relatively negatively by their peers, parents, and teachers; may have impaired peer relationships; and, in turn, may come to view themselves negatively (Celebi & Unal, 2021; Cueli et al., 2020).

Out in the schoolyard during recess, Christopher's difficulties continued. As the children lined up for turns on the slide, Christopher pushed to the head of the line, almost knocking one child off the ladder as he elbowed his way up. After going down the slide, Christopher barged into a game that some younger children were playing; he grabbed a ball away from one child and began trying to dribble it like a basketball, while another child yelled in frustration. The supervising teacher told Christopher to give the ball back, but Christopher kept dribbling, oblivious to her demands, the ball bouncing wildly off his feet and rolling across the playground, where another supervising teaching assistant picked it up and held onto it. Finally, with the ball no longer in his hands, Christopher became angry.

"Hey, I want that ball back!" he insisted.

"You took the ball from someone else," the teacher explained.

"But I want it back. That's not fair!" Christopher argued.

The teacher sent Christopher to sit on a bench, where he went back and forth from feeling angry about being mistreated to being anxious about whether the kids from the playground would ever be his friends.

This was a common day for Christopher at school. On some of his better days, he was less physically disruptive, but he still had his problems, particularly in attending to and completing his schoolwork. In a typical case, Ms. Freedman would give the class an assignment to work on, such as completing a couple of pages of arithmetic problems. While most of the children worked without supervision until the assignment was completed, Christopher was easily distracted. When he got to the end of the first page, he would lose his momentum and, rather than continuing, begin playing with any objects on his desk. Other times, if another child asked the teacher a question, Christopher would stop his own work to investigate the situation, getting up to view the other child's work and failing to complete his own. Or, Christopher would be distracted by an anxious thought that popped into his head and abandon the assignment to seek reassurance from Ms. Freedman.

Finally, at a parent–teacher conference, Ms. Freedman told Christopher's parents that she thought Christopher's problems might be attributable to attention-deficit/hyperactivity disorder. Concerned about Christopher's growing academic and social problems—not to mention feeling exhausted from continually having to remind, encourage, and threaten their son to get him to do the most elemental things—Shelley and Greg decided to seek professional assistance. They arranged for a consultation at the Ripple Center.

Symptoms of ADHD, particularly the hyperactive symptoms, are typically most pronounced during the elementary school years. They often become less conspicuous by early adolescence (APA, 2022, 2013).

Christopher in Treatment

After repeatedly observing a child's long-standing problems with inattention and recklessness, teachers or parents often conclude that the child suffers from attention-deficit/hyperactivity disorder (ADHD). However, 25 years of practice had

In order to accurately assess ADHD, a child's behaviors should be observed in multiple settings (school, home, friends), and a range of diagnostic interviews, rating scales, and psychological tests should be used. However, many children receive their diagnosis from pediatricians or family physicians rather than from a systematic mental health assessment (Krull, 2021a, 2019).

taught child psychiatrist Dr. Katherine Collins that such a conclusion is often premature and inaccurate, leading to incorrect and even harmful interventions. Thus, when Christopher's parents brought him to the Ripple Center, Dr. Collins was careful to conduct lengthy interviews with the child, his parents, and his teacher; to arrange for Christopher to be observed at home and at school by an intern; to set up a physical examination by a pediatrician to detect any medical conditions (for example, lead poisoning) that might be causing the child's symptoms; and to administer a battery of psychological tests. In addition to obtaining a description of Christopher's current problems and his history from his parents, Dr. Collins asked Christopher's mother to respond to questions from multiple assessment instruments: the Swanson, Nolan, and Pelham Checklist, which contains questions pertaining specifically to disruptive behavior problems, and the Conners Parent Rating Scale, which contains questions specifically for assessing ADHD. Similarly, Dr. Collins sent the teacher's versions of the Swanson, Nolan, and Pelham Checklist and the Conners scale to Ms. Freedman. These same measures would be administered again after treatment started to measure progress.

Christopher's battery of tests included the Wechsler Intelligence Scale for Children and the Wechsler Individual Achievement Tests (to provide scores in reading, mathematics, language, and written achievement). The results of these tests confirmed the impression already supplied by Christopher's parents and Ms. Freedman: Christopher's intelligence was above average, and his academic achievement was lower than his intelligence scores would predict. These findings established that Christopher's academic problems were not due to intellectual limitations. The report also noted how anxious he seemed to be throughout the testing, and that his anxiety might have adversely influenced test results.

After completing this comprehensive assessment, Dr. Collins was confident that Christopher's difficulties met the criteria in DSM-5-TR for a diagnosis of attention-deficit/hyperactivity disorder, combined type. Although she did not see evidence of a specific anxiety disorder, she believed that his anxiety also needed to be considered as part of the treatment plan. She explained to his parents that ADHD was the primary diagnosis. Christopher exhibited a majority of the symptoms listed both for inattention (for example, difficulty sustaining attention, failure to follow instructions, obliviousness to verbal commands, becoming distracted easily) and for hyperactivity-impulsivity (for example, difficulty remaining seated, excessive motor activity in inappropriate situations, difficulty waiting his turn). The symptoms were apparent before the age of 12, occurred both at home and school, and caused significant impairments in both the social and academic spheres.

Extensive studies indicate that ADHD is overdiagnosed among children in the United States and other parts of the world (Fresson et al., 2019).

Over the years, research has indicated that many children with ADHD respond well to either stimulant drugs or systematic behavioral treatment. Although some therapists prefer one of these approaches over the other, Dr. Collins had come to believe many of the studies that found a combination of the interventions increases a child's chances of recovery. By helping the child to focus better and slow down, the medications may help them profit from the procedures and rewards used in the behavioral program.

Stimulant drugs, which include *amphetamine/dextroamphetamine mixed salts* (Adderall), *methylphenidate* (Ritalin), *methylphenidate extended-release* (Concerta), *dextroamphetamine* (Dexedrine), and *pemoline* (Cylert), were first used to treat ADHD decades ago, when clinicians noted that the drugs seemed to have a "paradoxical" tranquilizing, quieting effect on these children. Subsequent research has shown that all children—both those with and those without ADHD—experience an increase in attentional capacity when taking stimulant drugs, resulting in behavior that is more focused and controlled. This may create the appearance of sedation, but the children are actually not sedated at all.

Unfortunately, the drugs are ineffective for some children, and only partially effective for others. And even when a drug is optimally effective, other areas of behavioral adjustment may still need to be addressed, because the child may have little practice in the more appropriate behaviors that they are now theoretically capable of producing. This is where behavioral programs may come into play.

In the ideal case, both parents and teachers are involved in implementing a behavior modification program, which is based on an ABC model of behavior. The A in the model denotes *antecedents,* the conditions that provide the occasion for an increased probability of a particular behavior; the B denotes the *behavior* itself; and the C denotes the immediate *consequences* of the behavior. Thus, a given behavior is seen as prompted by certain antecedents and maintained by its consequences. For example, Christopher's sprint to the window was prompted by the antecedent condition of a boring classroom exercise and the appearance of an exciting stimulus (the low-flying airplane seen through the classroom window). The behavior was maintained over time, according to the model, by its consequence—that is, the rewarding effect of viewing the airplane, which was much greater than the punishing effect of Ms. Freedman's warnings or even of being sent out of the room. In a behavior modification program, the usual strategy is to increase the rewards for engaging in alternative behaviors under the same antecedent conditions. Accordingly, if the reward for remaining seated can be made to exceed the reward for viewing the airplane, then, theoretically, the child will be more inclined to remain seated.

Learning alternative behaviors may involve more than just adjusting incentives or antecedents. Some skills may have to be taught directly. A child who has never practiced asking politely for a toy, as opposed to grabbing it, will need to learn this skill before they can respond to incentives to implement it. Direct *behavioral skills training* usually follows a standard sequence. First, the child receives an explanation of the skill; next, they observe a model demonstrating the skill; then, they practice performing the skill, first through role-playing in the training session and

More than 3 million children in the United States regularly take a stimulant drug for ADHD (CDC, 2020c).

then through real-life behavioral practice. After the skill is learned, both parents and teachers can prompt the child to employ it in a given situation. For example, after the skill of sharing is well learned, the parent can prompt the child to share in a situation calling for cooperation with another child, and then praise the child appropriately for so doing. The more the skill is employed and reinforced in a variety of appropriate circumstances, the more the child will use the skill spontaneously, receiving naturalistic positive reinforcement from the environment in the form of friendly or gratified reactions from others.

Thus, Dr. Collins outlined for Christopher's parents four primary treatment components: (1) stimulant medication, (2) parent training in the use of behavior modification principles, (3) social skills training for Christopher, and (4) a token economy in the school environment. She clarified that several components of the treatment plan, including the parent training, social skills training, and token economy, would each also include interventions designed to help reduce Christopher's anxiety. Because anxiety was not a primary diagnosis, she told Greg and Shelley that they could address his anxiety throughout the other parts of treatment. If needed, she explained, they could further consider additional interventions specifically for his anxiety. She also suggested that Shelley and Greg consider looking into a new digital therapeutic tool for attentional training, an app-based game that recently had been approved by the FDA for use in the treatment of ADHD.

Dr. Collins explained that stimulant medication was important for increasing Christopher's attention and impulse control; this, in turn, would enhance his capacity to do what was expected of him, both in general and in response to the behavior modification plan. The parent training, she explained, would acquaint Shelley and Greg with principles of behavior modification, allowing them to deal optimally with any remaining behavior problems, as well as with Christopher's behavior during periods when he might not be taking medication (so-called drug holidays). Social skills training seemed necessary, Dr. Collins said, in light of Christopher's problems in getting along with other children and in cooperating at home. Finally, she explained that, since a large portion of Christopher's difficulties occurred in the classroom, it would be helpful for both Christopher and Ms. Freedman to have a behavioral program operating in that environment. Dr. Collins spoke to Ms. Freedman about the matter, and the teacher agreed to institute a program provided it wasn't too burdensome; but given Christopher's problems up to now, Ms. Freedman said that almost anything seemed less burdensome than simply doing nothing.

Stimulant Medication After ruling out any physical problems (for example, motor tics) that might preclude the use of stimulant medication, Dr. Collins discussed the basic rationale for use of the medication with Christopher's parents. She explained that the medication had been used for years to treat children with

> Research suggests that children with ADHD may improve most when they receive a combination of drug therapy and behavioral therapy (Krull, 2021b; Pelham & Altszuler, 2020).

symptoms of inattention, impulsivity, and hyperactivity. She also explained that the medication is not a tranquilizer. On the contrary, the medication stimulates the central nervous system for 3 to 4 hours after it is ingested. This stimulant effect, she explained, seems to increase the capacity of children with ADHD to maintain their attention and to control their impulses. As a result, they are better able to be focused and skillful in responding to the demands and contingencies of school, home, and a social life.

In addition, she informed Christopher's parents that certain side effects can develop, including weight loss, slowed growth, dizziness, insomnia, and tics. Dr. Collins noted, however, that these effects usually are not severe and often disappear after the body becomes accustomed to the drug or whenever a drug holiday is scheduled. The clinician noted that since most children with ADHD respond well to Concerta without prohibitive side effects, she was inclined to try Concerta first.

Dr. Collins pointed out that the decision to take medication was not carved in stone. Indeed, the parents should consider the initial medication regimen as a trial period; if, during this time, they concluded that the medication was not worthwhile, then it should be discontinued. They could try a different medication, or they could rely on the behavioral methods alone. But research had been done for many years supporting the use of stimulant medication along with behavioral therapy. Greg and Shelley did not like the idea of putting their son on a stimulant. They worried about long-term effects. They questioned whether side effects would be harmful. They thought about their options, but in the end decided to follow Dr. Collins's suggestion.

Once Christopher began taking the medication, his behavior improved substantially, although not completely. In class, for example, Christopher still blurted out some answers and turned around to talk to his classmates during silent reading period, but he did these things only about one fourth as often as before. Most noticeable from Ms. Freedman's standpoint was that simply saying his name was often enough to get him to stop what he was doing. He was more focused than before—not perfect, but noticeably better.

Out in the schoolyard, Christopher was now less inclined to barge into other children's games or push others aside. Unfortunately, he still had difficulty socially. Either he wandered off by himself or, if he did join with others, he failed to abide by the rules consistently, which ended up causing arguments. For example, in joining a game of catch with four other children, Christopher would hold onto the ball after he received it. In spite of the other kids yelling at him to throw the ball back, he would hold onto it just long enough for one of them to get angry, or even chase after him.

At home, Christopher seemed less driven physically. He sat at the dinner table for the entire meal without constant requests to be excused and without getting up repeatedly to grab things or to play under the table. He also became more

According to some estimates, the use of stimulant drugs to treat children with ADHD has increased at least threefold since 1990 (Campez et al., 2021; Krull, 2021b). This increase in use also extends to preschoolers.

dependable in carrying out instructions. For example, if his parents sent him to wash up and sit at the table, they now could count on his following through 75% of the time (as opposed to 25% previously). Tendencies such as stubbornness and defiance remained a problem, however; it remained a struggle to get him to do chores, to get started on his homework, or to follow household rules in general. He continued to interrupt his mother when she was on the phone, shouting his insistent requests for snacks, toys, and videos. Overall, however, the medication seemed to have many advantages.

Parent Training   To gain some knowledge of behavioral management techniques, Christopher's parents enrolled in a training group for parents of children with ADHD (at about the same time that Christopher began taking medication). The group, led by psychologist Dr. Jay Mitchell, was designed to educate parents about both ADHD and the principles of behavior modification for managing it. Group sessions were held three times a month, and once a month Dr. Mitchell met alone with Christopher's parents to discuss their child's individual situation. In these individual appointments, Dr. Mitchell targeted anxiety reduction as part of a broader approach to behavioral management strategies.

At the first group session, Christopher's parents found comfort in learning that other parents' experiences closely paralleled their own. All the parents were able to share their experiences and found that they were all dealing with similar concerns. Many parents saw humor in some of the situations, and this helped to soften the impact of what they had all been going through. Some of the parents also commented on how their child's anxiety complicated things. This too helped reassure Christopher's parents that they were going through something many others were too. It felt good to have that sense of fellowship, of validation.

It also helped Shelley and Greg to know that some of their marital disputes were shared by the other parents. Like the others in the group, Christopher's parents often argued over how to deal with their child. Although it didn't solve the problem, it helped them to know that even their arguments were normal, given the circumstances.

In additional group sessions, Shelley and Greg were progressively introduced to the ABC principles of behavioral management. Among the points they found helpful was the idea that parents can become unduly focused on discouraging problem behaviors through criticism or punishments. It surprised them to learn that punishment, though common, only temporarily decreases the probability of a behavior. It is likely to return, and when it does, parents can feel resentful and guilty, failing to understand that no matter how stern or serious a punishment may be, it is unlikely to lead to long-term behavioral changes. A different approach, Dr. Mitchell explained, was to think in terms of the alternative behaviors (B) that

Although family conflict is often present in families with a child with ADHD, negative family interaction patterns are unlikely to cause the development of ADHD (APA, 2022, 2013).

parents would like their children to do under the same circumstances (A), and to provide genuine praise and natural rewards (C) accordingly.

Christopher's parents explored this principle in greater detail in individual sessions with the group leader, as they felt it applied particularly to the way they were handling many situations with their son. For example, a regular problem with Christopher was that he interrupted his mother when she was on the phone. She had to lock herself in the bedroom in order to have a coherent conversation with a pediatrician, contractor, friend, or relative. Often, even locking herself in was not enough to ensure peace and quiet, as Christopher might start pounding on the door in order to convey his demands in spite of repeated scolding.

To address the problem, the psychologist asked Christopher's parents to think of specific, alternative actions they would like Christopher to carry out under these conditions. At first, all Shelley and Greg could think of was "not interrupt," but Dr. Mitchell reminded them to think of a tangible alternative behavior for Christopher to carry out under the same circumstances. After some discussion, they came up with the idea of having Christopher write down his requests whenever his mother was on the phone. They noted that their son loved to write notes, so this might be a tangible thing he could do to satisfy his demands temporarily and allow him to resist interrupting. With further discussion, Christopher's parents and the psychologist worked out the following procedure: Before Shelley made a call or answered the phone, she would hand Christopher a special message pad, reminding him to write down any questions or problems that he had while she was talking; Shelley would then give prompt attention to Christopher's messages as soon as she was off the phone; finally, if Christopher succeeded in using the pad, instead of interrupting, for the majority of calls in a given week (his mother would keep a checklist to tabulate Christopher's compliance), he would be given a special reward on the weekend (such as eating out at his favorite restaurant).

This was the first behavioral plan that Christopher's parents put into effect, and after ironing out a few wrinkles, Christopher was able to follow the procedure, even to the point of getting the message pad himself whenever the phone rang. Eventually, he resisted interrupting almost entirely. The same approach was used to help reduce anxiety. They identified situations likely to increase anxiety, alternative behaviors they would like to reinforce, natural reinforcers for these more desirable behaviors, and a plan of action for training.

Other behavioral plans were then put into effect for other matters, such as household chores and homework completion. In both cases, Christopher's parents found an effective formula by reversing antecedent conditions and behavioral consequences. For example, they saw to it that video games would always follow the completion of homework rather than vice versa. Dr. Mitchell called it the Premack Principle, named after the person who noticed that to increase the likelihood of a low probability behavior (for example, homework), it must be followed by a high probability behavior (for example, video games). Eventually, with enough repetition, the probability of the less likely behavior will increase, because it is naturally reinforced by the higher probability and more pleasant behavior. Greg and Shelley both understood this in a simpler way. It was the same thing they learned when they were kids: to get your dessert, you have to eat your vegetables first. Eventually, vegetables get eaten without requiring dessert.

Social Skills Training   Shelley and Greg also enrolled their son in a class where he could learn skills for getting along better with other children. The class was composed of other children receiving treatment at the center for ADHD.

During each class the focus was on learning one particular social skill, such as sharing. First, the group leader explained the concept of sharing, and then asked the children their own opinions of what it meant. Next, she demonstrated the implementation of the skill with several children in different, contrived situations: sharing toys, sharing food, or sharing a seat. Then each child came up, one by one, and practiced sharing in each of these hypothetical circumstances. The group leader and the other children then gave corrective feedback on how well the child had shared. The group leader used modeling and positive reinforcement to increase the probability of a desirable behavior. Similar classes were devoted to other social skills, such as cooperating, speaking calmly, making polite requests, and following rules.

Christopher's parents and Ms. Freedman received written guidelines for discussing the social skills training sessions at home and in school and for guiding Christopher to use the skills in everyday situations. Many of the opportunities to help Christopher generalize his learning of new social skills from the group to his natural environment happened at home in his interactions with his younger sister and brother. With continued prompting, Christopher started to share things with them spontaneously on many occasions, which increased the harmony in the household.

Instructions from the group leaders also included skills to use to reduce anxiety. The group leader had taught every child to notice sensations in the body that are signs of feeling nervous, and to breathe through the belly to decrease these sensations. Christopher's parents and Ms. Freedman helped remind him to use these skills at home and in school, and eventually he started to do them on his own with little prompting.

Because of these successes, Shelley and Greg finally felt confident enough to invite one of Christopher's schoolmates over for a play date. The last time a child had come to their house, it had been a disaster, as Christopher had refused to relinquish any of his toys to his guest. Needless to say, no child was likely to return after such treatment. Although this play date was far from perfect and needed

> Almost 80% of all children and adolescents with ADHD receive treatment (CDC, 2020c).

Shelley's constant attention, it turned out to be reasonably pleasant. Christopher was less anxious, less impulsive, and better at cooperatively playing together with friends than his parents had ever seen.

Token Economy The token economy is an element of the ABC behavior modification system; it uses tokens, rather than immediate, tangible rewards, to reinforce desired behavior. The tokens are exchanged for an actual reward at a later time. Token reinforcement is particularly advantageous for children with ADHD, who can get so wrapped up in the attractiveness of the actual reward that they find it difficult to remain mindful of the behaviors that the reward is designed to encourage.

Christopher's teacher, Ms. Freedman, thought that some form of behavior modification might assist her in regulating several of his behaviors. Accordingly, she and the therapist decided to focus on encouraging three specific school behaviors in Christopher: raising his hand to speak in class (instead of blurting out his thoughts), staying in his seat during class, and finishing in-class assignments. As token reinforcers, Ms. Freedman would use dinosaur stickers affixed to a piece of paper, with the number of stickers in each of three columns reflecting Christopher's compliance with the three behavioral objectives. According to the plan (explained to Christopher in a meeting with his parents and Ms. Freedman), Ms. Freedman would keep track of Christopher's compliance separately for the morning period and the afternoon period, and award him one sticker if he achieved full compliance with a given behavioral objective in a given period. He would receive his morning stickers at lunchtime and his afternoon stickers upon dismissal. The stickers could then be redeemed at home for special privileges (going out to eat; going out to a movie; getting an extra half hour of television, time online, or gaming; and so forth).

Christopher liked the idea of getting stickers, so he agreed to the plan. On the first morning of the program, he received only one sticker: for finishing his assignment within the allotted time (he had blurted out a couple of answers and had gotten up and wandered around without permission). In the afternoon, however, he received two stickers: for staying in his seat and for finishing assignments.

After a few more days on the program, Christopher was showing substantial improvement in staying in his seat during lessons and finishing his in-class work on time, but he was still having some difficulties when it came to blurting out questions. Ms. Freedman noticed that Christopher's outbursts often seemed to be related to his anxious thoughts. When something in a lesson set Christopher off worrying, it seemed he had a hard time restraining himself from blurting out a question related to those worries. Ms. Freedman reminded Christopher to practice the breathing technique he had learned in his skills training. With this reminder, Christopher was eventually able to calm himself enough to raise his hand when

Many children with ADHD participate in eight-week therapeutic summer camps that apply systematic cognitive-behavioral principles and interventions (Low, 2021; Evans et al., 2019).

Children whose parents or other close relatives had ADHD are more likely than others to develop the disorder (APA, 2022, 2013).

he was worried about something rather than blurting out a question as soon as it came to him.

Within 2 months of the combined treatment program, Christopher had improved considerably. He was conforming to classroom rules by staying in his seat, not talking out of turn, and finishing his assignments most of the time. He was changing how he expressed his worries by asking questions more calmly. When he deviated, he required gentle reminders from Ms. Freedman to get back on track. Similarly, at home, he was less frenetic. He could carry out instructions more dependably, and he usually accepted his household responsibilities without too much argument. In peer relations, Christopher was still learning the culture of give and take, but with periodic guidance and further experience he was becoming increasingly effective. As a result, he was getting along better with his sister and brother, and he now had a couple of friends who would come over sometimes to play, and who invited him to their homes as well.

Unfortunately, after about 4 months of this improved functioning, Christopher began to slip into some of his old patterns both at home and at school. His parents felt that the problems had to be addressed, as he seemed to be losing ground. The recurrence of problems seemed to coincide with the family moving to a new house. In a discussion with Dr. Collins, Christopher's parents wondered whether their preoccupation with moving, and their consequent inability to implement many features of the behavioral program (including not following through on redeeming Christopher's dinosaur stickers), was responsible for the slippage in his progress. A renewed effort by the parents to apply the behavioral program, and an adjustment in the dosage of Christopher's medication, helped him to regain his previous achievements within a few weeks.

Epilogue

As many as 60% of individuals who have relatively severe symptoms of ADHD through adolescence continue to have ADHD as adults (Bukstein, 2021a, 2021b; Nylander et al., 2021). The symptoms of restlessness and overactivity are not usually as pronounced in adult cases.

After 18 sessions of group parent training (over a 6-month period), six sessions of individual parent training, six sessions of social skills training for Christopher, and four meetings at school with Christopher's teacher, his ADHD symptoms stabilized at an improved level, as measured by the same battery of questionnaires that were administered before treatment started.

Christopher reported that he was happier at school and enjoying time at home with his family. He was less anxious as well, as observed by his parents and Ms. Freedman. He still took medication and saw Dr. Collins for a checkup every 4 months. Christopher's parents planned to give Christopher a drug holiday in the summer and felt confident of their ability to manage his behavior during that time with just the behavioral techniques. They were a family again—sometimes laughing, sometimes crying—but, overall, enjoying their lives and activities together more than ever before.

Assessment Questions

1. When did Christopher's parents begin to suspect that Christopher's "dynamo" personality might be a psychological disorder?

2. Describe at least three behaviors that suggested Christopher's activity level was beyond what's normal for a child his age.

3. When did Christopher's family finally receive more objective feedback about his behavior?

4. How long did it take for Christopher's teachers to suggest professional consultation regarding his disruptive behavior?

5. Why did Dr. Collins, the psychiatrist at the Ripple Center, feel it was important to conduct a thorough assessment of Christopher before diagnosing ADHD?

6. Describe at least four different assessment techniques used by Dr. Collins to test for ADHD.

7. What were the assessment results that led Dr. Collins to diagnose ADHD for Christopher?

8. Why did Dr. Collins decide to use both medication and behavioral therapy to treat Christopher?

9. What are some potential problems with prescribing medication as the only treatment option for children with ADHD? What are some side effects of stimulant medications?

10. Describe the ABC model of behavioral therapy and give examples.

11. What were the four treatment components outlined for Christopher's treatment?

12. Why was it important for Christopher's parents to be a part of the treatment plan?

13. Describe the ABC plan that Christopher's parents developed to control his "interrupting" behaviors.

14. What other childhood psychological disorders often accompany ADHD?

15. Describe the concept of a token economy.

16. What event disrupted Christopher's progress?

17. What was the ultimate outcome after 18 sessions of group parent training?

CASE 17

Autism Spectrum Disorder

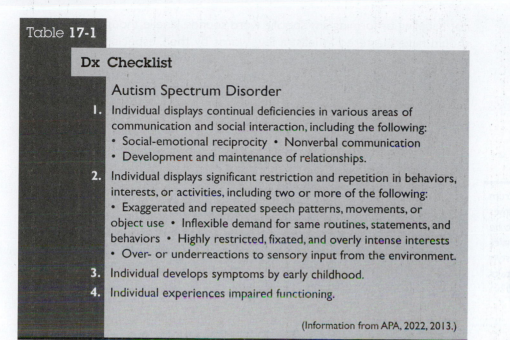

Table 17-1

Dx Checklist

Autism Spectrum Disorder

1. Individual displays continual deficiencies in various areas of communication and social interaction, including the following:
   • Social-emotional reciprocity • Nonverbal communication • Development and maintenance of relationships.

2. Individual displays significant restriction and repetition in behaviors, interests, or activities, including two or more of the following:
   • Exaggerated and repeated speech patterns, movements, or object use • Inflexible demand for same routines, statements, and behaviors • Highly restricted, fixated, and overly intense interests • Over- or underreactions to sensory input from the environment.

3. Individual develops symptoms by early childhood.

4. Individual experiences impaired functioning.

(Information from APA, 2022, 2013.)

Jameer was born into a middle-class young suburban family in a small town outside Fayetteville, Arkansas. His parents, both Black and from rural Arkansas, were Janelle, aged 23, and Antoine, aged 34. Janelle's pregnancy was full-term, the delivery was normal, and the baby weighed 8 pounds, 2 ounces. Janelle and Antoine also had another child, Jaquon, who was 6 years older than Jameer. Jameer was handsome, with brown hair, brown eyes, and a beautiful smile. The parents looked forward to an exciting future, filled with the dreams that having two children can inspire.

Jameer's development over the first year of his life was normal. He was able to sit without support by 7 months, crawl at 10 months, and stand alone by 12 months. He took his first independent step at 15 months and was walking everywhere within a week. All visits to the pediatrician went well, and immunizations were given at the appropriate times.

> At least 1 in 60 persons display autism spectrum disorder (Augustyn, 2020; Styles et al., 2020). Just two decades ago, the disorder was thought to affect 1 in 2,000 persons.

Jameer A Toddler with Troubles

After Jameer's first birthday party, to which several young children were invited, Janelle began to pay attention to some characteristics of her son's personality that just didn't seem to match those of the other children his age. Unlike the other toddlers, or even his brother when he had been a year old, Jameer was not babbling or forming any specific word sounds. Janelle thought that her son should have mastered at least a few words by then, especially after hearing other 1-year-olds say "mama" and "dada" and "cookie." Jameer could only produce a few noises, which he would utter randomly throughout the day. Janelle also noticed that these sounds were rarely directed toward anyone or anything. The child made no attempt to label people or objects; he would just make those noises.

At first, Janelle and Antoine attributed Jameer's language delay to the fact that he had an older brother who would speak for him and fulfill many of his needs without Jameer ever having to ask. But they soon became suspicious that a language delay was only part of the problem. At the birthday party and in other situations, Jameer seemed uninterested in playing with other children or even being around them socially. He seemed to enjoy everyone singing "Happy Birthday" to him, but he made no attempt to blow out the candles on the cake, even after others modeled this tradition for him. He was only a year old, but his indifference to the party bothered Janelle and Antoine.

Upon closer examination, his parents also noticed that Jameer had very few interests. He would seek out only one toy, even though his parents had purchased many for him, and his older brother had his as well. They shared a bedroom, so it was odd that Jameer never showed any interest in Jaquon's toys. If pushed to play with something new, he would sometimes throw intense, inconsolable tantrums. Often, he would take his favorite toy, a plastic dog, and stare it for a long time. His parents bought another one, then two more, so that he had four of these dogs. Sure enough, Jameer would play only with these toys, lining them up in a row, in the same order, and would not allow them to be removed until he decided he was finished with them. If someone attempted to rearrange or clear away the toys, he would again have a tantrum.

As her concern grew, Janelle decided to monitor her son's play habits more closely. She was both frightened and amazed at the meticulous way in which he manipulated the toys. On a few occasions, she realized that the order in which he aligned them matched the order in which they had been purchased. They were clean and free of any blemishes, and Jameer would take painstaking care in looking at all of their surface area each time he took them out.

He also had a marked preference for being with his mother. He had less of an interest in Antoine, Jaquon, or other people. In fact, Jameer might cry for hours if Janelle had to leave without him. Upon her return, he would stop crying but would not necessarily want to be with her. He would feel content knowing that she was home and go back to playing with his toys by himself. In addition, when called by either parent, Jameer often failed to respond to his name. And he displayed odd food preferences: He could not seem to get enough of some foods, and he simply could not tolerate the textures of others.

> Autism spectrum disorder is four times more likely to be diagnosed in males than females (Augustyn, 2020; Autism Speaks, 2020).

As the months went by and he remained unable to express his wants and needs, Jameer's tantrums became more frequent. If his mother did not understand his noises and gestures, he would grow angry at not being understood. The intensity of these episodes was also growing; Jameer was even beginning to hit his ears with his hands and cry for longer and longer periods. One of the most frightening aspects of this for Janelle was the fact that her misinterpretations of the episodes might sometimes endanger Jameer's health; she had no way of knowing if he had an upset stomach, a headache, or some other ailment.

Finally, when Jameer was 19 months old, Janelle took him to his pediatrician for some answers. The doctor agreed that there were some significant "delays" in Jameer's development, and he referred the child to a neurologist for a complete evaluation. The recommendation of a neurologist greatly upset Janelle and Antoine. They were now forced to confront their deepest fears. They found it extremely difficult to wait for the neurological evaluation, repeatedly dwelling on the terrible scenarios that the word *delay* evoked.

Prior to the appointment with the neurologist, the parents also followed up on the pediatrician's recommendation that they have Jameer's hearing formally tested. His hearing was found to be within normal range, and this news caused a mixed reaction in his parents. On one hand, they were happy that serious hearing deficits could be ruled out; on the other hand, where did that leave them? The results left many questions in their minds. Also prior to the neurological evaluation, Janelle and Antoine began to research the term *developmental delays* on the Internet; there, for the first time, they saw the word *disability*. When the time for Jameer's appointment with the neurologist finally arrived, they were extremely frightened, but they also still held out hope that Jameer's skills were just a little late in coming.

> Most of today's theorists believe that autism spectrum disorder is caused by biological factors, although many of the precise biological causes are not yet fully known (Ayub et al., 2021; Augustyn, 2020; Su et al., 2020).

Jameer Parents' Fears Confirmed

The neurologist was pleasant and very thorough. She reviewed the case history from pregnancy through birth, and then assessed Jameer's milestone achievements. She also completed physical, neurological, and motor examinations. Finally, she addressed his language delays and maladaptive behaviors by observing his lack of speech and his limited play skills. For all the weeks of waiting for this examination, it seemed to pass very quickly—almost too quickly, the parents believed, for the doctor really to get to know Jameer. In fact, she was able to gather a great deal of information, and she told Janelle and Antoine that Jameer seemed to have autism spectrum disorder.

Autism spectrum disorder is a neurodevelopmental disorder with a range of symptoms that can occur at various levels of severity. The neurologist cited several factors that led to her tentative diagnosis of autism spectrum disorder in Jameer: his deficits in social communication, including his nonverbal communication; his severely delayed receptive and expressive language skills; his lack of imaginative play with toys; and his history of repeated and rigid behaviors. In short, all of the things Janelle, Antoine, and several other family members had noticed were symptoms of this disorder.

A diagnosis of autism spectrum disorder had been his parents' worst fear, after having read so much about its different forms during their research. From the information they had gathered, they had formed a mental image of an aggressive or self-injurious child, locked in his own world and unable to communicate. Antoine began to tune out as the doctor described the typical features of the disorder. Too many questions were pounding inside his head: Should they get a second opinion? Could it possibly be as bad as she was describing? Whose fault was it? Why hadn't the pediatrician said something sooner? How would Janelle handle this? What would the rest of the family say? What was the cure?

By the time Antoine was able to focus again, the visit was over, and the neurologist was talking about her forthcoming report and discussing her recommendations. He heard her explain that, with appropriate early interventions and services, the disorder was "workable," and that because Jameer was starting treatment at such a young age, he had a great deal of potential for progress. Antoine couldn't imagine how this devastating problem might be workable. He knew that on the long car ride home he would have to be filled in on the missing pieces of the doctor's conversation with Janelle.

> Treatments for individuals with autism spectrum disorder tend to provide the most benefit when started early in the individual's life (Tseng et al., 2020).

Jameer Getting Started

Janelle took charge and played a more active role than Antoine in following up on the recommendations of the neurologist. In part this was because she stayed at home with the boys, while Antoine worked full-time at the county courthouse as a security officer. However, it was also because she felt she needed to stay busy to keep negative thoughts and mounting questions out of her mind. Antoine, who was feeling overwhelmed by the weight of the diagnosis, simply followed his wife's lead.

The first course of action was to have Jameer more fully and precisely evaluated and to have him begin early intervention services. And it was important that these services be provided by clinicians who specialized in the field of autism spectrum disorder. After consulting an advocacy group for individuals with developmental disabilities, Janelle learned of an early intervention center affiliated with the university. She scheduled an evaluation. Six weeks after seeing the neurologist, Jameer received a comprehensive evaluation and began treatment at the Kreutzman Child Development Center.

From this point forward, the family's lifestyle became a whirlwind of doctors' visits and a variety of therapies. The initial diagnostic evaluation itself was completed in 90 minutes. One clinician interviewed the parents, while a second took Jameer to a separate room for an individual assessment. They explained diagnostic and rating scales to the parents, including the DSM-5-TR criteria, the Modified Checklist for Autism in Toddlers—Revised, and the Childhood Autism Rating Scale. All of Jameer's delays and behaviors were specifically categorized and totaled to arrive at a detailed clinical picture and diagnosis.

Consistent with the DSM-5-TR criteria for autism spectrum disorder, Jameer showed impairment in social communication and social interaction, including marked impairment in the use of nonverbal behaviors such as eye-to-eye gaze; failure to develop peer relationships typical of his developmental level; and lack of social or emotional reciprocity. He also showed restricted and repetitive patterns of behavior, interests, and activities, including stereotyped motor movements (e.g., lining up toys); abnormal preoccupations and inflexible adherence to specific, nonfunctional routines or rituals; a strong attachment or preoccupation with unusual objects; and either hyperreactivity or hyporeactivity to sensory input or unusual interest in the sensory aspects of the environment (APA, 2022, 2013). His symptoms were present in early childhood, caused impairment in his life, and could not be accounted for by any other disorder.

Based on the Childhood Autism Rating Scale assessment, Jameer's autism spectrum disorder was rated between Level 1 ("requiring support") and Level 2 ("requiring substantial support"), in terms of social communication and restricted, repetitive behaviors. It was also specified in his diagnosis that Jameer's autism spectrum disorder was with accompanying intellectual impairment and with accompanying language impairment. He displayed a number of symptoms from the rating scale's 15 areas of assessment, including relating to people, imitation, emotional response, object use, visual and listening response, adaptation to change, verbal and nonverbal communication, and intellectual response. Slowly, these terms were starting to have more meaning to Janelle and Antoine. The diagnostic team at the center concluded that early intervention was certainly the treatment of choice at this point, and they helped the parents set up a variety of therapies for their son.

Jameer was enrolled in the center's *early intervention program*, which provided 3 hours of behavioral therapy each week: 2 hours at the center itself and 1 hour at home. The goal of these behavioral sessions was to help the child develop *learning readiness skills*—basic skills that one needs in order to be able to learn and acquire broader knowledge, behaviors, or skills. Jameer would be taught skills such as focusing his attention where directed, and following simple instructions. Again and again, in trial after trial, he would be rewarded whenever he performed these target behaviors or some approximation of them, and not rewarded if he failed to perform them. It was expected that through such efforts, the child would become increasingly able and willing to perform the behaviors across a

A diagnosis of autism spectrum disorder can feature a range of neurodevelopmental disturbances. Thus to help clarify an individual's particular pattern of the disorder, DSM-5-TR lists various *specifiers*—specific features of that individual's disorder that are to be cited as part of the diagnosis.

wide range of situations and, in turn, be more ready to learn broader behaviors and skills.

These sessions were to follow the principles of the *applied behavior analysis model*—a strict behavioral strategy that, according to research, helps many persons with autism spectrum disorder and other neurodevelopmental disorders. Jameer was also signed up for speech therapy 2 days a week and for occupational therapy 1 day a week. Ultimately, the three therapies all sought to increase his ability to engage new people. Janelle and Antoine felt incredibly grateful for their ability to access these services. In the rural town where they grew up, there were no such clinics or specialists. Antoine's job with the state government brought them to Fayetteville, where there were so many more resources to help them than they had back home. They were relieved, too, because his work enabled them to have high-quality health insurance, something they both knew was a privilege, having been raised on food stamps and enrolled in Medicaid as children.

> Applied behavior analysis is considered by most clinicians to be the single most efficacious intervention for autism spectrum disorder (Rodgers et al., 2021; Autism Speaks, 2020).

The child's life was turned upside down by the early intervention program. Strangers were now being thrown into his world on a rotating basis, and these people were placing demands on him and changing his routines. He was also being separated from his mother in a strange place for the first time ever. During the first few therapy sessions, Janelle wanted to run from the observation room into the treatment room to "rescue" him from the therapist. Jameer cried and threw tantrums throughout those sessions. The therapist continually had to reassure Janelle that the child would become less resistant as long as the sessions were carried out consistently. Otherwise, the distraught mother would have withdrawn him from the program and tried teaching him herself.

Slowly, Jameer's tears and tantrums lessened as his therapy sessions became a regular part of his weekly schedule. Janelle and Antoine began to notice, after 2 months, a slight increase in his eye contact and less resistance when they asked him to complete specific tasks within the home, such as clearing away his figurines after he was finished playing. Nevertheless, his progress felt unbearably slow to them, and they noticed no developments in the area of language, despite the speech therapist's positive reports. Jameer also remained unreceptive to all new toys, and his play skills continued to be very limited.

> In order to help children with autism spectrum disorder to speak, teachers often supplement their speech therapy with another form of communication, including sign language and simultaneous communication, a method that combines sign language and speech.

Janelle and Antoine decided to supplement the center's early intervention sessions by hiring therapists on a private basis to provide more learning trials at home, as well as scheduling additional speech therapy sessions. In fact, it was the speech therapy that was of most interest to the couple. They believed that if they could just help their son talk, they could better understand what he was feeling and, in turn, could more effectively resolve his other issues.

The in-home private therapy was difficult at first as Jameer could not bear having his home routine disrupted even more. But the in-home therapists persevered and tried to apply their services consistently. Like the center's program, the supplemental learning trials focused on learning readiness and on teaching Jameer to identify and manipulate various objects. In their work, the therapists selected objects that were particularly relevant to the child's home environment: chairs, eating utensils, and light switches, for example. When they incorporated dogs into the sessions, based on Jameer's special interest in dogs, the learning tended to go even better. Nevertheless, progress continued to be slow.

The speech therapists — those at the clinic and at home — worked together on several aspects of Jameer's speech. First, they did exercises with his mouth ("Open your mouth wide") and tongue ("Stick out your tongue") to strengthen muscles that are typically needed in speech. Second, they used imitation training to help Jameer create sounds, for example, the sounds "mmm" or "babababa." Finally, they sought to develop a working communication system that would enable him to convey his wants and needs. Everyone agreed that establishing a communication system for Jameer was the priority because if he could communicate better his needs could be better met and his tantrums would likely decrease. The speech therapists decided that it would be best to introduce a basic Picture Exchange Communication System — a system in which Jameer could point to or select pictures to help express himself.

At first his parents were opposed to this system. Antoine, in particular, feared that Jameer would come to rely solely on these pictures. He believed that unless his son were required to speak or at least make sounds in order to receive items, he would have little chance of learning to speak. The therapists explained, however, that many children with language processing problems like Jameer's initially learn better with a visual representation of the desired items. Eventually, the children come to appreciate that pictures of items can bring about the items themselves, and they grasp that there is a connection between their thoughts and their environment. Moreover, by helping the children to communicate their needs, the use of pictures reduces their frustrations and tantrums, thus creating a more positive environment for learning verbal skills. Although hesitant, Janelle and Antoine agreed to give the picture system a try.

At the same time, though, their worries continued to grow. Jameer was now 2 years old and continuing to grow physically but was without language and with only limited cognitive understanding. Their other son, Jaquon, had called for "mama" and "dada" long before his second birthday, and Jameer could not even imitate the "m" sound. Privately, they questioned how hard the therapists were really working and whether Jameer was being given enough hours of therapy. Maybe there was more that they could do with him at home. Before long, he would be 3 years old, and if this trend continued, they would have to seek placement in a specialized full-day program.

Clinicians and educators may also turn to *augmentative communication systems* for individuals with autism spectrum disorder, systems in which the persons are taught to express their needs and thoughts by pointing to pictures, symbols, letters, or words on a communication board or computer.

Janelle and Antoine What Else Can We Do?

Janelle began to investigate other interventions that she had heard about, just to see if anything out there could make a difference. One of the most talked about treatments that she came across was diet change—eliminating certain foods from Jameer's diet, foods with ingredients that some autistic children have trouble tolerating. In particular, Janelle read on the Internet that a gluten-free diet was helpful in many cases of autism spectrum disorder. Apparently, some children with autism spectrum disorder are unable to properly digest gluten (a protein found in wheat), leading many clinicians to speculate that gluten may contribute to inappropriate behaviors, perhaps by causing great discomfort. Janelle read that children like Jameer who eliminated most breads, pastries, crackers, snacks, and the like from their diets sometimes showed significant improvements in their behavior. Although she knew that the outcome of this approach would be uncertain, that it would be challenging to find appropriate foods that Jameer would tolerate, and that many children with autism spectrum disorder failed to respond to such diet changes, she felt that she must try everything in her power to reverse Jameer's delays. Otherwise, she would be failing him and perhaps missing the one intervention that could make a difference. Janelle and Antoine found a nutritionist familiar with the diet at the center. Wanting to be as objective as possible, they decided to give the dietary changes a year, with an assessment of his skills both before and after that year's time.

The whirlwind that their lives had become was continuing. Jameer's older brother, now 8 years old, was beginning to show signs of resentment for the amount of attention that his brother was receiving. Janelle and Antoine did their best to create special activities for Jaquon, but in fact, Jameer's therapies did take most of their time and energy. Time was passing, still with none of the vast improvements Janelle and Antoine were hoping for.

When Jameer reached 2½ years of age, the couple decided to sign him up for *auditory integration training*. They suspected that Jameer, like a number of children with autism spectrum disorder, might be *hypersensitive* in the auditory sphere. That is, he might have sensory-perceptual difficulties that cause certain sounds or tones to feel particularly unpleasant, making it difficult for him to listen to and process the words and noises within his environment. Auditory integration training is a procedure in which individuals wear headphones that actually alter (for example, soften) certain auditory inputs, making sounds more comfortable and, theoretically, improving the individuals' capacity to process what they are hearing. Although some children with autism spectrum disorder greatly improve their language capabilities with this training, Jameer showed no such improvement. Once again, his parents were disappointed. They were trying everything they could. "What else can we do?" Antoine would ask the doctors, his friends, even the pastor at their church.

Some people with autism spectrum disorder seem overstimulated by sights and sounds and try to block them out, while others seem understimulated and perform behaviors that may add to their stimulation, such as flapping their arms, cupping their hands so that they can scream in their ears, or rapidly moving their fingers before their eyes.

Bigger Child, Bigger Problems

Even with all of his interventions at the child development center and at home, Jameer continued to develop into a challenging child. His fascination with dogs remained strong and was now joined by an added interest in other animals. If he were left alone, animal toys would occupy him for hours, but again, he didn't play with them in the usual manner. The lining up of the toys continued, and the newer animals had to be carefully stacked according to how recently they were added to his collection, with the pattern always identical, from oldest to newest, right to left. His preference for certain routines and patterns became even stronger as he grew older; increasingly, these routines were dominating the family's schedule.

For example, Jameer was now in the habit of having his bath before going to sleep, and it had to be given by Janelle. For his first 2 years, this set procedure had been easy enough to carry out. But as Jameer's brother, Jaquon, grew older, he often needed his mother's help with homework. Moreover, Janelle had to attend more and more parent groups or conferences regarding Jameer. When someone other than Janelle had to give Jameer his bath, or if a bath had to be skipped altogether, he would throw a major tantrum, followed by poor sleep throughout the night. To avoid this situation, Janelle and Antoine found themselves scheduling as many activities, meetings, and outings as possible around the daily bath ritual. Recognizing that their lives had become thoroughly constrained by the child's rigid routines, the couple came to realize that they needed help with their son's home behaviors every bit as much as with his educational goals.

As Jameer grew older still and encountered new milestones, he revealed delays in yet other areas—producing further difficulties at home. Janelle was uncertain how to begin toilet training him, for example, since he showed no understanding regarding how and where to go. She was also unsuccessful in teaching him to brush his teeth. The first and last time she tried, Jameer became extremely upset and resistant, as his oral sensitivities to certain textures made the activity particularly uncomfortable for him. As his frustrations grew, Jameer's tantrums also got worse, both in intensity and in duration. Some days he would hit his ears so hard that Janelle feared he might be damaging them.

Still another difficulty for the family was their inability to manage their growing son's behaviors out in the community. They were unsure from one outing to the next how he would behave in a grocery store, mall, or restaurant. Sometimes, accidentally leaving a toy figurine at home would spark a tantrum so loud, upsetting, and embarrassing that Janelle and Antoine would be afraid to ever return to the store or restaurant. Family outings kept decreasing and eventually became a rarity—the very opposite of the family lifestyle the couple had always hoped for.

Jameer at 4 Beginning School

As Jameer approached 4 years of age, his parents realized that a full-day program was needed. Once again, it fell on Janelle's shoulders to find the best such program. Antoine was feeling depressed by his son's slow progress and by the position in which his family now found itself. This was not how he had envisioned his future. Since his wife seemed better able to handle everything, he decided that his role should be limited to that of breadwinner—working very hard to earn the extra income needed for all of Jameer's therapies. Thankfully, they lived in a state where their insurance company was mandated to include applied behavior analysis in their health insurance plan. And, to make things better, he was able to work a part-time job in security at a government facility on some weekends and evenings. Still, there was never enough money, and some of the health services needed were not covered by insurance, causing great financial strain. This meant that they could not have all of the things they wanted, or go to the places they wanted to go. The financial stress meant Jaquon was unable to attend camps in the summer, and was unable to have the things he wanted to have as a child. It was all taking an enormous toll on the family.

> In the 1940s and 1950s, it was believed that autism spectrum disorder was the result of "refrigerator parents." However, research has overwhelmingly failed to support a picture of rigid, cold, rejecting, or disturbed parents (Augustyn, 2020; Lerner et al., 2018).

Janelle insisted that Antoine accompany her on tours of full-day school programs for children with autism spectrum disorder. Although they focused primarily on preschool programs, they were also provided with information about how such programs would set the stage for Jameer's later years—if he were still to need services 5 years down the road. The more they spoke with professionals, the better equipped they became for Jameer's next few years. They started to see how the various early intervention services they had been providing would now come into play for their child as he entered a full-day program, and how the full-day services would help with later educational and vocational programs. They also learned about behavior management strategies that the family might be able to use to help deal with Jameer's increasing demands and routines. In fact, the discussions with professionals at the prospective schools helped Antoine emerge from his depressive state and take a few more steps toward acceptance of his son's disability.

The search for the best full-day program eventually led Antoine and Janelle to two schools. At each school, they were given a tour, an application form, and an appointment for an intake interview. The intake process was similar at each school: The director of the program would interview the parents, while three or four other professionals would take Jameer into a separate area to assess his skills and behaviors.

By this point, Janelle had already contacted her school district about Jameer's diagnosis and his need for specialized instruction. The district's officials had set up an appointment as well, completed their own assessment of Jameer, and assigned him a case manager and a child study team. The school district's involvement was necessary because it was they who would have to provide, or pay for, any special educational services that Jameer might need during his school years. The officials were supportive of Janelle's search for an appropriate outside program, as they themselves had a minimal number of preschool classrooms equipped for the special needs of students with autism spectrum disorder or other pervasive developmental disorders.

The school district's psychological and social profiles were added to the evaluations by the neurologist and the early intervention therapists to form a referral packet that Janelle took with her to interviews at the special preschool programs. She was pleased, and relieved, that this part of the process had gone so well, as she had heard many other parents describe the enormous difficulties they had encountered trying to convince their school districts' child study teams to find special programming.

The first school at which Janelle and Antoine made an appointment had an exceptional reputation and had been highly recommended by several other parents to whom they had grown close. The school's enrollment was small—a total of 30 students—and its teaching strategies followed the applied behavior analysis principles Janelle and Antoine had come to know so well from Jameer's early intervention therapists. Days at this school were very structured, and there was an ongoing effort to *mainstream* students into less-restrictive environments.

> **Mainstreaming** is the placement of children with special needs and disorders in regular school classes with children who do not have those special needs.

This first interview was the most difficult, since Jameer's parents had to convey all of their hopes and dreams for Jameer to a complete stranger. It was also painful for them to observe while Jameer had a tantrum when he was separated from them for his skills assessment. The director asked questions about Jameer's history, the family's history, and how the young child was responding to the early intervention services he was receiving. Janelle and Antoine tried to fit every piece of relevant information they could think of into the short hour of the interview, but left feeling as if there was much more to say.

For Jameer, this was yet another set of strangers placing demands on him in a completely new environment. The people assessing his skills at this first school included a special-education teacher, a speech therapist, and an occupational therapist. They completed a checklist of his skills, as well as his maladaptive behaviors. Their assessment agreed with previous findings that the absence of language or a formal communication system, along with Jameer's problematic behaviors, would necessitate a preschool program with special teaching techniques, including a continuation of the slow, trial-by-trial teaching program that Jameer had slowly been responding to with his early intervention therapists. An opening would be available at this school in September, and Janelle and Antoine were told that Jameer was among several candidates applying for this opening. The parents would be contacted within the next 3 weeks.

The interview at the second school was much like the first. This school, however, was run by the Kreutzman Child Development Center and so was closely affiliated with the early intervention program that Jameer had been attending for almost a year. Janelle and Antoine felt a bit more comfortable in this interview because they knew that Jameer's behavioral therapist at the center would be stopping in to check on his assessment, and because they had already met the director at one of the parent training sessions offered by the center a few months earlier.

Again, the interview seemed too short to convey Jameer's entire story, but Janelle and Antoine made sure to express their interest in a behavioral-based program that would address every aspect of Jameer's learning potential. By now, they recognized the value of learning programs in which tasks—all tasks, from toilet training to speaking—were broken down into the simplest possible steps to be learned one at a time. The consistent application of such learning programs over the past year had in fact produced some results. Jameer could now maintain eye contact and sit appropriately for longer periods, as opposed to the fleeting glances and constant movements of past times. He could wave hello and goodbye on command, a skill that helped bring him closer to his family. And his skill with the Picture Exchange Communication System was beginning to emerge; he was using pictures to convey five of his most desired items. Although the progress seemed a long time in coming and was far behind what Janelle and Antoine had expected of Jameer by the age of 4, the fact remained that his improvement had begun, and they wanted to see it continue.

When asked about Jameer's diet, the couple had mixed feelings. In Antoine's opinion, Jameer's special foods had not really brought about much change, and it was hard to keep him on these foods now that he was aware that his older brother was eating, and enjoying, different—often very tasty—foods. Food stealing had become a mealtime issue at home, and Antoine wondered whether it might be a problem at school lunches as well. On the opposite side, Janelle speculated that Jameer's steady, if slow, progress might be due in part to this special diet, and so she wanted to give it more time. The school was familiar with the gluten-free diet, as several students were currently following it. Thus, Janelle and Antoine's ultimate decision regarding the diet would not affect his placement at the school.

At this school, there were four candidates applying for the two openings available in September. Three of the four applicants had been receiving early intervention services at the center's associated program, and all had individual needs warranting specialized services. This decision would also be made within a few weeks, and once again Janelle and Antoine were forced to wait.

While awaiting the letters of acceptance or rejection, the parents reviewed the various scenarios they might be facing. They actually preferred the second school—the one run by the Kreutzman Child Development Center—because they were already familiar with the school's policies and staff members. They

> Studies indicate that many people with autism spectrum disorder have deficits in their ability to employ a *theory of mind*. That is, they have poor awareness that the other persons with whom they are interacting will base their behaviors on their own perspective rather than on the perspective of the individual with autism (Lecheler et al., 2020).

believed that the transition there would be the easiest for Jameer, as well as for them. On the other hand, they felt that if he were accepted at the first school as well, they might have to accept that placement, given the sterling reputation of that program. With either school, Antoine and Janelle knew that they would continue at least some of Jameer's in-home therapy. They were prepared to do whatever it took to help their son reach his potential during these early years. At the same time, they understood the risk of overloading a child once full-day programming started.

They didn't even want to think of the possibility of being rejected from both schools. If Jameer were not accepted by either program, the school district child study team, by law, would be responsible for finding an appropriate placement for him. Janelle and Antoine feared that the team might place him in a preschool program that was designed for children less impaired than Jameer. Although at the earlier meetings and evaluations, the team's case manager had seemed caring and aware of Jameer's severe limitations, Janelle remained on the alert, having heard so many horror stories from other parents.

The letters from both schools came within a day of each other, a rejection from the first school and then an acceptance from the Kreutzman Center. Janelle and Antoine were overjoyed and overwhelmed by the emotional roller coaster ride that they experienced within a 24-hour period. If asked 5 years before how rejection from one preschool program and acceptance at another would make them feel, they would completely have underestimated the effect it would have. They found it impossible to sleep the night between the receipt of those letters. But now, with Jameer's enrollment in the school that had links to his early intervention services, a school that already knew him, his parents felt a weight lifted off their shoulders.

For the first time in quite a while, they felt a sense of hope. They focused less on the many things that Jameer could not do and felt more empowered by the things that he might be able to do in a proper program. With full-day, trial-by-trial learning, behavioral management strategies, and one-to-one student-to-teacher ratios, Jameer was going to be given an opportunity to work through his disorder to reach his fullest potential. Although Janelle and Antoine were still far from fully accepting Jameer's disability, especially its lifelong implications, they were a step closer to understanding Jameer and enhancing his life.

His enrollment in the new program was only 2 months away, and a number of decisions had to be made. Janelle had some transportation concerns but was told that that responsibility fell to Jameer's case manager. That is, it was the responsibility of the school district to arrange Jameer's transportation to and from this school. She and Antoine decided to continue with Jameer's special diet for another 6 months and to then make a further decision about it after seeing how the new school was progressing. Finally, they decided to discontinue the behavioral

> The pattern of autism was first identified by the psychiatrist Leo Kanner in 1943.

therapy at home for 6 months after the new school program began. The behavioral program at the school would be intense, and additional behavioral therapy at home might create burnout and hinder Jameer's progress. On the other hand, they decided to continue his in-home speech therapy program, even though he would be receiving individual speech sessions four times a week at the new full-day program.

The month prior to enrollment, the school's program coordinator put together a parents' information and training session for Janelle and Antoine. This meeting provided them with an introduction to the school's executive director, a review of the school's policies and procedures, and a chance to meet their son's classroom teacher and teaching assistants. There would be five other students in the class, all between the ages of 3 and 6 years old. Janelle and Antoine learned that, in fact, a series of *parent-training* sessions would follow that at least one of them would be required to attend. The family would also be assigned a home-program consultant — a staff member who would visit their home on a regular basis to help them identify, prioritize, and manage home issues one at a time.

Jameer's enrollment in this school program also had an important advantage that Antoine and Janelle really didn't want to think much about at this point: the opportunity for *life-span services*. Although students with severe autism spectrum disorder graduate from school at age 21, they typically have needs that last a lifetime. Recognizing these potential needs, Jameer's new school had expanded its services. They offered workshop training and placement for adults with autism spectrum disorder. They also ran several *group homes* in which persons with autism spectrum disorder live in a house under the supervision of staff members. Their typical group home had eight residents and four supervisors. The needs of an adult Jameer were a long way off, and his parents decided that they would cross that bridge when they came to it. Nevertheless, it was reassuring to know that such services would be there when the time came.

> Individual therapy and support groups are also widely available to help the parents of children with autism spectrum disorder address their own emotions and needs, particularly those tied to their children's difficulties (Mills et al., 2020; Da Paz & Wallander, 2017).

Jameer at School A New Start

Jameer's first day of school came, and off he went on a school van. He always enjoyed car rides, so Janelle hoped that that his enjoyment would overcome his anxiety at being separated from her. She had also provided him with a new set of his favorite animal figurines to keep him occupied during the ride. She decided to follow the van on its 40-minute journey to the school, taking care to keep her distance so that Jameer would not spot her car. Once he arrived safely at the school, Janelle watched as his teacher took him off the bus and escorted him into the building.

All day she expected a phone call saying that she would have to retrieve Jameer because his tantrums were inconsolable or because he was too disruptive in the class. But no phone call came, and the van dropped Jameer off at the end of the day. The note from his teacher described a typical first day — with some tears and some smiles. The note also indicated that Jameer had been able to successfully carry over some of the behaviors and skills that he had acquired in the early intervention program. Janelle felt reassured that she had underestimated her son's coping abilities; at least the first day of school was a positive experience.

The first few months were ones of transition. Jameer's sleep pattern was disrupted for a while. He had to wake up an hour earlier than he was used to; this caused him to nap on the bus ride home, making it hard for him to fall asleep at the proper time later in the evening. But with the consistent application of his new schedule and the assistance of the home-program consultant assigned to the family, he came to accept his new routine, and the family was able to move on to other issues.

The next few months of Jameer's full-day school program were devoted primarily to helping him carry over gains that he had made previously in the early intervention program. The new school program also introduced several self-care skills during the early months. Jameer's teacher even introduced toilet training within 2 weeks of his starting at the school, wanting to establish this skill as early as possible. He started what the school called a "5-minute schedule." He was directed to sit on a potty seat for 1 to 2 minutes, then was returned to a regular session of activity for 5 minutes, then directed back to the potty seat, and so on. Throughout the procedure, he was given extra fluids, which meant that he would have many opportunities to go to the bathroom. Whenever Jameer successfully used the potty, he was rewarded with his favorite cookie. Over time, the number of toilet successes increased and the number of accidents decreased, and the teacher was able to slowly expand the length of the intervals between potty sittings. Jameer was on his way to being toilet trained.

> Despite continuing claims in some circles, virtually all relevant research conducted in this century has argued against the theory that autism spectrum disorder is caused by the measles, mumps, rubella (MMR) vaccine (Augustyn, 2020).

In October, Janelle and Antoine met with all of the key persons in Jameer's school program to discuss the goals and objectives for the coming year. The participants at the meeting included Jameer's case manager, the psychologist from his school district, his special-education teacher, his speech therapist, his occupational therapist, and the director of the school. All programs and goals were reviewed, and questions from all parties were discussed. The teacher indicated that the program for the following year would center on developing a consistent communication system for Jameer and on teaching him learning readiness skills and self-care skills, including maintaining eye contact; appropriate sitting; imitation skills; following simple one- and two-step directions; matching colors, shapes, and letters; pre-handwriting; waiting; appropriate play skills; hand washing; brushing his teeth; and getting dressed.

Antoine asked whether mainstreaming would be included in Jameer's program. The teacher indicated that at this point it was important for the child to spend a great deal of his time increasing his beginning skills through the behavioral therapy. Throughout the year there would be several community experiences and field trips for Jameer's class, where he would have the opportunity to play with other children, but mainstreaming would not be a central part of his school program for this first year. At the same time, she noted, there were extracurricular activities in which other parents often enrolled their children that could provide mainstreaming experiences. Examples included toddler gymnastics sessions, music and movement classes, and specialized horseback riding lessons. More and more disciplines were becoming sensitive to working with children with special needs and offered special sessions devoted to enhancing the socialization skills of these children.

Epilogue

As the school personnel laid out their plans and hopes for Jameer, Janelle and Antoine felt reassured. They sensed that he, and they, were in good hands. It was comforting to know that they were no longer in this alone, and that Jameer would have the opportunity to work every weekday with people who knew how to manage this difficult situation.

At the same time, they knew, and the staff members reminded them, that they were at the beginning, not the end, of a long and difficult and confusing journey. Although school programs such as this one were considered state-of-the-art they rarely helped children with severe autism spectrum disorder to reach a high level of functioning. Nor could such programs guarantee particular gains or achievements. They could, at best, help children with severe autism spectrum disorder reach their full potential, a potential that remained limited and somewhat unpredictable. Thus, Janelle and Antoine settled in for the continued journey—with feelings of fear, depression, and also anger that Jameer would not have the life they had originally imagined for him. They prepared for a long journey in which their son would continue to grow and learn in his own way, with everyone involved—his teachers, his parents, and his brother—working to find the techniques and reinforcements that would challenge him and move him forward, step by step. Surely, Jameer's life, and the lives of his parents, did not have to be devoid of joy, satisfaction, or accomplishment. But, just as surely, the satisfactions and accomplishments that awaited them would be very different from the ones that Janelle and Antoine had envisioned just a few years ago. It was now time for Jameer to become Jameer.

> "No two people with autism are the same. Its precise form of expression is different in every case."
> —Oliver Sacks (1993)

Assessment Questions

1. What is the prevalence rate of autism spectrum disorder, and what are some of the current statistics regarding the long-term prognosis of individuals diagnosed with autism spectrum disorder?

2. What were some behaviors that Jameer demonstrated that concerned his mother when she compared his behavior with the behavior of the other children at his birthday party and with the development of his older brother?

3. List two categories of symptoms that are hallmarks of autism spectrum disorder.

4. On the basis of the DSM-5-TR diagnostic criteria, the Childhood Autism Rating Scale, and the Modified Checklist for Autism for Toddlers—Revised, what level of severity was given to Jameer's diagnosis, and which features and symptoms of the disorder were particularly specified in Jameer's case?

5. Why was it important to involve Jameer in an early intervention program as soon as possible?

6. What is the preferred therapeutic intervention for children with autism spectrum disorder?

7. Why did Jameer's parents decide to add home therapy to his treatment program?

8. Speech therapy is an important aspect of treatment for many children with autism spectrum disorder. Describe three of the techniques the speech therapists used to assist Jameer in furthering his communication skills.

9. How did Jameer's disorder affect the family? Give some examples.

10. What were the advantages of a full-day program for Jameer?

11. Why might it be important for Jameer's family members to themselves take advantage of individual counseling or a support group?

12. Why is the quote by Oliver Sacks important to remember in cases of autism spectrum disorder?

CASE 18

The Case of Greta: You Decide

This case is presented in the voices of Greta and her roommate, Irina. As you're reading, you'll be asked to consider a number of issues and to arrive at various decisions, including diagnostic and treatment decisions. After completing this case, go to the next chapter, *Case 18 Appendix*, for Greta's probable diagnosis, the DSM-5-TR criteria, clinical information, and possible treatment directions.

Greta Trying to Live Up to Expectations

I grew up in a northwestern suburban town, and I've lived in the same house for my entire life. My father works as an IT technician, and my mother is the manager of several hotels in the area. My sister, Molly, is 4 years younger than I am.

My parents have been married for almost 25 years. Aside from the usual sort of disagreements, they get along well. In fact, I would say that my entire family gets along well. We're not particularly touchy-feely; it's always a little awkward when we have to hug our grandparents on holidays, because we just never do that sort of thing at home. That's not to say that my parents are uninterested or don't care about us. Far from it; even though they both have busy work schedules, one of them would almost always make it to my soccer and volleyball games and to Molly's field hockey games. My mother, in particular, has always tried to keep on top of what's going on in our lives.

In high school, I took advanced-level classes and earned good grades. I also got along quite well with my teachers and ended up graduating in the top 10 percent of my class. I know this made my mother really proud. She would get worried that I might not be doing my best and "working to my full potential." All through high school, she tried to keep on top of my homework assignments and test schedules. She liked to look over my work before I turned it in and would make sure that I left myself plenty of time to study for tests.

In addition to schoolwork, the soccer and volleyball teams were a big part of high school for me. I had started playing soccer in elementary school because my parents wanted me to do something athletic, and I was never graceful enough to be good at ballet or dance. I was always a little bit chubby when I was a kid. I don't know if I was actually overweight, but everyone used to tease me about my baby fat. Soccer seemed like a good way to lose that extra weight; it was hard at first, but I gradually got better, and by high school I was one of the best players on the team. Schoolwork, soccer, and volleyball didn't leave me much time for anything else. I got along fine with the other kids at school, but I basically hung out with just a few close friends. When I was younger, I used to get teased for being a "goody two-shoes," but that had died down by high school. I can't remember anyone with whom I ever had serious problems.

I did go to the prom, but I didn't date very much in high school. My parents didn't like me hanging out with boys unless it was in a group. Besides, the guys

Describe the family dynamics and school pressures experienced by Greta. Under what circumstances might such family and school factors become problematic or set the stage for psychological problems?

I had crushes on were never the ones who asked me out. So any free time was mostly spent with my close girlfriends. We would go shopping or to the movies, and we frequently spent the night at one another's houses. It was annoying that, although I never did anything wrong, I had the earliest curfew of my friends. Also, I was the only one whose parents would text me throughout the night just to check in. I don't ever remember lying to them about what I was doing or whom I was with. Although I felt like they didn't trust me, I guess they were just worried and wanted to be sure that I was safe.

Greta Coping with Stress

Now I am 18 years old and in the spring semester of my first year at college. I was awarded a scholar-athlete full scholarship. I'm not sure of the exact cause of my current problems, but I know a lot of it must have to do with college life. I have never felt so much pressure before. Because my scholarship depends both on my staying on the soccer team and on my maintaining a 3.6 grade point average, I've been stressed out much of the time. Academic work was never a problem for me in the past, but there's just so much more expected of you in college.

It was pressure from my coach, my teammates, and myself that first led me to dieting. During the first semester, almost all my girlfriends in college experienced the "freshman 15" weight gain—it was a common joke among everyone when we were up late studying and someone ordered a pizza. For some of them it didn't really matter if they gained any weight, but for me it did. I was having trouble keeping up during soccer practices. I even had to sit out of a couple of games because I felt so awful and out of shape. I couldn't catch my breath, and I'd get terrible cramps. And my performance on the field was suffering. I was getting deked out easily, letting players from the opposing teams get past me with their speed, and generally not keeping up with the level of play. I know that my coach was really disappointed in me. He called me aside about a month into the season. He wanted to know what I was eating, and he told me the weight I had gained was undoubtedly hurting my performance. He said that I should cut out snacks and sweets of any kind, and stick to things like salads to help me lose the extra pounds and get back into shape. He also recommended some additional workouts.

Was the advice from Greta's coach out of line, or was it her overreaction to his suggestions that caused later problems?

I was all for a diet—I hated that my clothes were getting snug. In addition, I was feeling left out of the rest of the team. As a freshman, I was self-conscious and not very close with any of the girls on the team at the beginning of the year, and I certainly wasn't proving myself worthy of being on the team. At that point, I was 5'6" and weighed 145 pounds. When I started college I had weighed 130 pounds. Both of these weights fell into the "healthy" body mass index range of 18.5 to 25, but 145 pounds was on the upper end of normal for my height.

Dieting was surprisingly easy. The dining hall food bordered on inedible anyway, so I didn't mind sticking to salads, cereal, or yogurt. Occasionally I'd allow myself pasta, but only without sauce. I completely eliminated dessert, except for fruit on occasion. If anyone commented on my small meals, I just told them that I was in training and gearing up for the big games at the end of the season. I found ways to ignore the urge to snack between meals or late at night when I was studying. I'd go for a quick run to burn off some calories, check Snapchat or TikTok, or take a nap—whatever it took to distract myself. Sometimes I'd drink water or Diet Coke and, if absolutely necessary, I'd munch on a carrot.

Once I started dieting, the incentives to continue were everywhere. My speed on the field improved, so my coach was pleased. I felt more a part of the team and less like an outsider. My clothes were less snug, and when my parents saw me at my games they said I looked great. I even received an invitation to a party given by a fraternity that only invited the most attractive first-year women. After about a month, I was back to my typical weight of 130 pounds.

At first, my plan was to get back down to 130 pounds, but it happened so quickly that I didn't have time to figure out how to re-adjust my diet to include some of the things that I had been leaving out. Things were going so well that I figured it couldn't hurt to stick to the diet a little longer. I was on a roll. I remembered all the people whom I had seen on television who couldn't lose weight even after years of trying. I began to think of my frequent hunger pangs as badges of honor, symbols of my ability to control my bodily urges.

I set a new weight goal of 115 pounds. I figured if I hit the gym more often and skipped breakfast altogether, it wouldn't be hard to reach that weight in another month or so. Of course this made me even hungrier by lunchtime, but I didn't want to increase my lunch size. I found it easiest to pace myself with something like crackers. I would break them into several pieces and only allow myself to eat one piece every 15 minutes. The few times I did this in the dining hall with friends I got weird looks and comments. I finally started eating lunch alone in my room. I would simply say that I had some readings or a paper to finish before afternoon class. I also made excuses to skip dinner with people. I'd tell my friends that I was eating with my teammates, and tell my teammates that I was meeting my roommate. Then I'd go to a dining hall on the far side of campus that was usually empty, and eat by myself.

I remember worrying about how I would handle Thanksgiving. Holidays are a big deal in my family. We get together with my aunts and uncles and grandparents, and of course there is a huge meal. I couldn't bear the stress of being expected to eat such fattening foods. I felt sick just thinking about the stuffing, gravy, and pies for dessert. I told my mother that there was a team Thanksgiving dinner for those who lived too far away to go home. That much was true, but then I lied and told her that the coach thought it would be good for team morale if we all attended.

Many eating disorders follow a period of intense dieting. Is dieting inevitably destructive? Are there safeguards that can be taken during dieting that can head off the development of an eating disorder?

I know it disappointed her, but I couldn't deal with trying to stick to my diet with my family all around me, nagging me to eat more.

Greta Things Get Worse

I couldn't believe it when the scale said I was down to 115 pounds. I still felt that I had excess weight to lose. Some of my friends were beginning to mention that I was actually looking too thin, as if that's possible. I wasn't sure what they meant—I was still feeling chubby when they said I was too skinny. I didn't know who was right, but either way I didn't want people seeing my body. I began dressing in baggy clothes that would hide my physique. I thought about the overweight people my friends and I had snickered about in the past. I couldn't bear the thought of anyone doing that to me. In addition, even though I was playing some of my best soccer, I knew there was still room for improvement.

Look back at Case 9, Bulimia Nervosa. How are Greta's symptoms similar to those of the individual in that case? How are her symptoms different?

Around this time, I started to get really stressed about my schoolwork. I had been managing to keep up throughout the semester, but your final grade basically comes down to the final exam. It was never like this in high school, when you could get an A just by turning in all your homework assignments. I felt unbearably tense leading up to exams. I kept replaying scenarios of opening the test booklet and not being able to answer a single question. I studied nonstop. I brought notes with me to the gym to read on the treadmill, and I wasn't sleeping more than an hour or two at night. Even though I was exhausted, I knew I had to keep studying. I found it really hard to be around other people. Listening to my friends talk about their exam schedules only made me more frantic. I had to get back to my own studying.

The soccer season ended, and my workouts became less intense. Instead of practicing with the team, we were expected to create our own workout schedule. Constant studying left me little time for the amount of exercise I was used to. Yet I was afraid that cutting back on my workouts would cause me to gain weight. It seemed logical that if I couldn't keep up with my exercise, I should eat less in order to continue to lose weight. I carried several cans of Diet Coke with me to the library. Hourly trips to the lounge for coffee were the only study breaks I allowed myself. Aside from that, I might have a bran muffin or a few celery sticks, but that would be it for the day. Difficult though it was, I believed that this regimen was working out well for me. I did fine on my exams. At that point, I weighed 103 pounds and my body mass index was 16.6, which is considered underweight. However, I didn't think of myself as being too thin.

Based on your reading of either DSM-5-TR or your textbook, what disorder might Greta be displaying? Which of her symptoms suggest this diagnosis?

After finals, I went home for winter break for about a month. It was strange to be back home with my parents after living on my own for the semester. I had established new routines for myself and I didn't like having to answer to anyone else about them. Right away, my mother started in; she thought I spent too much time at the gym every day and that I wasn't eating enough. When I told her that I was doing the same thing as everyone else on the team, she actually called my coach and told him that she was concerned about his training policies! More than once she commented that I looked too thin, like I was a walking skeleton. She tried to get me to go to a doctor, but I refused.

Dinner at home was the worst. My mother wasn't satisfied when I only wanted a salad—she'd insist that I have a "well-balanced meal" that included some protein and carbohydrates. We had so many arguments about what I would and wouldn't eat that I started avoiding dinnertime altogether. I'd say that I was going to eat at a friend's house or at the mall. When I was at home I felt like my mother was watching my every move. Although I was worried about the upcoming semester and indoor soccer practice, I was actually looking forward to getting away from my parents. I just wanted to be left alone—to have some privacy and not be criticized for working out to keep in shape.

Since I've returned to school, I've vowed to do a better job of keeping on top of my classes. I don't want to let things pile up for finals again. With my practice schedule, I realize that the only way to devote more time to my schoolwork is to cut back on socializing with friends. So, I haven't seen much of my friends this semester. I don't go to meals at all anymore; I grab coffee or a soda and drink it on my way to class. I've stopped going out on the weekends as well. I barely even see my roommate. She's asleep when I get back late from studying at the library, and I usually get up before her to go for a morning run. Part of me misses hanging out with my friends, but they had started bugging me about not eating enough. I'd rather not see them than have to listen to that and defend myself.

Even though I think that I'm playing better on the field than I was when I first got to school and I'm finally able to stick to a diet, everyone thinks I'm not taking good enough care of myself. I know that my mother has called my coach and my roommate. She must have called the dean of student life, because that's who got in touch with me and suggested that I go to the health center for an evaluation. I hate that my mother is going behind my back after I told her that everything was fine. I realize that I had a rough first semester, but everyone has trouble adjusting to college life. I'm doing my best to keep in control of my life, and I wish that I could be trusted to take care of myself.

> Was there a better way for Greta's mother to intervene? Or would any intervention have brought similar results?

> Greta seems to be the only person who is unaware that she has lost too much weight and developed a destructive pattern of eating. Why is she so unable to look at herself accurately and objectively?

Irina Losing a Roommate

When I first met Greta back in August, I thought we would get along great. She seemed a little shy but like she'd be fun once you got to know her better. She was really cool when we were moving into our room. Even though she arrived first, she waited for me so that we could divide up furniture and closet space together. Early on, a bunch of us in the dorm started hanging out together, and Greta would join us for meals or parties on the weekends. She's pretty and lots of people would hit on her, but she never seemed interested. The rest of us would sit around and gossip about people we met and who liked who, but Greta just listened.

From day one, Greta took her academics seriously. She was sort of an inspiration to the rest of us. Even though she was busy with practices and games, she always had her readings done for class. But I know that Greta also worried constantly about her studies and staying in game shape. She'd talk about how frustrating it was to not be able to compete at the level she knew she was capable of. She would get really nervous before games. Sometimes she couldn't sleep, and I'd wake up in the middle of the night and see her pacing around the room. When she told me her coach suggested a new diet and training regimen, it sounded like a good idea.

How might high schools and universities better identify individuals with serious eating disorders? What procedures or mechanisms has your school put into operation?

I guess I first realized that something was wrong when she started avoiding our group of friends. She stopped going out with us on weekends, and we almost never saw her in the dining hall anymore. A couple of times I even caught her eating by herself in a dining hall on the other side of campus. She explained that she had a lot of work to do and found that she could get some of it done while eating if she had meals alone. When I did see her eat, it was never anything besides vegetables. She'd take only a tiny portion, and then she wouldn't even finish it. She didn't keep any food in the room except for cans of Diet Coke and a bag of baby carrots in the fridge. I also noticed that her clothes were starting to look baggy and hang off her. A couple of times I asked her if she was doing okay, but this only made her defensive. She claimed that she was playing some of her best soccer, and since she didn't seem sick, I figured that I was overreacting. When I talked to another girl on the team, I learned that some of Greta's teammates were worried about how much weight she had lost. They also shared that Greta's weight loss was not making her a better soccer player. In contrast, I learned that she was getting pushed around physically on the field, losing battles for the ball that she normally would win. She was indeed fast but was not performing well.

Still, I kept believing that she was basically okay—until I returned from Thanksgiving. It was right before final exams, so everyone was pretty stressed out. Greta had been a hard worker before, but now she took things to new extremes. She dropped off the face of the earth. I almost never saw her, even though we shared a room. I'd get up around 8:00 or 9:00 in the morning, and she'd already be gone. When I went to bed around midnight, she still wasn't back. Her side of the room was immaculate: bed made, books and notepads stacked neatly on her desk. When I did bump into her, she looked awful. She was way too thin, with dark circles under her eyes. She seemed like she had wasted away; her skin and hair were dull and dry. I was pretty sure that something was wrong, but I told myself that it must just be the stress of the upcoming finals. I figured that if there were a problem, her parents would notice it and do something about it over winter break.

Why was Irina inclined to overlook her initial suspicions about Greta's behaviors? Was there a better way for the roommate to intervene?

When we came back to campus in January after break, I was surprised to see that Greta looked even worse than during finals. When I asked her how her vacation had been, she mumbled something about being sick of her mother and happy to be back at school. As the semester got under way, Greta further distanced herself from us. There were no more parties or hanging out at meals for her. She was acting the same way she had during finals, which made no sense because classes had barely gotten going. We were all worried, but none of us knew what to do. One time, Greta's mother sent me a direct message on Instagram and asked me if I had noticed anything strange going on with Greta. I wasn't sure what to write back. I felt guilty, like I would be tattling on her, but I also realized that I was in over my head and that I needed to be honest.

I wrote her mother about Greta's odd eating habits, how she was exercising a lot and how she had gotten pretty antisocial. Her mother wrote me back and said she had spoken with their family doctor. Greta was extremely underweight, even though she still saw herself as chunky and was afraid of gaining weight.

A few days later, Greta approached me. Apparently she had just met with one of the deans, who told her that she'd need to undergo an evaluation at the health center before she could continue practicing with the team. She asked me pointblank if I had been talking about her to anyone. I told her how her mother had contacted me and asked me if I had noticed any changes in Greta over the past several months, and how I honestly had told her mother yes. She stormed out of the room, and I haven't seen her since. I know how important the team is to Greta, so I am assuming that she'll be going to the health center soon. I hope that they'll be able to convince her that she's taken things too far and that they can help her to get better.

> How might the treatment approaches used in Case 2 (Obsessive-Compulsive Disorder), Case 4 (Posttraumatic Stress Disorder), and Case 9 (Bulimia Nervosa) be applied to Greta? How should they be altered to fit Greta's problems and personality? Which aspects of these treatments would not be appropriate? Should additional interventions be applied?

Reader Alert!

Now that you've read about Greta, considered important issues, and made key decisions, go to the next chapter, *Case 18 Appendix*, for Greta's probable diagnosis, the DSM-5-TR criteria, clinical information, and possible treatment directions.

CASE 18 Appendix
The Case of Greta: Diagnosis, Information, and Treatment

In the previous chapter, *The Case of Greta: You Decide,* you were asked to consider a number of issues and to arrive at various decisions, including diagnostic and treatment decisions. How did you do? This chapter presents Greta's probable diagnosis, the DSM-5-TR criteria, relevant clinical information, and possible treatment directions.

Diagnosis

Greta's pattern would receive a diagnosis of **anorexia nervosa.**

Dx Checklist

Anorexia Nervosa

1. Individual purposely takes in too little nourishment, resulting in body weight that is very low and below that of other people of similar age and gender.

2. Individual is very fearful of gaining weight, or repeatedly seeks to prevent weight gain despite low body weight.

3. Individual has a distorted body perception, places inappropriate emphasis on weight or shape in judgments of herself or himself, or fails to appreciate the serious implications of their low weight.

(Information from APA, 2022, 2013)

Clinical Information

1. Approximately 0.6% of all people in Western countries develop anorexia disorder in their lifetime, and many more display at least some of its symptoms (Halmi, 2020; NEDA, 2020; NIMH, 2021b, 2020c, 2017e). Approximately 75% of all cases occur among women and adolescent girls (ANAD, 2020).

2. Although anorexia nervosa can occur at any age, the peak age of onset is between 14 years and 20 years (ANAD, 2020).

3. Researchers have identified *body dissatisfaction* as a significant factor in the development of eating disorders (Klein & Attia, 2021).

4. Anorexia nervosa typically begins after a person who is slightly overweight or of normal weight has been on a diet (Mitchell & Peterson, 2020).

5. Individuals with anorexia nervosa often also struggle with other psychological symptoms such as depression, anxiety, low self-esteem, substance abuse, and/or clinical perfectionism (Munn-Chernoff et al., 2021; Halmi, 2020; Marzola et al., 2020).

6. Surveys of both adolescents and young adults have directly tied eating disorders and body dissatisfaction to social networking, Internet activity, and television browsing (Ioannidis et al., 2021; Latzer, Katz, & Spivak, 2011).

7. Research suggests that as many as half of the families of people with anorexia nervosa or bulimia nervosa have a long history of emphasizing thinness, physical appearance, and dieting. The mothers in these families are more likely to diet themselves and to be generally perfectionistic than are the mothers in other families (Halmi, 2020; NEDA, 2020).

8. Studies have found that performers, models, and athletes are more prone than others to develop anorexia nervosa and bulimia nervosa, partly because thinness is especially emphasized in these professions (Caceres, 2020).

9. As many as 60% of elementary school girls express concern about their weight and becoming overweight. The number of girls under the age of 12 years who develop a full eating disorder is growing (Ekern, 2020; NEDA, 2020).

10. For most of the twentieth century, non-Hispanic white American women were more likely than women of other racial and ethnic groups to experience body dissatisfaction and develop eating disorders. However, current research suggests that young women of color in the United States now express body dissatisfaction to at least the same degree as young non-Hispanic white American women (Halmi, 2020; NEDA, 2020). Eating disorders also appear to be rising among young Asian American women (Javier & Belgrave, 2019).

11. Although most people with anorexia nervosa recover, as many as 6% of them become so seriously ill that they die, usually from medical problems brought about by starvation or from suicide (Fairburn & Murphy, 2020; Halmi, 2020).

Treatment Overview and Strategies

Around one-third of those with anorexia nervosa receive treatment (NIMH, 2021b, 2020c, 2017e). The immediate aims of treatment are to help people regain their lost weight, recover from malnourishment, and eat normally again (McElroy et al., 2020). The longer-term goals are to help them to make psychological and perhaps family changes to lock in those eating gains (Fitzsimmons-Craft & Pike, 2021;

Cooper & Mitchell, 2020). Therapists typically use a combination of education, psychotherapy, and family therapy to reach these broader goals (Mitchell & Peterson, 2020).

A highly regarded treatment strategy developed by psychiatric researcher Christopher Fairburn combines cognitive-behavioral interventions with several other techniques. Research has found this approach to be helpful in many cases of anorexia nervosa, enabling many individuals to overcome their disorder and to also avoid relapse (Fairburn & Murphy, 2020; Fairburn et al., 2013, 2008; Grave et al., 2013; Cooper & Fairburn, 2011). The strategy includes three phases:

1. First step: Help to increase the individual's readiness and motivation for change (called motivational interviewing) (Yager, 2020, 2019; Zhu et al., 2020).

2. Second step: When the clients are ready or if their medical condition dictates, increase caloric intake to regain weight while simultaneously addressing the underlying eating disorder psychopathology, particularly the individual's extreme concerns about shape and weight (McElroy et al., 2020).

3. Third step: Focus on *relapse prevention* by helping clients develop personalized strategies for identifying and immediately correcting any setbacks.

CASE 19

The Case of Hector: You Decide

This case is presented in the voices of Hector and his wife, Miranda. As you're reading, you'll be asked to consider a number of issues and to arrive at various decisions, including diagnostic and treatment decisions. After completing this case, go to the next chapter, *Case 19 Appendix*, for Hector's probable diagnosis, the DSM-5-TR criteria, clinical information, and possible treatment directions.

Miranda "My Husband's Brain Stopped Working Properly"

About 8 years ago, my life changed completely. The reason? My husband's brain stopped working properly. We had been married 34 years, and Hector was 67 years old. He had worked for the same construction company in Union City, New Jersey, for 32 years, first as a laborer, then as a security supervisor and union leader. He was a strong man, both mentally and physically; a good husband; and a good father to our son, Gabriel. Together, we had managed to make a decent living with him in construction and me supplementing our income as a substitute teacher. Life was good. But then Hector's brain started to let him down.

The problems seemed small at first, hardly noticeable really. Sometimes, when telling me about his day at work, Hector would talk about the foreman, Jimmy, driving a "tractor" when he meant "bulldozer," or he'd say that he had made a "revision" instead of "decision." Little stuff. And he'd catch himself. I didn't worry too much about it, but it was odd. It doesn't sound like much, but it wasn't like him. I even thought, "Oh, well, the old boy's slipping," and would laugh to myself. But when he forgot the anniversary of our first date, well . . . I knew something was wrong. I gave him all kinds of hell for that — I accused him of having an affair, I cried, I really let him have it. But I was also scared. I mean, maybe an anniversary like that doesn't mean much to other people, but for us — well, over the years, he'd taken me to Atlantic City for shows and to dinners in expensive restaurants. Once, after Gabriel was grown, he even got us a hotel room in the Catskills for a weekend. There was always some sort of surprise. So, 8 years ago, in anticipation of a special evening, I got all dressed up. When he got home from work that night and sat down on the sofa, I knew he'd forgotten; and when he saw the disappointment in my eyes, he realized the same thing pretty quickly. In fact, he felt terrible about it and took me out to a very fancy restaurant after I calmed down. But it was a bad sign. That year turned out to be a rough one.

It wasn't as if he suddenly forgot everything, but it seemed like he was forgetting a bunch of things that he'd never forgotten before. I had always been the one with my head in the clouds, forgetting dates and losing car keys. Hector would be the one keeping me organized, nagging about the bills or a doctor's appointment for Gabriel. Of course, I'd joke, "Why don't we switch jobs and you'll see who's got it tougher," but he definitely had a sharper head, no denying that. Now, suddenly, he

> Forgetfulness is universal, and increases in forgetfulness are a normal part of aging. How might we distinguish normal forgetting or normal aging from the symptoms of a clinical disorder?

was losing his wallet and we'd find it later in the study, where he'd sworn he hadn't been in days. Or he would leave half-full glasses of juice on the floor of the living room, and when I'd chide him about it he'd say, "Oh, I'm sorry," and change the subject. This was Mr. Neat Freak who, in the past, couldn't stand it if a dirty dish sat on the kitchen table more than a half hour after dinner.

He also had little accidents, spilling food on himself, or knocking over a pile of papers or the jar of pencils from the counter. Then he started asking me to drive him to work all the time. He said that he'd caught himself veering off the road a few times and had just barely avoided an accident. "It's all the stress," he'd tell me. "We've got a new contract coming up and I don't think it's gonna go our way. I've just got too much on my mind."

As the forgetfulness and unusual behavior mounted, it couldn't be ignored any more. Yet I didn't want to believe there was anything seriously wrong. I told myself that this was all just a normal part of getting older. Then, one day, he missed a meeting with an important contractor—just didn't show up. Instead, he went to his office like it was any other day. The company lost the contract and a lot of money, and it was bad for their image. Actually, by that point in time, I wasn't all that surprised by his error. This responsible and organized man, who had taken care of everything for so many years, was by then becoming a different person, and I was now taking care of him. That's when I told him that he must see a doctor. And Hector did something I'd never seen him do: He burst into tears.

Despite his emotional outpouring that evening, Hector managed to put off medical treatment for nearly a year. Eventually, however, the incidents caught up with him—for example, leaving his glasses in the mailbox or mowing only half the lawn—and he went for a neuropsychological exam. The results of a battery of tests revealed significant problems, and the neuropsychologist, Dr. Schoenfeld, broke the news to us that he was suffering from a neurocognitive disorder. The doctor explained to us that we would be facing a very difficult battle—that Hector would become less and less able to take care of himself. He also told us that very little could be done to stem the progress of Hector's condition. Hector was going to have to rely on the support of his loved ones, particularly me, to see him through this.

Hector had already planned to retire, as his position in the company had been scaled down drastically after the contract debacle. The doctor's diagnosis simply made it official in our minds. Within 3 months, he was thrown a retirement party by his coworkers, many of whom he had mentored. By then he was having trouble remembering people's names, but that party meant a lot to him. He knew just how lucky he was to have so many caring friends and colleagues. He was still embarrassed about having lost that contract, but everybody tried their best to show him that they had nothing but gratitude for his years of service. He wasn't walking too well by then, either, so I helped him to a chair, where he sat for most

What might be the most difficult aspects of observing a spouse, parent, or other close relative gradually lose their memory or other cognitive faculties?

Neurocognitive disorders include a group of organic syndromes, marked by major problems in cognitive functioning, such as memory and learning, attention, visual perception, planning and decision making, language ability, or social awareness. Based on your reading of either DSM-5-TR or your textbook, what form of neurocognitive disorder might Hector be displaying? Which of his symptoms suggest this diagnosis?

of the party, sometimes crying quietly to himself because he no longer had full control of his emotions. I think that was really his last great experience, the last time he had a really special night out.

At the party, Hector gave a short talk to his coworkers, thanking them for the event. He had been worried about this speech for days. He feared attempting to reminisce or trying to be too specific, because he'd been having so much trouble remembering things. But he didn't want to read a written speech, so he just kept it short. It broke my heart when I heard him say, "This is really a special night. I want to thank you all for this and for helping me out the way you've done the last few months. I'm not the kinda guy who talks a lot and makes big speeches to his friends. And that's what you are—my friends. That's why I've had a great time all these years. That's why I've loved my job, and going to work in the morning. We've had a lot of good times, and I'll miss you, my friends."

It was more than a retirement speech; it was a farewell speech. But, as painful as that was, the impromptu speech that he gave to me alone just 2 days later hurt even more. He was lucid that day. He was clear and organized and sharp as a tack, just like the old Hector. And he was hurting.

The close family members and friends who provide care for persons with neurocognitive disorders typically must expend enormous amounts of time and energy and concern for their stricken relative or friend, which can lead to a range of psychological problems for the caregivers. What kinds of problems would you expect caregivers to develop?

Hector "Preparing for a Trip to Nowhere"

I'm mad, I'm frustrated, I'm everything in between. It sure is embarrassing, Mandy, it sure is. Can you imagine what it's like to have to think for 2 whole minutes before remembering our own grandchild's name? A child I held in my arms when he was born, and said, "This boy is a perfect child." I watched him grow and played ball with him, and I can see his face in front of me as if he was in the room with me, but when I reach for his name, there's nothing there. Blank. How do I convince an 8-year-old child that his *abuelo* loves him and cares about him when I can't even remember his name?

I spend my whole life trying to be sharp, but I end up a failure. I'm a 69-year-old man who needs a woman to take care of him like he's 90. What use am I? I provided for my family. I earned money. I did my job to help keep Wellstone Construction running. And now that's all gone. All gone. I can't do any of it anymore. I lie in bed or sit in a chair all day. My wife and son provide for me. The company takes care of me. I'm a drain. No one will ever again think of trusting me with anything. Anything. "No, it would be too taxing for the poor guy." That's what they'll say, but what they'll mean is, "He'll just screw it up, like he screws everything up."

Think back to Case 5 (Major Depressive Disorder). Did Hector show any symptoms of clinical depression as his disorder unfolded? Did Miranda? Would any of the treatment techniques described in Case 5 be helpful to either of them?

Sometimes, all of a sudden, I don't know what time of day it is, or even what day of the week it is. I don't even know what I had for breakfast this morning. If I want to go over there to pick up that book off that table, I have to ask you to help me walk. I can't walk without leaning on someone. Otherwise, I'll fall or have to stop and sit down.

Why should I even want to get up in the morning? Being up isn't all that different from being asleep, only a bit more confusing. Nothing in the world is more infuriating than knowing that you know the thing you can't remember. Knowing that you're not stupid, but that everything you once knew is being stripped away from you, little by little. God knows how long I'll even know who you are, Mandy. How long will it be before it's all just shapes and colors? How long before everyone else is making plans for me. Putting me in a home, putting me out to pasture, putting me to sleep. I feel like I'm preparing for a trip to nowhere.

I don't even know if I'll mind that so much. When I don't remember anything, it won't be so hard. Probably then I won't feel so stupid. I won't realize how much I am forgetting. That's what gets me—the forgetting. It gets me mad, but it gets me scared, too. I reach for a pen that I thought I was just writing with and I realize that it's not there. I look for it and then I realize that I'm not writing anything. Now I can't find the pen, and I don't even remember why I'm looking for it, and nothing makes any damned sense. It's like this dream that's real upsetting because I don't know what's going on, but I know I should know. Oh, God!

When this all started, you know, I didn't believe it. A man can get used to a lot if he can convince himself that nothing is wrong. Every time I'd forget something, or lose something, or drive off the road, it bothered me for exactly 5 minutes. I'd be scared for 5 minutes and I'd admit to myself for those 5 minutes that there was a serious problem—that these things were happening more and more and that something was very wrong and that I should get this taken care of somehow. But after those 5 minutes, I would laugh it off and decide that everything was fine—everyone forgets things, everyone loses concentration driving, everyone misplaces things—and I'd be fine. I'd come home, and I wouldn't think about it until the next thing happened. Then I'd be upset for another 5 minutes.

I want you to put me away, Mandy—you know what I mean—let me go, if I ever don't remember who you are. I don't want to forget my beautiful wife, and if I don't know who you are anymore, have them just inject me or give me whatever is necessary in order to get this life over with. Don't worry about whether it's the right thing, because it is. I'm afraid that you won't do this, that you'll let me go on when I'm not myself anymore. I don't want you to have to see me and not know that I love you and need you with me. I don't want you to doubt my love for you because of this damned disease. Please, Mandy, don't let that happen. Please promise me.

Miranda "A Long Goodbye"

I heard versions of that speech from Hector several other times during the next 2 years. But of course I couldn't make that promise. Eventually, he became less clear and less interested, and less able, and he stopped saying those things. The last

> If you were to lose your memory and other cognitive faculties, bit by bit, how would you feel? What fears and worries do you think you would experience?

> Why would Hector and Miranda have tried to overlook his symptoms, even as they were worsening?

Unlike most of the other disorders in this casebook, Hector's problem was organic, progressive, and largely irreversible. What role might psychological treatments play in disorders of this kind?

What role might psychotherapists play in helping close relatives cope with the deterioration of a loved one? What therapy approaches described throughout this casebook might be particularly helpful to such relatives?

4 years really have been a long goodbye for us. As the years have passed, Hector has been less and less able to do for himself. He has been increasingly unsteady on his feet. Furthermore, he lost control of his motor functions and is now unable to feed or clothe himself, or to use the bathroom on his own. At first, this was very upsetting to Hector; he was still aware enough to feel that his incapacitation made him ridiculous in some way, and he often lashed out at me in anger—even accusing me at times of trying to drug him so that he couldn't take care of himself. Later, he would tearfully apologize after these outbursts.

About 4 years ago, I bought him a walker to make it easier for him to get around. But a year later, he fell while trying to walk across the hall to take a bath. He broke his hip and couldn't leave his bed for 4 months. Hector became more and more depressed and began spending days staring at the wall or the bed sheets, refusing to talk even when I tried to speak to him. After his hip had healed, he still remained in bed, refusing to try to walk. He even began hearing voices and seeing people who weren't really in the room. Sometimes he would believe that long-gone relatives were in front of him and talking to him. Eventually, it seemed like it was just too taxing for him to try to distinguish the real from the imagined, and Hector began to treat everyone and everything around him with indifference or doubt. He treated real people who were talking to him as though they might be figments of his imagination and just turned away.

Our son, Gabriel, visited regularly, at least once every other weekend, from his New Hampshire home. Even so, Gabriel was always surprised by the speed of Hector's deterioration. After breaking his hip, Hector, who had always looked so forward to Gabriel's visits, often failed to get out of bed to greet our son, sometimes sleeping through the entire visit. Gabriel noticed that his father appeared to get less pleasure from the visits. He tried to prepare himself for the ravages of Hector's condition, but as his father deteriorated more and more, Gabriel became very shaken.

During one visit, Hector looked Gabriel in the eye, then turned to me and asked, "Who is this, Mandy? Who's he? Is that your brother Mateo? What's he doing here?" Gabriel faced his father and said in a quiet voice, "Dad, it's me. Your son, Gabriel. And I love you." As he said this, however, Hector fell asleep, and Gabriel left the room feeling dejected. Later, after Gabriel and I ate lunch, Hector awoke again, and called out. When Gabriel entered the room and stood over his father's bed, Hector touched his hand to Gabriel's face and after a minute said, quietly and hoarsely, "Son . . ." And they held hands without saying a word for an hour. I almost couldn't bear it.

Also, about 3 years ago, Hector started having violent nightmares, and he would sometimes wake me with his screaming. During and after some of the nightmares, he seemed like a completely different person, with a crazed passion behind his frightened eyes. He was growing more and more convinced that I was plotting against him. During one of our visits to the neuropsychologist, he complained to the doctor, "She's stealing things from me. She steals my clothes so that she can make me feel foolish when I can't find them. I was eating a banana, and she wanted the banana. I put it down and turned my back for a minute, and that banana was gone. She's taking my food. This is all her fault. I know it is."

It's now been 8 years of taking care of him. At this point, I have to feed him and help him use the bathroom. I bathe him and I take him to the doctor. Thanks to his retirement package, we're okay financially. Still, I need to spend every penny we have on Hector's care. I can't work myself, since I have to be with him. The worst part is when he looks at me and I know he doesn't know who I am, yells at me as if I'm an enemy, and accuses me of stealing his things. At other times, however, he looks at me and his eyes say, "Thanks, Mandy," and I know he hasn't forgotten—even if he's remembering for only a moment.

Hector's decline seemed to reach a new level beginning around 6 months ago. Since then, he has been completely incontinent and barely able to speak. He has also been unable to leave our bedroom. He hasn't shown any recognition of Gabriel during his visits, and he has barely even acknowledged me. About 3 weeks ago, he developed a cold that would not go away, and last week I took him to the hospital. He's still there, with a respiratory infection, using a ventilator to breathe. He is in such a weakened condition that the doctors are not sure he will live out the week.

I suspect that Gabriel and I each privately hope that the doctors' prognoses are accurate and Hector will die within the week. Neither of us has dared express this to the other, but I think we will both be relieved at some level when Hector is gone—that is, the bedridden Hector whose true spirit has already left us. Because, when he is gone, we will all finally be delivered from this long ordeal. And Gabriel and I will be able to think of our beloved Hector again as he once was—strong of mind and body.

Reader Alert!

Now that you've read about Hector, considered related issues, and made key decisions, go to the next chapter, *Case 19 Appendix*, for Hector's probable diagnosis, the DSM-5-TR criteria, clinical information, and possible treatment directions.

People with a disorder such as Hector's often become angry, suspicious, and accusatory. What are some of the potential reasons for such reactions and personality changes?

After a long ordeal such as Hector's, it is common for close relatives to find themselves almost wishing for or looking forward to the person's death. What factors might explain such feelings and reactions?

CASE 19 Appendix
The Case of Hector: Diagnosis, Information, and Treatment

In the previous chapter, *The Case of Hector: You Decide,* you were asked to consider a number of issues and to arrive at various decisions, including diagnostic and treatment decisions. How did you do? This chapter presents Hector's probable diagnosis, the DSM-5-TR criteria, relevant clinical information, and possible treatment directions.

Diagnosis

Hector's pattern would receive a diagnosis of ***major neurocognitive disorder due to Alzheimer's disease.***

> ### Dx Checklist
>
> #### Major Neurocognitive Disorder Due to Alzheimer's Disease
>
> 1. Individual displays substantial, progressive, and gradual decline and impairment in memory and learning and at least one other area of cognitive function as well, such as attention, planning and decision making, perceptual-motor skills, language ability, and social awareness.
>
> 2. Cognitive deficits interfere with the individual's independence in everyday activities.
>
> 3. Symptoms are not due to other types of disorders or medical problems.
>
> (Information from APA, 2022, 2013)

Clinical Information

1. Approximately 1% to 2% of people 65 years of age suffer from some kind of neurocognitive disorder, a number that increases to as many as 50% of all people older than 85 (Heflin, 2020).

2. Alzheimer's disease is the most common form of major neurocognitive disorder, accounting for at least two-thirds of all cases of the disorder (Emmady & Tadi, 2020).

3. Around 6 million people in the United States currently have Alzheimer's disease, a number that is expected to be 14 million by the year 2050 (Alzheimer's Association, 2020).

4. Women are twice as likely as men to develop Alzheimer's disease. Black Americans and Hispanic Americans are twice as likely as non-Hispanic white Americans to develop it (Alzheimer's Association, 2020). The reasons for this significant racial and ethnic difference are not known.

5. Alzheimer's disease sometimes appears in middle age but most often occurs after the age of 65, particularly among people in their late 70s and early 80s.

6. Although some people with Alzheimer's disease may survive for as many as 20 years, the time between onset and death is typically less than 9 years (Kumar et al., 2020; Wolk & Dickerson, 2020).

7. People with Alzheimer's disease may at first deny that they have a problem, but they may soon become anxious or depressed; many also become agitated. As many as 40% of them develop a depressive disorder (ALZRA, 2020).

8. Structural changes in the brains of people with Alzheimer's disease include an excessive number of *neurofibrillary tangles* (twisted protein fibers found within the neurons of the hippocampus and certain other brain structures) and of *senile plaques* (sphere-shaped deposits of a small molecule known as the beta-amyloid protein that form between neurons in the hippocampus, cerebral cortex, and certain other brain regions).

9. Alzheimer's disease often has a genetic basis, although other factors, such as environmental, lifestyle, and stress-related factors, may also have a significant impact on its development (Latimer et al., 2021; Alzheimer's Association, 2020).

10. Victims of Alzheimer's disease usually remain in fairly good health until the later stages of the disease, when they may become significantly less active (Cote et al., 2021). With less activity, they may become prone to illnesses such as pneumonia, which can result in death.

11. Alzheimer's disease is the sixth leading cause of death in the United States overall, resulting in 122,000 deaths each year throughout the country—a number more than 50% higher than it was a decade ago (CDC, 2021a, 2019b).

Treatment Overview and Strategies

1. No single approach or set of approaches is highly effective in all cases of Alzheimer's disease, and no intervention actually stops the progression of the disease (Cummings, 2021; Wolk & Dickerson, 2020).

2. The drugs currently prescribed for Alzheimer's patients are designed to affect *acetylcholine* and *glutamate*, neurotransmitters that play important roles in memory (Alzheimer's Association, 2020). The short-term memory and reasoning ability of some Alzheimer's patients who take these drugs improve modestly, as do their use of language and their ability to cope under pressure (Cummings, 2021; Zhang et al., 2020).

3. There is evidence that regular physical exercise may help reduce the risk of developing Alzheimer's disease and improve its symptoms (Yu et al., 2021; Alzheimer's Association, 2020; Thomas et al., 2020). Similarly, cognitive activities, including computer-based cognitive stimulation programs, sometimes help prevent or delay the onset of Alzheimer's disease (Alzheimer's Association, 2020).

4. Behavior-focused interventions may be used to help change everyday patient behaviors that are stressful for the family, such as wandering at night, loss of bladder control, demands for attention, and inadequate personal care (Press, 2021; Press & Alexander, 2021).

5. The needs of the caregivers must also be met via psychoeducation, psychotherapy, support groups, and regular time-outs (Friedman & Kennedy, 2021; CDC, 2021b, 2019a).

6. Alzheimer's disease *day-care facilities* (providing outpatient treatment programs and activities during the day) are becoming common. In addition, many *assisted-living facilities* are being built—apartments that provide supervision and are tailored to the needs and limitations of people with diseases such as Alzheimer's disease. And a growing number of *practical devices*, such as wrist bands or shoes containing GPS trackers, can help family members keep track of where their confused relative may be or have wandered off to (Press, 2021; Press & Alexander, 2021; Alzheimer's Association, 2020).

CASE 20

The Case of Shaylynn:
You Decide

This case is presented in the voices of Shaylynn and her mother, Tanya. As you're reading, you'll be asked to consider a number of issues and to arrive at various decisions, including diagnostic and treatment decisions. After completing this case, go on to the next chapter, *Case 20 Appendix*, for Shaylynn's probable diagnosis, the DSM-5-TR criteria, clinical information, and possible treatment directions.

Shaylynn A Harmful Pattern Unfolds

I don't know when I started doing it. I guess I've always hated school and I've always been really nervous about things. A lot of the time, even before college, I used to pinch or scratch my skin; the more nervous I became, the more it happened. But I didn't think there was anything unusual about it. You know, everyone has nervous habits that they turn to when they get stressed out, right?

My parents were super worried. They thought maybe I had some kind of psychosis. I can see why they thought that. When I was stressed out, I would stare blankly at my arms for long periods of time, inspecting them. I probably looked like I was seeing things, like I was hallucinating or something, the way I would intensely and relentlessly scan my skin, moving my hands over the surface and slowly touching, looking, sometimes pinching. It could go on for long periods of time, especially when I was in a bad mood.

It didn't help that my parents were hard on me. They were always making me feel like I didn't do well enough. "Couldn't you have gotten an A? Couldn't you play on the varsity basketball or soccer team? Couldn't you have been the best? What could you have done to prepare for the test better? What can we learn from this? Why don't you have a boyfriend? Maybe if you dressed differently? You know, we just want you to be happy."

I guess this whole thing really started a long time ago. When I was in seventh grade, I used to pluck out my eyelashes. I can't remember how it started, but I remember that it used to relax me when I was tense. One time, I pulled out all of my eyelashes. It felt really relieving, but when my older brother saw me the next morning, he saw what I had done and laughed at me. He called me a freak and said I needed to go talk to my older sister and see if she had any false eyelashes. She did, thankfully, but I swore I would not pull out my eyelashes or any other hair on my body again. It was humiliating. After my eyelashes grew back, I never went after them again.

Another time while studying with my friend, I started to pinch my skin. We were talking about a test that was coming up in chemistry. She was far more prepared than me, but she was talking like she was going to fail the exam. I hate when people do that. Like, come on, you know you are going to do well, and yet you're making me reassure you when I'm feeling way behind? It was making me anxious and very annoyed. I tried to change the topic, but she kept on

Many loving parents are described as being "overconcerned" about their children, or "overcontrolling" or "overinvolved." Where do such patterns of behavior come from? What can parents do to avoid crossing the line in their efforts to guide and protect their maturing children?

it, so I gave up trying and just sat there while she rambled on and on about her insecurities. I felt tension building in my body. My heart was beating faster. I was feeling my muscles tighten in my arms. I didn't even realize what I was doing until I felt a sharp pain on my hand. I looked down, and saw that I was pinching the skin on the top of my hand, secretly so she didn't notice. As a result, I didn't feel as anxious anymore, and I stopped paying attention to what she was saying. The tension had vanished. From that point forward, whenever I was in a situation that I couldn't escape from and that was irritating me, I would pinch my skin until it hurt. Somehow, it took the edge off.

A few years later, while studying for the SAT — or maybe it was the ACT — I think that was when I first started to *pick* my skin as a way to deal with stress. I hated taking the practice exams for those tests. My parents would always wait until I finished and then pounce on me after, trying to pretend like they were casually interested in how I performed. Even when I got my highest practice score, a 1450 on the SAT, they seemed disappointed and critical. Nothing was ever good enough. Anyway, while studying, I found myself avoiding taking a practice test and inspecting my skin for blemishes instead. I felt a few bumps on my elbow; however, I couldn't see them easily, so I used my hand to feel around carefully. Time slowed down, like I was fixated or mesmerized by the subtleties of the sensations on my elbow. I probably looked like I was cut off from reality, absorbed completely by the way it felt to move my fingernail with precision across each millimeter of skin. But I wasn't hallucinating or having any delusions. No, I was obsessively focused, searching for feelings of pain and relief to displace my stress about that damn practice test!

My elbows were smooth, so their various imperfections stood out. I scraped around methodically, feeling tiny bumps but not knowing what they were. I was really stressed, and I started to pick at every place where skin was raised. I remember thinking that maybe I had some minute bug bites. But, at the same time, I recognized that the little pain of running my fingernail across the skin was something I liked, like when you have an itch and you need to scratch it. I kept going, and then moved to the other elbow. Then to other parts of my arms. I found lots of places to pick and dig into my skin. It felt oddly satisfying. As I approached each new spot, I would get nervous and think that maybe I shouldn't dig into that location. But then, when I was picking, I would get a small rush of anticipation, knowing I would soon feel the quick prick of pain followed by instant relief when the skin came off. And after it was over, I felt relieved, all of my nervousness gone. I looked at the skin I had picked, obsessively staring at it, thinking about nothing in particular.

After several episodes of this kind, I developed small red marks on my elbows from picking. But no one seemed to notice, so I concluded that it wasn't a big deal. Maybe I wasn't really doing anything harmful, I thought. Maybe I was just picking skin that was already hanging off, ready to be shed anyway. Maybe I'm just sensitive to how it feels because I keep thinking about it so much. Over time, my picking started to bleed, and then scabs began forming. Of course, I couldn't help but notice that the red marks and scabs were growing in size as I kept on picking when stressed. Also, my elbows were hurting all the time.

One night after an upsetting conversation at dinner, my mom came up to my room to talk to me about some test or another and caught me off-guard, in the middle of picking. She screamed out, "What happened to your elbows?" That was so embarrassing! I wanted my parents to just go away. They wouldn't understand why I had to do it. I just wanted to crawl into a hole and die. I promised my mom that I would stop, but that promise was easier said than done. Time and again, I'd catch myself—or should I say Mom would catch me?—doing it, picking my arms instinctively whenever I got stressed out.

My embarrassment kept growing, until eventually it became so great that it helped me to stop. Whenever I would reach for my arms, I was able to catch myself before I touched them. My scabs went away, and my elbows weren't as irritated all the time. After a few months, I didn't even have to think about it anymore. When I did think back on my behavior, I couldn't believe that I had quickly caused so many scabs and red marks on my elbows. It didn't make sense anymore, and it seemed so unnatural. I was glad I had stopped, but I didn't want to think about it too much because I didn't want to consider the possibility that I wasn't normal.

After I had stopped skin picking, I developed some other problematic patterns in response to school and the other stresses in my life. Throughout my senior year, I bit my nails. And I would often stay up all night worrying myself to the point of tears, then walk around with a headache, half asleep the next day.

For months and months, I was desperately concerned about which schools I would get into for college. Then, after I received a bunch of acceptances and decided where to go, I worried about all the preparations I would eventually have to make. All this while at the same time trying to finish my senior year in good standing. Then of course the time did eventually arrive when I had to get ready to move away from home. And amidst all these events and concerns, I kept worrying in the back of my mind that there was something different about me from everyone else. I really didn't get along that well with most people; I just got too nervous around them; and relationships with boys never seemed to go anywhere. In fact, I wasn't sure in high school whether I was even interested in boys, despite my mom constantly telling me how she was had already started dating my father when she was my age.

> Entering college is a major life stress that seems to trigger or exacerbate psychological difficulties for many persons. Why might this be such a difficult period in life?

Shaylynn Away at College

When I first got to college, I was really scared. I'd never been away from home for more than a couple of weeks, and never so far from my parents. I was from a rural part of Canada, in southern Alberta. Now I was away at a huge university in

California. Even though I couldn't wait to get away from my parents, I didn't know how I was going to get through life without them telling me how to do everything and how to get by in the real world. My next-door neighbor in the dorm suite, Srishti, was a big help. She was from India and seemed so confident and sure of herself. She showed me how to be assertive and less judgmental of myself. We did everything together. It was really a lot of fun; we made a little family out of our suite. Srishti and I spent tons of time together, and I was happy that I had wound up with her; it seemed like a stroke of luck.

Then one day she kissed me. Gosh, it seems so simple just to say it like that: "She kissed me." But that was how it happened. And I didn't think twice; I just kissed her back, even though I had never kissed a girl before. Not like that. I had always wondered what that would be like. How would it feel? But it felt wonderful — so right, so natural. I wasn't very experienced sexually, and I thought of myself as open to loving anyone, man or woman, cisgender or transgender, if they were the right person for me. I was so happy with Srishti, and when we were together, I was feeling things that I had never experienced before. She had not come out to her family yet, and she shared with me that she never felt safe to show her sexuality openly to her family. She felt liberated with me. And even though we kept our relationship secret from our other suite mates, she seemed so happy being with me. Those days were amazing. Then things changed.

One day, after about a month, Srishti suddenly told me she thought we shouldn't be doing what we were doing anymore. She said it just like that, and just like that it was all over. She talked about expanding our horizons, exploring other relationships, and other such things. She told me she wasn't ready to be open about her sexuality, that she felt morally corrupt being with me, and that I couldn't tell anyone about our relationship, ever. None of it made much sense or comforted me. I was totally devastated. And I was shocked by the suddenness with which the relationship ended. That alone would have been enough to crush me, but there was more. Srishti wouldn't even talk to me or hang out with me anymore. It was a nightmare. I knew she had another girl over and was sleeping with her — a reminder of how undesirable I was, of my failure at love, of my loss. I felt terrible about myself because Srishti didn't love me like I loved her, and terrible because I had loved her in the first place. I was so depressed that I stopped going to my early morning classes and my biology lab. It didn't take long before I started failing a couple of courses.

I think it was around this time, about midway through that semester, that I first became aware that I was picking my skin again. I say "first became aware," because I have no idea how long I'd actually been doing it. I just suddenly noticed, while in the middle of picking at my arm, that there were already a few droplets of blood forming.

I realized immediately that the picking was back because I was so depressed and stressed. I didn't feel so much the itchy, irritated feeling, but I would feel very

Everyone has certain habits they exhibit when they are under stress. Only occasionally do such habits blossom into a disorder such as Shaylynn's. Are there ways of distinguishing innocent bad habits from signs of problems to come?

uncomfortable. If I tried not to do it, I'd get really nervous and tense. I'd get this cramped, tight feeling in my stomach, and I'd worry that something bad was going to happen. By picking, I would feel that wonderfully familiar surge of relief. Especially when I picked a scab, the tension in my body would pass and my mind would clear. I could lean back in my chair or bed and breathe much more easily. Unfortunately, this feeling of relief wouldn't last for long. The picking behavior occurred more and more. In fact, it would happen so often that I usually didn't know I was doing it — I would sometimes simply catch myself in the act.

Recalling the picking I did in high school, I'd say to myself, "Remember that was just a phase. You didn't have any trouble stopping," and I'd feel reassured. But of course, it had actually been a lot harder to stop back then than I was willing to remember. As I paid more attention to my picking, I observed that I had also started to pick from my face or the side of my head, with my right hand. But I honestly couldn't be sure that that was the only hand I ever used.

A month or two after I first noticed what I was doing, I was in the shower and felt a little patch of skin exposed around my newest favorite picking spot, at the nape of my neck near the hairline, usually covered by my long hair. I think I was running the shampoo through my hair and I was rubbing it through my scalp. When I felt the patch where there was a scab, I picked it and looked at my hands to see the skin, noticing that the shampoo was red with blood. It was bleeding profusely. I panicked. What was I doing? I hadn't even been stressed. I was taking a shower all calm and picking out chunks of my skin, making myself bleed. What is wrong with me? I thought, here I am doing this bizarre and perverse thing that no one else does; I must be a freak. The thought swept through me that everyone must know, and I just wanted to run and hide. At that moment, I started breathing heavily, and I silently promised myself that I would never do this horrible thing again — I was immature and stupid and disgusting, and I had to stop! I rinsed out my hair, toweled it off, then, terrified, I moved to the mirror to see just how bad I looked.

Peeking from between squinted eyelids, I couldn't see a difference at first. Then I opened my eyes wide and saw that there were red spots and scabs in about a dozen places across my body. I sobbed. What was wrong with me? I couldn't go home to my family failing courses and covered in bloodied scabs. And what if these scabs left permanent scars? I felt humiliated and vowed to stay away from my suite mates and friends until the scabs healed and marks went away. I could cover some of them with makeup, but some were too big. The scabs had to go away on their own. It was a horribly distressing time in my life. Miserable emotionally, failing classes, unable to cope with stress without skin picking, incapable of being loved, and avoiding friends and classes — I had never been so low in my life.

When I went home for the winter break, I was terrified. I didn't want to risk my parents seeing any blemishes on their "perfect" little daughter. For the entire time

Based on your reading of either DSM-5-TR or your textbook, what disorder might Shaylynn be displaying? Which of her symptoms suggest this disorder?

during winter break, I kept repeating to myself, "Don't pick. Don't pick. Don't pick." Then I'd think, when the urge had its grip on me, "Well, break is short anyway." And so, I'd pick at my skin. I couldn't control myself. The problem was as bad as ever when I went back to school. To calm myself, I took an Ativan I had stolen from my parents' medicine cabinet and I slept the whole flight back, trying not to allow any urges to pick my skin.

I went back to school, and I predictably continued to pick my skin. My arms looked so bad I gave up on trying to find a romantic partner. It wasn't until 2 more years of this that I finally decided to try therapy. I've been in counseling for 6 months now. I've come to appreciate that I have a lot of anxiety issues, as well as problems with myself and my parents, and that's probably a lot of the reason I do this—at least in part. At the same time, my therapist has explained that many people have this disorder. I couldn't believe that at first; I really thought I was the only one.

I'm going to graduate this coming spring, and I'm doing better at school. Mom and Dad are so happy! I haven't picked my skin in close to 4 months, and I'm not feeling the urge much anymore, which is great. I feel better about the way I look. I've also started seeing Briana, an accepting and easygoing Black woman from Louisville. Our relationship is going great, although, after the disaster with Srishti, I'm trying to take it slow. All in all, things are pretty good, but I do wonder whether I am now prone to picking and whether I'll start doing it again. Will I revert to this whenever I face a crisis? That worries me, and for now that's why I am continuing to go to therapy.

A Mother's View "You've Got to Stop This"

I think Shaylynn was about 16 when I first noticed that she had a truly major problem dealing with stress. We were sitting at the dinner table and talking about her joining the future leaders of Canadian industry club in school. She was telling us that she'd been picked to be the club vice president. Rick and I were happy about that, but asked her who was elected president. We'd been encouraging Shay to lobby to be the club president. It would look better on her college applications. She started to cry, and when we'd ask her what was wrong, she said, "I don't know," and "School is really hard." Rick and I talked about it and thought she might need to get involved in a different extracurricular activity.

When I saw how upset she was getting, I wanted to give my little girl a big hug. When I leaned in, I thought something looked peculiar about how she was holding herself. Her body was angled oddly, with her hand crossed over her body and held close to her abdomen. I hugged her and told her that I was so proud of my little girl. Rick said nothing and simply watched as we hugged. Later, after dinner I went upstairs to check on her in her bedroom. We were talking about her test the next

Shaylynn's disorder is listed as one of several *obsessive-compulsive-related* disorders in DSM-5-TR, disorders related to obsessive-compulsive disorder but technically separate from it. How are Shaylynn's symptoms similar to those of someone with obsessive-compulsive disorder? How are they different?

How might some of the treatments used in Case 2 (Obsessive-Compulsive Disorder) and Case 5 (Major Depressive Disorder) be applied in Shaylynn's case? Which aspects of these approaches would likely not be appropriate for her? Should additional interventions be applied?

Are the family, school, and social pressures described by Shaylynn particularly unusual? Why might they have led to so much dysfunction in Shaylynn's case, but not in the lives of other persons?

day in social studies and how much studying she still needed to do. At one point, she looked up, and that's when I noticed it.

"What happened to your elbow? It's bleeding! And there's blood on your bed sheets!" I exclaimed, before I could stop myself. Shaylynn turned her head away and muttered, "I don't know." But I said, "Rick, come upstairs and look at this! Shay is bleeding!"

He came upstairs, leaned over Shay, and said, "You're right. What's going on here, Shay?" She took a deep breath and said she sometimes picks her arms. She didn't know why she did it. She said she just did—they itched her, maybe. I figured it was some sort of nervous habit, and I told her she had to stop. I told her it wasn't normal. She got upset but finally promised she would try to stop doing it. I then sought to give her some more incentive. "You're so beautiful," I told her, "but you will look strange with scabs all over you! You could look so much better. You've got to stop this, okay?"

For a while after that, I'd see her rubbing her elbows where the scabs were. Rick and I tried to help out by stopping her whenever we saw her scratching or touching her arms. After a while, and with some effort, things seemed to get better. Her scabs went away, and she didn't seem to be picking anymore. Rick and I forgot all about it after a few years.

When Shaylynn went off to college in California, the last thing on my mind was the way she had picked her elbows when she was younger. Rick and I had been hoping she would go to a top school, but she didn't do as well on her SATs as she needed to. Anyway, the school she went to was fine, and we were proud that Shay was heading off to college.

She never called us when she first went away. I guess it was the excitement of being somewhere new. Anyway, girls are like that at that age. When we would call her to see how she was doing in her classes, she never seemed to want to talk—she would talk very softly, say things were fine, and yes, she was making friends. She would then rush off the phone; one time, I was sure that she was holding back tears.

When she came home for her first winter break, she seemed like an emotional wreck. She was tense, distant, and wore much heavier makeup than she ever had before. She stayed in her room most of the time over break, and whenever she was out she was covered from head to toe with clothes. She never came out of her room with shorts or short sleeves. It was always yoga pants and long sleeve shirts. Rick and I could not help but notice how much she had changed, and we thought it was for the worse. I asked her why she dressed like that and wore so much makeup in the house, and she just said she liked it that way. After she'd been home a few weeks, she let her guard down, and when she tilted her head sideways once, right before she quickly brushed the hair back over, I saw it—the back of her scalp! A horrifying, huge bloodied spot. I asked her what was wrong.

"Are you sick?" But she just got really serious and said she didn't want to talk about it. Then she left the room.

Later, she admitted that she had started picking again. She said she didn't know why she did it, but she was considering going into therapy, for that and for a lot of other things. She explained that the picking—and feelings of stress—were similar to what she was doing and feeling in high school, and I thought, "Of course, it all makes sense now." This is really strange, but she told me that it wasn't my problem and I should just let her try to work on it herself.

After that, once she was back at school, whenever I would ask her on the phone how she was doing with the picking problem, she would mumble a short answer like "Fine." Sometimes she wouldn't come home at all on vacations. But I guess now that she's a senior, she's made things right and put it all behind her. She was home just last month, and she certainly seemed to be fine. But I don't really know for sure how well she is doing.

On the surface, Shaylynn and her mother had a close and loving relationship, but they also had some significant problems in their interactions. What were some of these problems, and how might they have contributed to Shaylynn's disorder?

Reader Alert!

Now that you've read about Shaylynn, considered important issues, and made key decisions, go to the next chapter, *Case 20 Appendix*, for Shaylynn's probable diagnosis, the DSM-5-TR criteria, clinical information, and possible treatment directions.

CASE 20 Appendix
The Case of Shaylynn: Diagnosis, Information, and Treatment

In the previous chapter, *The Case of Shaylynn: You Decide,* you were asked to consider a number of issues and to arrive at various decisions, including diagnostic and treatment decisions. How did you do? This chapter presents Shaylynn's probable diagnosis, the DSM-5-TR criteria, relevant clinical information, and possible treatment directions.

Diagnosis

Shaylynn's pattern would receive a diagnosis of **excoriation disorder (skin-picking disorder).**

Dx Checklist

Excoriation Disorder (Skin-Picking Disorder)

1. Individuals repeatedly pick off parts of their skin, causing skin lesions.
2. Despite attempts to stop, individuals are unable to stop this practice.
3. Significant distress or impairment.

(Information from APA, 2022, 2013)

Clinical Information

Although studies of excoriation disorder have been limited in number, investigators have been able to gather a body of important information about it (Park & Koo, 2021; APA, 2022, 2013).

1. At least 1.6% of adults exhibit excoriation disorder at some point in their lives. Females with the problem seem to heavily outnumber males by a ratio of 8:1.

2. Excoriation disorder may emerge between puberty and 45 years of age.

3. For those with the disorder, episodes of skin picking are often triggered by anxiety or boredom, preceded by growing tension, and followed by feelings of relief or pleasure. The overall syndrome sometimes begins for individuals when they are grappling with a dermatological condition like acne.

4. Excoriation disorder may come and go for an individual — lasting days, weeks, months, or years each time.

5. Medical complications of repeated skin picking may include tissue damage, scarring, and/or infection.

6. DSM-5-TR lists excoriation disorder as one of the obsessive-compulsive-related disorders, a group of disorders marked by particular patterns of repetitive and excessive behavior that greatly disrupt the lives of individuals.

7. Some clinicians believe that the disorder is actually a form of obsessive-compulsive disorder, because the skin picking, like the compulsions found in obsessive-compulsive disorder, is compulsive in nature, feels involuntary, and is recognized by the individual as senseless.

8. On the other hand, there seem to be some distinct contrasts between skin picking and the compulsions that usually characterize obsessive-compulsive disorder. For example, compulsions are most often performed in response to obsessions, aimed at preventing some dreaded event, done with full awareness by the patient, and span beyond a single behavior.

9. People with excoriation disorder often also exhibit another psychological disorder, either concurrently or at another point in their lives. Depressive disorders, trichotillomania (hair-pulling) disorder, and obsessive-compulsive disorder are among the most common such disorders.

Treatment Overview and Strategies

Clinicians often treat people with excoriation disorder by applying the kinds of treatments used in cases of obsessive-compulsive disorder (Park & Koo, 2021; Taylor et al., 2020). The following interventions are commonly part of treatment:

1. Self-help groups, including ones on the Internet

2. Certain antidepressant medications

3. Cognitive-behavioral therapy, featuring:

   a. Self-monitoring of skin-picking behaviors

   b. Exposure to situations that usually trigger skin picking

    c. Performance of alternative or competing behavior during such exposure, until the urge to pick skin passes

    d. Identification and alteration of maladaptive beliefs about the nature of stress, the need for immediate relief, counterproductive ways to cope, or the like that may be contributing to the skin-picking behavior

4. Psychotherapy for any feelings of depression that may accompany excoriation disorder

5. Relapse-prevention strategies

References

AA (Alcoholics Anonymous). (2020). *AA around the world.* Retrieved from https://www.aa.org.

AAMFT (American Association for Marriage and Family Therapy). (2021a, July 17). *Substance abuse and intimate relationships.* Alexandria, VA: AAMFT. Retrieved from https://www.aamft.org/Consumer_Updates.

AAMFT (American Association for Marriage and Family Therapy). (2021b, July 18). *Children of alcoholics.* Alexandria, VA: AAMFT. Retrieved from https://www.aamft.org/Consumer_Updates.

ADAA (Anxiety and Depression Association of America). (2020). *Facts & statistics.* Silver Spring, MD: Author.

Adler, J. (1998, May 4). Take a pill and call me tonight. *Newsweek,* p. 48.

Alarcón, R. D., & Palmer, B. A. (2020). Personality disorders: Epidemiology and clinical course. In J. R. Geddes, N. C. Andreason, & G. M. Goodwin (Eds.), *New Oxford textbook of psychiatry* (3rd ed., Ch. 119). New York: Oxford University Press.

Álvarez-García, D., González-Castro, P., Núñez, J. C., Rodríguez, C., & Cerezo, R. (2019). Impact of family and friends on antisocial adolescent behavior: The mediating role of impulsivity and empathy. *Frontiers in Psychology, 10,* 2071.

Alzheimer's Association. (2020). *2020 Alzheimer's disease facts and figures: On the front lines: Primary care physicians and Alzheimer's care in America.* Chicago, IL: Author.

ALZRA (Alzheimer's Research Association). (2020). *Depression.* St. Clair Shores, MI: ALRA. Retrieved from https://www.alzra.org.

ANAD (National Association of Anorexia Nervosa and Associated Disorders). (2020). *Eating disorder statistics.* Chicago: Author.

APA (American Psychiatric Association). (2013). *Diagnostic and statistical manual of mental disorders* (5th ed.). Washington, DC: Author.

APA (American Psychiatric Association). (2020a). *What is depression?* Washington, DC: Author.

APA (American Psychological Association). (2020b). *Telehealth guidance by state during COVID-19.* Retrieved from https://www.apaservices.org:practice :legal:technology:state-telehealth-guidance%3F_ga=2.38552288.258586707 .1587402602-161748745.1584460934.

APA (American Psychiatric Association). (2022). *Diagnostic and statistical manual of mental disorders, fifth edition text revision (DSM-5-TR).* Washington, DC: Author.

Artoni, P., Chierici, M. L., Arnone, F., Cigarini, C., De Bernardis, E., Galeazzi, G. M., . . . Pingani, L. (2020, March 2). Body perception treatment, a possible way to treat body image disturbance in eating disorders: A case–control efficacy study. *Eating and Weight Disorders: Studies on Anorexia, Bulimia and Obesity.* [Epub ahead of print]

Ashbaugh, A. R., McCabe, R. E., & Antony, M. M. (2020). Social anxiety disorder. In M. M. Antony & D. H. Barlow, *Handbook of assessment and treatment planning for psychological disorders* (3rd ed., Ch. 7). New York: Guilford Press.

Augustyn, M. (2020, May 4). Autism spectrum disorder: Terminology, epidemiology, and pathogenesis. *UpToDate.* Retrieved from https://www.uptodate.com.

Autism Speaks. (2020). *Autism statistics and facts.* New York: Autism Speaks Org.

Ayub, R., Sun, K. L., Flores, R. E., Lam, V. T., Jo, B., Saggar, M., & Fung, L. K. (2021). Thalamocortical connectivity is associated with autism symptoms in high-functioning adults with autism and typically developing adults. *Translational Psychiatry, 11*(1), 93.

Azevedo, J., Vieira-Coelho, M., Castelo-Branco, M., Coelho, R., & Figueiredo-Braga, M. (2020). Impulsive and premeditated aggression in male offenders with antisocial personality disorder. *PLoS One, 15*(3), e0229876.

Bajaj, V., Gadi, N., Spihlman, A. P., Wu, S. C., Choi, C. H., & Moulton, V. R. (2021). Aging, immunity, and COVID-19: How age influences the host immune response to coronavirus infections. *Frontiers in Physiology, 11,* 571416.

Balderrama-Durbin, C. M., Abbott, B. V., & Snyder, D. K. (2020). Couple distress. In M. M. Antony & D. H. Barlow (Eds.), *Handbook of assessment* *and treatment planning for psychological disorders* (3rd ed., Ch. 13). New York: Guilford Press.

Baldessarini, R. J., Vázquez, G. H., & Tondo, L. (2020). Bipolar depression: A major unsolved challenge. *International Journal of Bipolar Disorders, 8*(1), 1.

Baldwin, D. S., & Huneke, T. M. (2020). Treatment of anxiety disorders. In J. R. Geddes, N. C. Andreason, & G. M. Goodwin (Eds.), *New Oxford textbook of psychiatry* (3rd ed.). New York: Oxford University Press.

Bates, G. W., Thompson, J. C., & Flanagan, C. (1999). The effectiveness of individual versus group induction of depressed mood. *Journal of Psychology, 133*(3), 245–252.

Beeney, J. E., Forbes, E. E., Hipwell, A. E., Nance, M., Mattia, A., Lawless, J. M., . . . Stepp, S. D. (2020, May 25). Determining the key childhood and adolescent risk factors for future BPD symptoms using regularized regression: Comparison to depression and conduct disorder. *Journal of Child Psychology and Psychiatry, and Allied Disciplines.* [Epub ahead of print]

Begley, S. (2020, March 3). Who is getting sick, and how sick? A breakdown of coronavirus risk by demographic factors. *STAT.* Retrieved from https://www.statnews.com.

Behenck, A. da S., Wesner, A. C., Guimaraes, L. S. P., Manfro, G. G., Dreher, C. B., & Heldt, E. (2020, July 9). Anxiety sensitivity and panic disorder: Evaluation of the impact of cognitive-behavioral group therapy. *Issues in Mental Health Nursing, 42*(2), 112–118. https://doi.org/10.1080/01612840.2020.1780527.

Bernal, G., Adames, C., Mariani, K., & Morales, J. (2018). Cognitive behavioral models, measures, and treatments for anxiety disorders in Latinos: A systematic review. In E. C. Chang, C. A. Downey, J. K. Hirsch, & E. A. Yu (Eds.), *Cultural, racial, and ethnic psychology book series. Treating depression, anxiety, and stress in ethnic and racial groups: Cognitive behavioral approaches* (pp. 149–177). Washington, DC: American Psychological Association.

Billard, T. J. (2018). Attitudes toward transgender men and women: Development and validation of a new measure. *Frontiers in Psychology, 9,* 387.

Black, D. W. (2020, November 12). Treatment of antisocial personality disorder. *UpToDate.* Retrieved from https://www.uptodate.com.

Blair, R. J. R., Meffert, H., Hwang, S., & White, S. F. (2019). Psychopathy and brain function: Insights from neuroimaging research. In C. J. Patrick (Ed.), *Handbook of psychopathy* (2nd ed., Ch. 17, pp. 401–421). New York: Guilford Press.

BLS (Bureau of Labor Statistics). (2021, April 21). *Employment characteristics of families—2020.* Retrieved from https://www.bls.gov/news.release/famee.nr0.htm.

Boskey, E. (2020, March 30). The 7 best online transgender support groups of 2020. *Verywellmind.* Retrieved from https://www.verywellmind.com.

Bränström, R., & Pachankis, J. E. (2019, October 4). Reduction in mental health treatment utilization among transgender individuals after gender-affirming surgeries: A total population study. *American Journal of Psychiatry, 177*(8), 727–734.

Bressert, S. (2018). Who gets bipolar disorder? *Psych Central.* Retrieved from https://psychcentral.com.

Bristow, G. C., Thomson, D. M., Openshaw, R. L., Mitchell, E. J., Pratt, J. A., Dawson, N., & Morris, B. J. (2020). 16p11 duplication disrupts hippocampal-orbitofrontal-amygdala connectivity, revealing a neural circuit endophenotype for schizophrenia. *Cell Reports, 31*(3), 107536.

Brooks, S. K., Webster, R. K., Smith, L. E., Woodland, L., Wessely, S., Greenberg, N., & Rubin, G. J. (2020). The psychological impact of quarantine and how to reduce it: Rapid review of the evidence. *The Lancet, 395*(10227), 912–920.

Bukstein, O. (2021a, February 24). Pharmacotherapies for attention deficit hyperactivity disorder in adults. *UpToDate.* Retrieved from https://www.uptodate.com.

Bukstein, O. (2021b, March 26). Attention deficit hyperactivity disorder in adults: Epidemiology, pathogenesis, clinical features, course, assessment, and diagnosis. *UpToDate.* Retrieved from https://www.uptodate.com.

Burton, C., Fink, P., Henningsen, P., Löwe, B., & Rief, W. (2020). Functional somatic disorders: Discussion paper for a new common classification for research and clinical use. *BMC Medicine, 18*(1), 34.

Business Wire. (2019, February 25). The $72 billion weight loss & diet control market in the United States, 2019–2023: Why meal replacements are still booming, but not OTC diet pills. *Business Wire.* Retrieved from https://www.researchandmarkets.com.

Business Wire. (2020, June 4). United States weight loss market in 2020: Effects of the COVID-19 pandemic. *Business Wire.* Retrieved from https://www.researchandmarkets.com.

Bustillo, J., & Weil, E. (2019, April 30). Psychosocial interventions for schizophrenia. *UpToDate.* Retrieved from https://www.uptodate.com.

Butler, R. M., & Heimberg, R. G. (2020). Exposure therapy for eating disorders: A systematic review. *Clinical Psychology Review, 78,* 101851.

Buzzell, G. A., Morales, S., Bowers, M. E., Troller-Renfree, S. V., Chronis-Tuscano, A., Pine, D. S., . . . Fox, N. A. (2021). Inhibitory control and set shifting describe different pathways from behavioral inhibition to socially anxious behavior. *Developmental Science, 24*(1), e13040. https://doi.org/10.1111/desc.13040.

Caceres. V. (2020, February 14). Eating disorder statistics. *U.S. News.* Retrieved from https://health.usnews.com.

Campez, M., Raiker, J. S., Little, K., Altszuler, A. R., Merrill, B. M., Macphee, F. L., . . . Pelham, W. E. (2021, January 21). An evaluation of the effect of methylphenidate on working memory, time perception, and choice impulsivity in children with ADHD. *Experimental and Clinical Psychopharmacology.* [Epub ahead of print]

Capasso, A., Jones, A. M., Ali, S. H., Foreman, J., Tozan, Y., & DiClemente, R. J. (2021, April). Increased alcohol use during the COVID-19 pandemic: The effect of mental health and age in a cross-sectional sample of social media users in the U.S. *Preventive Medicine, 14,* 106422.

Carroll, N. M., & Banks, A. (2020, January 28). Health care for female trauma survivors (with posttraumatic stress disorder or similarly severe symptoms). *UpToDate.* Retrieved from http://www.uptodate.com.

Carvalho, A. F., Firth, J., & Vieta, E. (2020). Bipolar disorder. *The New England Journal of Medicine, 383*(1), 58–66.

Castleman, M. (2017, August 1). Surprise: Men enjoy—and want—foreplay. *Psychology Today.*

CDC (Centers for Disease Control and Prevention). (2019a, July 31). *Alzheimer's disease and healthy aging: Supporting caregivers.* Atlanta, GA: CDC.

CDC (Centers for Disease Control and Prevention). (2019b, June 3). *Disease or condition of the week: Alzheimer's disease.* Atlanta, GA: CDC.

CDC (Centers for Disease Control and Prevention). (2020a). *The drug overdose epidemic: Behind the numbers.* Atlanta, GA: CDC.

CDC (Centers for Disease Control and Prevention). (2020b). Overdose deaths accelerating during COVID-19. Retrieved from https://www.cdc.gov/media/releases/2020/p1218-overdose-deaths-covid-19.html.

CDC (Centers for Disease Control and Prevention). (2020c, November 16). *Data and statistics about ADHD.* Atlanta, GA: CDC.

CDC (Centers for Disease Control and Prevention). (2021a, February 3). *Disease or condition of the week: Alzheimer's disease.* Atlanta, GA: CDC.

CDC (Centers for Disease Control and Prevention). (2021b, November 21). *Alzheimer's disease and healthy aging: Supporting caregivers.* Atlanta, GA: CDC.

Celebi, F., & Ünal, D. (2021, January 21). Self esteem and clinical features in a clinical sample of children with ADHD and social anxiety disorder. *Nordic Journal of Psychiatry,* 1–6.

Cénat, J. M., Blais-Rochette, C., Kokou-Kpolou, C. K., Noorishad, P.-G., Mukunzi, J. N., McIntee, S.-E., Dalexis, R. D., Goulet, M.-A., & Labelle, P. R. (2021). Prevalence of symptoms of depression, anxiety, insomnia, posttraumatic stress disorder, and psychological distress among populations affected by the COVID-19 pandemic: A systematic review and meta-analysis. *Psychiatry Research, 295,* 113599. https://doi.org/10.1016/j.psychres.2020.113599.

Chapman, A. L., & Dixon-Gordon, K. L. (2020. May 12). *Dialectical behavior therapy* (Theories of Psychotherapy Series, 1st ed.) Washington, DC: American Psychological Association.

Chapman, J., Jamil, R. T., & Fleisher, C. (2021, August 1). Borderline personality disorder. *StatPearls.*

Churchill, G. C., Singh, N., & Berridge, M. J. (2020). Basic mechanisms of and treatment targets for bipolar disorder. In J. R. Geddes, N. C. Andreasen, & G. M. Goodwin (Eds.), *New Oxford textbook of psychiatry* (3rd ed., Ch. 69). New York: Oxford University Press.

Connolly, S. L., Stolzmann, K. L., Heyworth, L., Weaver, K. R., Bauer, M. S., & Miller, C. J. (2020, September 14). Rapid increase in telemental health within the Department of Veterans Affairs during the COVID-19 pandemic. *Telemedicine Journal and e-Health.* [Epub ahead of print]

Cooper, Z., & Fairburn C. G. (2011). The evolution of "enhanced" cognitive behavior therapy for eating disorders: Learning from treatment nonresponse. *Cognitive and Behavioral Practice, 18*(3), 394–402.

Cooper, Z., & Mitchell, K. S. (2020). Eating disorders. In M. M. Antony & D. H. Barlow (Eds.), *Handbook of assessment and treatment planning for psychological disorders* (3rd ed., Ch. 12). New York: Guilford Press.

Correll, C. U., & Schooler, N. R. (2020). Negative symptoms in schizophrenia: A review and clinical guide for recognition, assessment, and treatment. *Neuropsychiatric Disease and Treatment, 16,* 519–534.

Coryell, W. (2020, April 26). Unipolar depression in adults: Course of illness. *UpToDate.* Retrieved from http://www.uptodate.com.

Cote, A. C., Phelps, R. J., Kabiri, N. S., Bhangu, J. S., & Thomas, K. K. (2021). Evaluation of wearable technology in dementia: A systematic review and meta-analysis. *Frontiers in Medicine, 7,* 501104.

Cowan, R. G., Blum, C. R., Szirony, G. M., & Cicchetti, R. (2020). Supporting survivors of public mass shootings. *Journal of Social, Behavioral, and Health Sciences, 14,* 169–182.

Craske, M. G. (2021, May 11). Psychotherapy for panic disorder with or without agoraphobia in adults. *UpToDate.* Retrieved from https://www.uptodate.com.

Craske, M. G., & Barlow, D. H. (1993). Panic disorder and agoraphobia. In D. H. Barlow (Ed.), *Clinical handbook of psychological disorders* (2nd ed., pp. 1–47). New York: Guilford Press.

Craske, M. G., Wolitzky-Taylor, K., & Barlow, D. H. (2021). Panic disorder and agoraphobia. In D. H. Barlow (Ed.)., *Clinical handbook of psychological disorders* (6th ed., Ch. 1). New York: Routledge.

Cueli, M., Rodríguez, C., Cañamero, L. M., Núñez, J. C., & González-Castro, P. (2020, April). Self-concept and inattention or hyperactivity-impulsivity symptomatology: The role of anxiety. *Brain Sciences, 10*(4).

Cummings, J. (2021). New approaches to symptomatic treatments for Alzheimer's disease. *Molecular Neurodegeneration, 16*(1), 2.

Cyrkot, T., Szczepanowski, R., Jankowiak-Siuda, K., Gawęda, Ł., & Cichoń, E. (2021, January 18). Mindreading and metacognition patterns in patients with borderline personality disorder: Experimental study. *European Archives of Psychiatry and Clinical Neuroscience.* [Epub ahead of print]

D'Souza, R. S., & Hooten, W. M. (2020a). Somatic syndrome disorders. *StatPearls.*

D'Souza, R. S., & Hooten, W. M. (2020b). Extrapyramidal symptoms (EPS). *StatPearls.*

Da Paz, N. S., & Wallander, J. L. (2017). Interventions that target improvements in mental health for parents of children with autism spectrum disorders: A narrative review. *Clinical Psychology Review, 51,* 1–14.

Davey, G. C. L. (2019, December 3). The psychology of OCD. *Psychology Today.*

DBSA (Depression and Bipolar Support Alliance). (2020). *Depression statistics.* Chicago: Author.

DeRubeis, R. J., Zjecka, J., Shelton, R. C., Amsterdam, J. D., Fawcett, J., Xu, C., . . . Hollon, S. D. (2020). Prevention of recurrence after recovery from a major depressive episode with antidepressant medication alone or in combination with cognitive behavioral therapy: A phase 2 randomized clinical trial. *JAMA Psychiatry, 77*(3), 237–245.

Desormeau, P. A., Walsh, K. M., & Segal, Z. V. (2020). Mindfulness-based stress reduction and mindfulness-based cognitive therapy. In K. L. Harkness & E. P. Hayden (Eds.), *The Oxford handbook of stress and mental health* (Ch. 31, pp. 689–704). New York: Oxford University Press.

DF. (2020). *DrFirst survey: 44% of Americans have used telehealth services during coronavirus pandemic but some admit not paying attention.* Rockville, MD: DrFirst.

Dishman, R. K., McDowell, C. P., & Herring, M. P. (2021). Customary physical activity and odds of depression: A systematic review and meta-analysis of 111 prospective cohort studies. *British Journal of Sports Medicine.*

Douglas, K. S., Vincent, G. M., & Edens, J. F. (2019). Risk for criminal recidivism: The role of psychopathy. In C. J. Patrick (Ed.), *Handbook of psychopathy* (2nd ed., Ch. 28, pp. 682–709). New York: Guilford Press.

Dozois, D. J. A., Wilde, J. L., & Dobson, K. S. (2020). Depressive disorders. In M. M. Antony & D. H. Barlow (Eds.), *Handbook of assessment and treatment planning for psychological disorders* (3rd ed., Ch. 11). New York: Guilford Press.

Duek, O., Pietrzak, R. H., Petrakis, I., Hoff, R., & Harpaz-Rotem, I. (2021). Early discontinuation of pharmacotherapy in U.S. veterans diagnosed with PTSD and the role of psychotherapy. *Journal of Psychiatric Research, 132,* 167–173.

Duncan, P. M. (2020, November 26). *Substance use disorders: A biopsychosocial perspective* (1st ed.). New York: Cambridge University Press.

Ekern, J. (2020). *Anorexia nervosa: Causes, symptoms, signs and treatment help.* Retrieved from https://www.eatingdisorderhope.com/information.

Ekman, P., O'Sullivan, M., & Frank, M. G. (1999). A few can catch a liar. *Psychological Science, 10*(3), 263–266.

Elaut, E., & Heylens, G. (2020). Gender dysphoria. In J. R. Geddes, N. C. Andreasen, & G. M. Goodwin (Eds.), *New Oxford textbook of psychiatry* (3rd ed., Ch. 116). New York: Oxford University Press.

Ellickson-Larew, S. A., Carney, J. R., Coady, A. T., Barnes, J. B., Grunthal, B., & Litz, B. T. (2020). Trauma- and stressor-related disorders. In M. M. Antony & D. H. Barlow (Eds.), *Handbook of assessment and treatment planning for psychological disorders* (3rd ed., Ch. 10). New York: Guilford Press.

Emery, L. R. (2018, September 24). The 10 most common things people do right after sex, according to a new survey. *Bustle.* Retrieved from https://www.bustle.com.

Emmady, P. D., & Tadi, P. (2020). Dementia. *StatPearls.*

Endocrine Society. (2017, September). *Gender dysphoria/gender incongruence guideline resources.* Washington, DC: Author.

Endocrine Society. (2020). *Transgender medicine and research.* Washington, DC: Author.

Engel, S., Steffen, K., & Mitchell, J. E. (2021, May 10). Bulimia nervosa in adults: Clinical features, course of illness, assessment, and diagnosis. *UpToDate.* Retrieved from https://www.uptodate.com.

Evans, S. W., Owens, J. S., & Power, T. J. (2019). Attention-deficit/ hyperactivity disorder. In M. J. Prinstein, E. A. Youngstrom, E. J. Mash, & R. A. Barkley (Eds.), *Treatment of disorders in childhood and adolescence* (4th ed.). New York: Guilford Press.

Fairburn, C., & Murphy, R. (2020). The eating disorders. In J. R. Geddes, N. C. Andreason, & G. M. Goodwin (Eds.), *New Oxford textbook of psychiatry* (3rd ed., Ch. 101). New York: Oxford University Press.

Fairburn, C. G., Cooper, Z., Doll, H. A., O'Connor, M. E., Palmer, R. L., & Dalle Grave, R. (2013). Enhanced cognitive behaviour therapy for adults with anorexia nervosa: A UK–Italy study. *Behaviour Research and Therapy, 51*(1), R2–R8.

Fairburn, C. G., Cooper, Z., Shafran, R., & Wilson, G. T. (2008). Eating disorders: A "transdiagnostic" protocol. In D. H. Barlow (Ed.), *Clinical handbook of psychological disorders: A step-by-step treatment manual* (4th ed.). New York: Guilford Press.

Fariba, K., Gupta, V., & Kass, E. (2021, June 9). Personality disorder. *StatPearls.*

Farrell, M., Larance, B., & Breen, C. (2020). Opiates: Heroin, methadone, buprenorphine. In J. R. Geddes, N. C. Andreason, & G. M. Goodwin (Eds.), *New Oxford textbook of psychiatry* (3rd ed., Ch. 51). New York: Oxford University Press.

Fernandes, V., Al-Sukhni, M., Lawson, A., & Chandler, G. (2020). Lithium prescribing and therapeutic drug monitoring in bipolar disorder: A survey of current practices and perspectives. *Journal of Psychiatric Practice, 26*(5), 360–366.

Ferrando, C., & Thomas, T. N. (2020, January 27). Transgender surgery: Male to female. *UpToDate.* Retrieved from https://www.uptodate.com.

Ferrando, C., Zhao, L. C., & Nikolavsky, D. (2020, March 20). Transgender surgery: Female to male. *UpToDate.* Retrieved from https://www.uptodate.com.

Firth, J., Solmi, M., Wootton, R. E., Vancampfort, D., Schuch, F. B., Hoare, E., . . . Stubbs, B. (2020). A meta-review of "lifestyle psychiatry": The role of exercise, smoking, diet and sleep in the prevention and treatment of mental disorders. *World Psychiatry, 19*(3), 360–380.

Fischer, B. A., & Buchanan, R. W. (2020a). Schizophrenia in adults: Clinical manifestations, course, assessment, and diagnosis. *UpToDate.* Retrieved from https://www.uptodate.com.

Fischer, B. A., & Buchanan, R. W. (2020b). Schizophrenia in adults: Epidemiology and pathogenesis. *UpToDate.* Retrieved from https://www.uptodate.com.

Fisher, K. A., & Hany, M. (2021, May 21). Antisocial personality disorder. *StatPearls.*

Fitzsimmons-Craft, E., & Pike, K. (2021, December 15). Anorexia nervosa in adults: Cognitive-behavioral therapy (CBT). *UpToDate.* Retrieved from https://www.uptodate.com.

Forcier, M., & Olson-Kennedy, J. (2020a, June 22). Gender development and clinical presentation of gender diversity in children and adolescents. *UpToDate.* Retrieved from http://www.uptodate.com.

Forcier, M., & Olson-Kennedy, J. (2020b, September 17). Lesbian, gay, bisexual, and other sexual minoritized youth: Epidemiology and health concerns. *UpToDate.* Retrieved from http://www.uptodate.com.

Fountoulakis, K. N., Apostolidou, M. K., Atsiova, M. B., Filippidou, A. K., Florou, A. K., Gousiou, D. S., . . . Chrousos, G. P. (2021). Self-reported changes in anxiety, depression and suicidality during the COVID-19 lockdown in Greece. *Journal of Affective Disorders, 279,* 624–629. https://doi.org/10.1016/j.jad.2020.10.061

Fresson, M., Meulemans, T., Dardenne, B., & Geurten, M. (2019). Overdiagnosis of ADHD in boys: Stereotype impact on neuropsychological assessment. *Applied Neuropsychology Child, 8*(3), 231–245.

Friedman, E. M., & Kennedy, D. (2021, February 15). Typologies of dementia caregiver support networks: A pilot study. *The Gerontologist.* [Epub ahead of print]

Gindt, M., Fernandez, A., Battista, M., & Askenazy, F. (2021, January 8). [Psychiatric consequences of Covid 19 pandemic in the pediatric population.] *Neuropsychiatrie De l'enfance et de l'adolescence.* [Epub ahead of print]

Gottesman, I. I. (1991). *Schizophrenia genesis.* New York: Freeman.

Graham, C., & Bancroft, J. (2020). The sexual dysfunction and paraphilias. In J. R. Geddes, N. C. Andreason, & G. M. Goodwin (Eds.), *New Oxford textbook of psychiatry* (3rd ed.). New York: Oxford University Press.

Grave, R., Calugi, S., Conti, M., Doll, H., & Fairburn, C. G. (2013). Inpatient cognitive behaviour therapy for anorexia nervosa: A randomized controlled trial. *Psychotherapy and Psychosomatics, 82*(6), 390–398.

Grinspoon, P. (2021, October 7). *5 myths about using soboxone to treat opiate addiction.* Retrieved from https://www.health.harvard.edu/blog.

Guzmán-González, M., Barrientos, J., Saiz, J. L., Gómez, F., Cárdenas, M., Espinoza-Tapia, R., . . . Giami, A. (2020). [Mental health in a sample of transgender people.] *Revista Medica De Chile, 148*(8), 1113–1120.

Halmi, K. A. (2020). Epidemiology and primary prevention of feeding and eating disorders. In J. R. Geddes, N. C. Andreason, & G. M. Goodwin (Eds.), *New Oxford textbook of psychiatry* (3rd ed., Ch. 103). New York: Oxford University Press.

Halverson, J. L. (2019, October 7). What is the suicide rate among persons with depressive disorder (clinical depression)? *Medscape.* Retrieved from https://medscape.com/answers/286759-14675.

Hancock, L., & Bryant, R. A. (2020). Posttraumatic stress, stressor controllability, and avoidance. *Behaviour Research and Therapy, 128*, 103591.

Hany, M., Rehman, B., Azhar, Y., & Chapman, J. (2020). Schizophrenia. *StatPearls.*

Harned, M. S., Fitzpatrick, S., & Schmidt, S. C. (2020, March 26). Identifying change targets for posttraumatic stress disorder among suicidal and self-injuring women with borderline personality disorder. *Journal of Traumatic Stress.* [Epub ahead of print]

He, H., Cao, H., Huang, B., He, M., Ma, C., Yao, D., . . . Duan, M. (2021, January 4). Functional abnormalities of striatum are related to the season-specific effect on schizophrenia. *Brain Imaging and Behavior.* [Epub ahead of print]

Heflin, M. (2020, March 9). Geriatric health maintenance. *UpToDate.* Retrieved from https://www.uptodate.com.

Herman, J. L., Brown, T. N. T., & Haas, A. P. (2019). *Suicide thoughts and attempts among transgender adults: Findings from the 2015 U.S. Transgender Survey.* Los Angeles: Williams Institute, University of California Los Angeles.

Hofmann, S. G. (2021, November 17). Psychotherapy for social anxiety disorder in adults. *UpToDate.* Retrieved from https://www.uptodate.com.

Holm, M., Taipale, H., Tanskanen, A., Tiihonen, J., & Mitterdorfer-Rutz, E. (2021). Employment among people with schizophrenia or bipolar disorder: A population-based study using nationwide registers. *Acta Psychiatrica Scandinavica, 143*(1), 61–71.

Hyland, P., Murphy, J., Shevlin, M., Vallières, F., McElroy, E., Elkit, A., . . . Cloitre, M. (2017). Variation in post-traumatic response: The role of trauma type in predicting ICD-11 PTSD and CPTSD symptoms. *Social Psychiatry and Psychiatric Epidemiology, 52*, 727–773.

Hyland, P., Shevlin, M., Fyvie, C., Cloitre, M., & Karatzias, T. (2020). The relationship between ICD-11 PTSD, complex PTSD and dissociative experiences. *Journal of Trauma & Dissociation, 21*(1), 62–72.

Ioannidis, K., Hook, R. W., Grant, J. E., Czabanowska, K., Roman-Urrestarazu, A., & Chamberlain, S. R. (2021). Eating disorders with over-exercise: A cross-sectional analysis of the mediational role of problematic usage of the internet in young people. *Journal of Psychiatric Research, 132*, 215–222.

Jauhar, S., Laws, K. R., & Young, A. H. (2021). Mindfulness-based cognitive therapy and depression relapse-evaluating evidence through a meta-analytic lens may indicate myopia. *Acta Psychiatrica Scandinavica, 143*(1), 3–5.

Javier, S. J., & Belgrave, F. Z. (2019). "I'm not White, I have to be pretty and skinny": A qualitative exploration of body image and eating disorders among Asian American women. *Asian American Journal of Psychology, 10*(2), 141–153.

Jibson, M. D. (2021, February 23). Second-generation antipsychotic medications: Pharmacology, administration, and side effects. *UpToDate.* Retrieved from https://www.uptodate.com.

Johns, M. M., Beltran, O., Armstrong, H. L., Jayne, P. E., & Barrios, L. C. (2018, April 26). Protective factors among transgender and gender variant youth: A systematic review by socioecological level. *Journal of Primary Prevention, 39*(3), 263–301.

Johnston, L. D., Miech, R. A., O'Malley, P. M., Backman, J. G., Schulenberg, J. E., & Patrick, M. E. (2020). *Monitoring the Future national survey results on drug use 1975–2019: Overview, key findings on adolescent drug use.* Ann Arbor: Institute for Social Research, University of Michigan.

Jones, N., Gius, B., Daley, T., George, P., Rosenblatt, A., & Shern, D. (2020). Coordinated specialty care discharge, transition, and step-down policies, practices, and concerns: Staff and client perspectives. *Psychiatric Services, 71*(5), 487–497.

Jørgensen, M. S., Bo, S., Vestergaard, M., Storebø, O. J., Sharp, C., & Simonsen, E. (2021, January 11). Predictors of dropout among adolescents with borderline personality disorder attending mentalization-based group treatment. *Psychotherapy Research: Journal of the Society for Psychotherapy Research,* 1–12. [Epub ahead of print]

Juvonen, J., & Ho, A. Y. (2008). Social motives underlying antisocial behavior across middle school grades. *Journal of Youth and Adolescence, 37,* 747.

Kanner, L. (1943). Autistic disturbances of affective contact. *Nervous Child, 2,* 217.

Kaplan, H. S. (1987). *The illustrated manual of sex therapy* (2nd ed.). New York: Brunner/Mazel.

Kaya, S., Yildirim, H., & Atmaca, M. (2020). Reduced hippocampus and amygdala volumes in antisocial personality disorder. *Journal of Clinical Neuroscience: Official Journal of the Neurosurgical Society of Australasia, 75,* 199–203.

Keitner, G. (2021, August 12). Unipolar depression in adults: Family and couples therapy. *UpToDate.* Retrieved from https://www.uptodate.com.

Kessing, L. V. (2020). Epidemiology of mood disorders. In J. R. Geddes, N. C. Andreasen, & G. M. Goodwin (Eds.), *New Oxford textbook of psychiatry* (3rd ed., Ch. 67). New York: Oxford University Press.

Khera, M. (2021, July 28). Treatment of male sexual dysfunction. *UpToDate.* Retrieved from https://www.uptodate.com.

Khoury, J. E., Pechtel, P., Andersen, C. M., Teicher, M. H., & Lyons-Ruth, K. (2019). Relations among maternal withdrawal in infancy, borderline features, suicidality/self-injury, and adult hippocampal volume: A 30-year longitudinal study. *Behavioural Brain Research, 374,* 112139.

Kleberg, J. L., Högström, J., Sundström, K., Frick, A., & Serlachius, E. (2021). Delayed gaze shifts away from others' eyes in children and adolescents with social anxiety disorder. *Journal of Affective Disorders, 278,* 280–287. https://doi.org/10.1016/j.jad.2020.09.022.

Klein, D., & Attia, E. (2021, June 4). Anorexia nervosa in adults: Clinical features, course of illness, assessment, and diagnosis. *UpToDate.* Retrieved from https://www.uptodate.com.

Kolla, N. J., Boileau, I., Karas, K., Watts, J. J., Rusjan, P., Houle, S., & Mizrahi, R. (2021). Lower amygdala fatty acid amide hydrolase in violent offenders with antisocial personality disorder: An [11C]CURB positron emission tomography study. *Translational Psychiatry, 11*(1), 57.

Korte, K. J., Jiang, T., Koenen, K. C., & Gradus, J. (2020, August 30). Trauma and PTSD: Epidemiology, comorbidity and clinical presentation in adults. In D. Forbes, J. I. Bisson, C. M. Monson, & L. Berliner (Eds.), *Effective treatments for PTSD* (3rd ed., Ch. 2). New York: Guilford Press.

Kriegel, D. L., & Azrak, A. (2020). Benzodiazepines for panic disorder in adults. *American Family Physician, 101*(7). [Online].

Krishnan, R. (2020, April 17). Unipolar depression in adults: Epidemiology, pathogenesis, and neurobiology. *UpToDate.*

Krishnan, R. (2021a, January 6). Unipolar depression in adults: Epidemiology. *UpToDate.* Retrieved from https://www.uptodate.com.

Krishnan, R. (2021b, January 6). Unipolar depression: Pathogenesis. *UpToDate.* Retrieved from https://www.uptodate.com.

Krishnan, R. (2021c, March 8). Unipolar depression: Neurobiology. *UpToDate.* Retrieved from https://www.uptodate.com.

Krull, K. R. (2019, November 27). Attention deficit hyperactivity disorder in children and adolescents: Clinical features and diagnosis. *UpToDate.* Retrieved from https://www.uptodate.com.

Krull, K. R. (2021a, October 29). Attention deficit hyperactivity disorder in children and adolescents: Epidemiology and pathogenesis. *UpToDate.* Retrieved from https://www.uptodate.com.

Krull, K. R. (2021b, May 13). Attention deficit hyperactivity disorder in children and adolescents: Treatment with medications. *UpToDate.* Retrieved from https://www.uptodate.com.

Kulz, A. K., Landmann, S., Schmidt-Ott, M., Zurowski, B., Wahl-Kordon, A., & Voderholzer, U. (2020). Long-term follow-up of cognitive-behavioral therapy for obsessive-compulsive disorder: Symptom severity and the role of exposure 8–10 years after inpatient treatment. *Journal of Cognitive Psychotherapy, 34*(3), 261–271.

Kumar, A., Sidhu, J., Goyal, A., & Tsao, J. W. (2020, April 20). Alzheimer disease. *StatPearls.*

Lai, C.-H. (2020). Task MRI-based functional brain network of anxiety. *Advances in Experimental Medicine and Biology, 1191,* 3–20.

LaRosa, J. (2019, October 16). $1.2 billion U.S. meditation market growing strongly as it becomes more mainstream. *Market Research.* Retrieved from https://blog.marketresearch.com.

Latimer, C. S., Lucot, K. L., Keene, C. D., Cholerton, B., & Montine, T. J. (2021). Genetic insights into Alzheimer's disease. *Annual Review of Pathology, 16,* 351–376.

Lawrence, A. A. (2010). Sexual orientation versus age of onset as bases for typologies (subtypes) for gender identity disorder in adolescents and adults. *Archives of Sexual Behavior, 39,* 514–545.

Latzer, Y., Katz, R., & Spivak, Z. (2011). *Facebook users more prone to eating disorders.* University of Haifa, Israel. [Unpublished manuscript]

Lebow, J. L., & Kelly, S. (2020). Couple therapies. In S. B. Messer & N. J. Kaslow (Eds.), *Essential psychotherapies: Theory and practice* (4th ed., Ch. 10, pp. 333–368). New York: Guilford Press.

Lecheler, M., Lasser, J., Vaughan, P. W., Leal, J., Ordetx, K., & Bischofberger, M. (2020, January 10). A matter of perspective: An exploratory study of a theory of mind autism intervention for adolescents. *Psychological Reports, 124*(1), 39–53.

Leonard, J. (2019, May 31). What is learned helplessness? *Medical News Today.*

Lerner, M. D., Mazefsky, C. A., White, S. W., & McPartland, J. C. (2018). Autism spectrum disorder. In J. N. Butcher & J. M. Hooley (Eds.), *APA handbook of psychopathology: Vol. 2. Psychopathology in children and adolescents* (Ch. 20). Washington, DC: American Psychological Association.

Levenson, J. L. (2020, January 8). Somatic symptom disorder: Epidemiology and clinical presentation. *UpToDate.* Retrieved from https://www.uptodate.com.

Liang, T.-W., & Tarsy, D. (2021, June 16). Tardive dyskinesia: Prevention, treatment, and prognosis. *UpToDate.* Retrieved from https://www.uptodate.com.

Lilienfeld, S. O. (2017). Microaggressions: Strong claims, inadequate evidence. *Perspectives on Psychological Science, 12*(1), 138–169.

Linehan, M. M. (2020, January 7). *Building a life worth living: A memoir.* New York: Random House Publishing.

Liu, N., Zhang, F., Wei, C., Jia, Y., Shang, Z., Sun, L., . . . Liu, W. (2020). Prevalence and predictors of PTSS during COVID-19 outbreak in China hardest-hit areas: Gender differences matter. *Psychiatry Research, 287,* 112921.

Liu, S., Yang, L., Zhang, C., Xiang, Y.-T., Liu, Z., Hu, S., & Zhang, B. (2020). Online mental health services in China during the COVID-19 outbreak. *The Lancet Psychiatry, 7*(4), e17–e18.

Lobato, M. I., Soll, B. M., Brandelli Costa, A., Saadeh, A., Gagliotti, D. A. M., Fresán, A., Reed, G., & Robles, R. (2019). Psychological distress among transgender people in Brazil: Frequency, intensity and social causation—an ICD-11 field study. *Brazilian Journal of Psychiatry, 41*(4), 310–315.

Lopez-Duran, N. L., Micol, V. J., &. Roberts, A. (2020). Neuroendocrinological models of stress and psychopathology. In K. L. Harkness & E. P. Hayden (Eds.), *The Oxford handbook of stress and mental health* (Ch. 21, pp. 463–486). New York: Oxford University Press.

Low, K. (2021, February 2). Summer camps for kids with ADHD. *Verywellmind.* Retrieved from https://www.verywellmind.com.

Lykken, D. T. (2019). Psychopathy, sociopathy, and antisocial personality disorder. In C. J. Patrick (Ed.), *Handbook of psychopathy* (2nd ed., Ch. 2, pp. 22–32). New York: Guilford Press.

Lyness, J. M. (2020, September 29). Unipolar minor depression in adults: Epidemiology, clinical presentation, and diagnosis. *UpToDate*. Retrieved from http://www.uptodate.com.

Lyness, J. M. (2021, October 4). Unipolar depression in adults: Assessment and diagnosis. *UpToDate*. Retrieved from https://www.uptodate.com.

Marchetti, D., Musso, P., Verrocchio, M. C., Manna, G., Kopala-Sibley, D. C., De Berardis, D., De Santis, S., & Falgares, G. (2021). Childhood maltreatment, personality vulnerability profiles, and borderline personality disorder symptoms in adolescents. *Development and Psychopathology*, 1–14.

Marsh, S. (2017, August 11). Viagra prescriptions on NHS triple in 10 years as stigma fades. *The Guardian*.

Marzola, E., Porliod, A., Panero, M., De-Bacco, C., & Abbate-Daga, G. (2020). Affective temperaments and eating psychopathology in anorexia nervosa: Which role for anxious and depressive traits? *Journal of Affective Disorders, 266*, 374–380.

Masters, W. H., & Johnson, V. E. (1970). *Human sexual inadequacy.* Boston: Little, Brown.

McCrady, B. S. (1990). The marital relationship and alcoholism treatment. In R. L. Collins, K. E. Leonard, B. A. Miller, & J. S. Searles (Eds.), *Alcohol and the family: Research and clinical perspectives* (pp. 338–355). New York: Guilford Press.

McCrady, B. S., Epstein, E. E., & Holzhauer, C. (2022). Couple therapy in the treatment of alcohol problems. In D. K. Snyder & J. Lebow (Eds.), *Clinical handbook of couple therapy* (6th ed.). New York: Guilford Press.

McElroy, S. L., Guerdjikova, A. I., Mori, N., Houser, P. L., & Keck, P. E., Jr. (2020). Management and treatment of feeding and eating disorders. In J. R. Geddes, N. C. Andreason, & G. M. Goodwin (Eds.), *New Oxford textbook of psychiatry* (3rd ed., Ch. 106). New York: Oxford University Press.

McGuire, A. P., Hayden, C. L., Zambrano-Vazquez, L., & Connolly, K. M. (2021). Examining the link between intolerance of uncertainty and positive and negative urgency in veterans with comorbid posttraumatic stress disorder and substance use disorders. *The Journal of Nervous and Mental Disease, 209*(1), 82–84.

McLaughlin, K. A., & Nolen-Hoeksema, S. (2011). Rumination as a transdiagnostic factor in depression and anxiety. *Behaviour Research and Therapy, 49*(3), 186–193.

MHA (Mental Health America). (2020). *Lesbian/gay/bisexual/transgender communities and mental health.* Retrieved from https://www.mhanational.org/issues.

Miller, K. J., Goncalves-Bradley, D. C., Areerob, P., Hennessy, D., Mesagno, C., & Grace, F. (2020). Comparative effectiveness of three exercise types to treat clinical depression in older adults: A systematic review and network meta-analysis of randomised controlled trials. *Ageing Research Review, 58,* 100999.

Mills, A. S., Vimalakanthan, K., Sivapalan, S., Shanmugalingam, N., & Weiss, J. A. (2020, May 16). Brief report: Preliminary outcomes of a peer counselling program for parents of children with autism in the south Asian community. *Journal of Autism and Developmental Disorders, 51*(1), 334–340.

Mitchell, J. E. (2021, July 7). Bulimia nervosa in adults: Cognitive-behavioral therapy (CBT). *UpToDate.* Retrieved from https://www.uptodate.com.

Mitchell, J. E., & Peterson, C. B. (2020). Anorexia nervosa. *New England Journal of Medicine, 382*(14), 1343–1351.

Mobach, L., Klein, A. M., Schniering, C. A., & Hudson, J. L. (2020). Specificity of dysfunctional beliefs in children with social anxiety disorder: Effects of comorbidity. *Journal of Clinical Child & Adolescent Psychology.* [Epub ahead of print]

Mondimore, F. M. (2020). *Bipolar disorder: A guide for you and your loved ones* (4th ed.). Baltimore, MD: Johns Hopkins University Press.

Morissette, S. B., Lenton-Brym, A. P., & Barlow, D. H. (2020). Panic disorder and agoraphobia. In M. M. Antony & D. H. Barlow, *Handbook of assessment and treatment planning for psychological disorders* (3rd ed., Ch. 6). New York: Guilford Press.

Muhlheim, L. (2020, January 28). Relapses in bulimia recovery. *Verywellmind.* Retrieved from https://www.verywellmind.com.

Munn-Chernoff, M. A., Johnson, E. C., Chou, Y.-L., Coleman, J. R. I., Thornton, L. M., Walters, R. K., . . . Agrawal, A. (2021). Shared genetic risk between eating disorder- and substance-use-related phenotypes: Evidence from genome-wide association studies. *Addiction Biology, 26*(1), e12880.

NCTE (National Center for Transgender Equality). (2020). *Additional help.* Washington, DC: NCTE.

NEDA (National Eating Disorders Association). (2020). *Statistics and research on eating disorders.* New York: Author.

Neufeld, C. B., Palma, P. C., Caetano, K. A. S., Brust-Renck, P. G., Curtiss, J., & Hofmann, S. G. (2020). A randomized clinical trial of group and individual cognitive-behavioral therapy approaches for social anxiety disorder. *International Journal of Clinical and Health Psychology, 20*(1), 29–37.

Newton-Howes, G., & Mulder, R. (2020). Treatment and management of personality disorder. In J. R. Geddes, N. C. Andreason, & G. M. Goodwin (Eds.), *New Oxford textbook of psychiatry* (3rd ed., Ch. 121). New York: Oxford University Press.

NIAAA (National Institute on Alcohol Abuse and Alcoholism). (2021a). *College drinking.* Bethesda, MD: NIAAA.

NIAAA (National Institute on Alcohol Abuse and Alcoholism). (2021b). *Alcohol problems in intimate relationships: Identification and intervention.* Bethesda, MD: NIAAA.

NIDA (National Institute on Drug Abuse). (2019). *Genetics and epigenetics of addiction.* Bethesda, MD: NIDA. Retrieved from https://www.drugabuse.gov/publications.

NIDA (National Institute on Drug Abuse). (2020a, April). *Opioid overdose crisis.* Bethesda, MD: NIDA.

NIDA (National Institute on Drug Abuse). (2020b). *Misuse of prescription drugs research report: What is the scope of prescription drug misuse?* Bethesda, MD: NIDA.

NIDA (National Institute on Drug Abuse). (2020c, August). *Genetics and epigenetics of addiction.* Bethesda, MD: NIDA.

Niles, J. K., Gudin, J., Radcliff, J., & Kaufman, H. W. (2021). The opioid epidemic within the COVID-19 pandemic: Drug testing in 2020. *Population Health Management, 24*(1).

NIMH (National Institute of Mental Health). (2017a). *Panic disorder among adults.* Bethesda, MD: Author.

NIMH (National Institute of Mental Health). (2017b). *Obsessive-compulsive disorder (OCD).* Bethesda, MD: Author.

NIMH (National Institute of Mental Health). (2017c). *Social anxiety disorder.* Bethesda, MD: Author.

NIMH (National Institute of Mental Health). (2017d). *Bipolar disorder.* Bethesda, MD: Author.

NIMH (National Institute of Mental Health). (2017e). *Eating disorders.* Bethesda, MD: Author.

NIMH (National Institute of Mental Health). (2020a). *Panic disorder.* Bethesda, MD: Author.

NIMH (National Institute of Mental Health). (2020b). *Obsessive-compulsive disorder (OCD).* Bethesda, MD: Author.

NIMH (National Institute of Mental Health). (2020c). *Statistics: Eating disorders.* Bethesda, MD: Author.

NIMH (National Institute of Mental Health). (2020d, January). *Bipolar disorder.* Bethesda, MD: Author.

NIMH (National Institute of Mental Health). (2020e). *Schizophrenia.* Bethesda, MD: Author.

NIMH (National Institute of Mental Health). (2021a, October). *Major depression.* Bethesda, MD: Author.

NIMH (National Institute of Mental Health). (2021b, December). *Eating disorders: Overview, signs and symptoms.* Bethesda, MD: Author.

Nolan, I. T., Kuhner, C. J., & Dy, G. W. (2019). Demographic and temporal trends in transgender identities and gender confirming surgery. *Translational Andrology and Urology, 8*(3), 184–190.

NSC (National Safety Council). (2020a). *Impairment begins with the first drink.* Retrieved from https://www.nsc.org/road-safety.

Nurnberger, J. I., Jr (2021). New analyses provide supportive evidence for specific genes related to bipolar disorder. *Bipolar Disorders. 23*(3), 295–296. https://doi.org/10.1111/bdi.13044

Nylander, E., Floros, O., Sparding, T., Rydén, E., Hansen, S., & Landén, M. (2021). Five-year outcomes of ADHD diagnosed in adulthood. *Scandinavian Journal of Psychology, 62*(1), 13–24.

Olivares-Olivares, P. J., Ortiz-González, P. F., & Olivares, J. (2019). Role of social skills training in adolescents with social anxiety disorder. *International Journal of Clinical and Health Psychology, 19*(1), 41–48.

Olson-Kennedy, J., & Forcier, M. (2020, June 22). Management of transgender and gender-diverse children and adolescents. *UpToDate.* Retrieved from http://www.uptodate.com.

Ornell, F., Schuch, J. B., Sordi, A. O., & Kessler, F. H. P. (2020, June). "Pandemic fear" and COVID-19: Mental health burden and strategies. *Brazilian Journal of Psychiatry, 42*(3). [Epub ahead of print]

Orpana, H., Giesbrecht, N., Hajee, A., & Kaplan, M. S. (2020). Alcohol and other drugs in suicide in Canada: Opportunities to support prevention through enhanced monitoring. *Injury Prevention.* [Epub ahead of print]

Park, K. K., & Koo, J. (2021, October 28). Skin picking (excoriation) disorder and related disorders. *UpToDate.* Retrieved from https://www.uptodate.com.

Pastor, Y. (2020). Psychosocial determinants of depression and maladaptive behaviour in adolescence: Two tested models. *Journal of Child & Adolescent Mental Health, 32,* 11–22.

Peavy, K. M. (2021, November 29). Psychosocial interventions for opioid use disorder. *UpToDate.* Retrieved from https://www.uptodate.com.

Pelham, W. E., & Altszuler, A. R. (2020). Combined treatment for children with attention-deficit/hyperactivity disorder: Brief history, the Multimodal Treatment for Attention-Deficit/Hyperactivity Disorder Study, and the past 20 years of research. *Journal of Developmental and Behavioral Pediatrics, 41,* S88–S98.

Peterson, A. L., Foa, E. B., Resick, P. A., Hoyt, T. V., Straud, C. L., Moore, B. A., . . . Strong Star Consortium. (2020). A nonrandomized trial of prolonged exposure and cognitive processing therapy for combat-related posttraumatic stress disorder in a deployed setting. *Behavior Therapy, 51*(6), 882–894.

Phillips, K. (2015). Obsessive-compulsive and related disorders. In A. Tasman, J. Kay, J. A. Lieberman, M. B. First, & M. Riba (Eds.), *Psychiatry* (4th ed., 2 vols., pp. 1093–1128). Hoboken, NJ: Wiley-Blackwell.

Phillips, M. L., & Drevets, W. C. (2020). Neuroimaging of bipolar disorder. In J. R. Geddes, N. C. Andreasen, & G. M. Goodwin (Eds.), *New Oxford textbook of psychiatry* (3rd ed., Ch. 71). New York: Oxford University Press.

Pina, A. A., Gonzales, N. A., Mazza, G. L., Gunn, H. J., Holly, L. E., Stoll, R. D., . . . Tein, J.-Y. (2020). Streamlined prevention and early intervention for pediatric anxiety disorders: A randomized controlled trial. *Prevention Science, 21*(4), 487–497.

Polanczyk, G. V. (2020). Epidemiology of attention deficit hyperactivity disorder and the implications for its prevention. In J. R. Geddes, N. C. Andreason, & G. M. Goodwin (Eds.), *New Oxford textbook of psychiatry* (3rd ed., Ch. 33). New York: Oxford University Press.

Poore, H. E., & Waldman, I. D. (2020). The association of oxytocin receptor gene (Oxtr) polymorphisms antisocial behavior: A meta-analysis. *Behavior Genetics, 50*(3), 161–173.

Post, R. M. (2021, June 4). Bipolar disorder in adults: Choosing maintenance treatment. *UpToDate.* Retrieved from https://www.uptodate.com.

Press, D. (2021, December 22). Management of the patient with dementia. *UpToDate.* Retrieved from https://www.uptodate.com.

Press, D., & Alexander, M. (2021, June 21). Cholinesterase inhibitors in the treatment of dementia. *UpToDate.* Retrieved from https://www.uptodate.com.

Psychiatric Rehabilitation Consultants. (1991). *Modules for training and independent living skills for persons with serious mental disorders.* Available from Dissemination Coordinator, Camarillo-UCLA Research Center, Box 6022, Camarillo, CA 93011-6022.

Quidé, Y., Bortolasci, C. C., Spolding, B., Kidnapillai, S., Watkeys, O. J., Cohen-Woods, S., . . . Green, M. J. (2021). Systemic inflammation and grey matter volume in schizophrenia and bipolar disorder: Moderation by childhood trauma severity. *Progress in Neuro-Psychopharmacology & Biological Psychiatry, 105,* 110013.

Rakicevic, M. (2019, July 12). 27 meditation statistics that you should be aware of. *Disturbmenot.* Retrieved from https://disturbmenot.com.

Rappaport, L. M., Hunter, M. D., Russell, J. J., Pinard, G., Bleau, P., & Moskowitz, D. S. (2021). Emotional and interpersonal mechanisms in community SSRI treatment of social anxiety disorder. *Journal of Psychiatry & Neuroscience: JPN, 46*(1), E56–E64. https://doi.org/10.1503/jpn.190164

Reid, M. A. (2021). Glutamate and gamma-aminobutyric acid abnormalities in antipsychotic-naïve patients with schizophrenia: Evidence from empirical and meta-analytic studies using magnetic resonance spectroscopy. *Biological Psychiatry, 89*(3), e1–e3.

Ren, S.-Y., Gao, R.-D., & Chen, Y.-L. (2020). Fear can be more harmful than the severe acute respiratory syndrome coronavirus 2 in controlling the coronavirus disease 2019 epidemic. *World Journal of Clinical Cases, 8*(4), 652–657.

Retz, W., Ginsberg, Y., Turner, D., Barra, S., Retz-Junginger, P., Larsson, H., & Asherson, P. (2021). Attention-deficit/hyperactivity disorder (ADHD), antisociality and delinquent behavior over the lifespan. *Neuroscience and Biobehavioral Reviews, 120,* 236–248.

Riggs, D. S., Tate, L., Chrestman, K., & Foa, E. B. (2020). Prolonged exposure. In D. Forbes, J. I. Bisson, C. M. Monson, & L. Berliner (Eds.), *Effective treatments for PTSD* (3rd ed., Ch. 12). New York: Guilford Press.

Rodgers, M., Simmonds, M., Marshall, D., Hodgson, R., Stewart, L. A., Rai, D., . . . Couteur, A. L. (2021, January 22). Intensive behavioural interventions based on applied behaviour analysis for young children with autism: An international collaborative individual participant data meta-analysis. *Autism: The International Journal of Research and Practice.* [Epub ahead of print]

Rose, G. M., & Tadi, P. (2021, January 31). Social anxiety disorder. *StatPearls.*

Rosen, R. C., & Khera, M. (2021, May 27). Epidemiology and etiologies of male sexual dysfunction. *UpToDate.* Retrieved from https://www.uptodate.com.

Rosenberg, D. (2021, May 12). Treatment of obsessive-compulsive disorder in children and adolescents. *UpToDate.* Retrieved from https://www.uptodate.com.

Roy-Byrne, P. P. (2020, January 20). Pharmacotherapy for panic disorder with or without agoraphobia in adults. *UpToDate.* Retrieved from http://www.uptodate.com.

Rutherford-Morrison, L., & Polish, J. (2020, March 31). 8 statistics that prove why Transgender Day of Visibility is so crucial. *Bustle.* Retrieved from https://www.bustle.com.

Sacks, O. (1993, December 27). An Anthropologist on Mars. *The New Yorker.* Retrieved from: https://www.newyorker.com/magazine/1993/12/27/anthropologist-mars.

Saitz, R. (2021, October 21). Alcohol use disorder: Psychosocial treatment. *UpToDate.* Retrieved from https://www.uptodate.com.

Salkovskis, P. M., & Harrison, J. (1984). Abnormal and normal obsessions—a replication. *Behaviour Research and Therapy, 22*(5), 549–552.

Salters-Pedneault, K. (2020, January 21). Borderline personality disorder statistics. *Verywellmind.* Retrieved from https://verywellmind.com.

SAMHSA (Substance Abuse and Mental Health Services Administration). (2019). *Results from the 2019 National Survey on Drug Use and Health: Detailed Tables.* Rockville, MD: SAMHSA.

SAMHSA (Substance Abuse and Mental Health Services Administration). (2021). *2018 National Survey of Drug Use and Health (NSDUH) releases.* Rockville, MD: SAMHSA.

Sareen, J. (2021, February 4). Posttraumatic stress disorder in adults: Epidemiology, pathophysiology, clinical manifestations, course, assessment, and diagnosis. *UpToDate.* Retrieved from https://www.uptodate.com.

Sareen, J., Afifi, T. O., McMillan, K. A., & Asmundson, G. J. G. (2011). Relationship between household income and mental disorders: Findings from a population-based longitudinal study. *Archives of General Psychiatry, 68*(4), 419–426.

Sato, K. (2021). Why is lithium effective in alleviating bipolar disorder? *Medical Hypotheses, 147,* 110484.

Schneeberger, A. R., Huber, C. G., Lang, U. E., Muenzenmaier, K. H., Castille, D., Jaeger, M., . . . Link, B. G. (2017). Effects of assisted outpatient treatment and health care services on psychotic symptoms. *Social Science & Medicine, 175,* 152–160.

Schneier, F. R. (2021, May 26). Social anxiety disorder in adults: Epidemiology, clinical manifestations, and diagnosis. *UpToDate.* Retrieved from https://www.uptodate.com.

Schreiber, J., & Culpepper, L. (2021, May 24). Suicidal ideation and behavior in adults. *UpToDate.* Retrieved from https://www.uptodate.com.

Seelman, K. L, Miller, J. F., Fawcett, Z. E. R., & Cline, L. (2018, April 30). Do transgender men have equal access to health care and engagement in preventing health behaviors compared to cisgender adults? *Social Work in Health Care, 57*(7), 502–525.

Seligman, N. S., Cleary, B. J., & Berghella, V. (2021, December 1). Methadone and buprenorphine pharmacotherapy of opioid use disorder during pregnancy. *UpToDate.* Retrieved from https://www.uptodate.com.

Selkie, E., Adkins, V., Masters, E., Bajpai, A., & Shumer, D. (2020). Transgender adolescents' uses of social media for social support. *Journal of Adolescent Health, 66*(3), 275–280.

Shapero, B. G., Gibb, B. E., Archibald, A., Wilens, T. E., Fava, M., & Hirshfeld-Becker, D. R. (2021). Risk factors for depression in adolescents with ADHD: The impact of cognitive biases and stress. *Journal of Attention Disorders, 25*(3), 340–354.

Sherrill, A. M., Maples-Keller, J. L., Yasinski, C. W., Loucks, L. A., Rothbaum, B. O., & Rauch, S. A. M. (2020). Perceived benefits and drawbacks of massed prolonged exposure: A qualitative thematic analysis of reactions from treatment completers. *Psychological Trauma: Theory, Research, Practice, and Policy.* [Epub ahead of print]

Shifren, J. L. (2020, February 24). Overview of sexual dysfunction in women: Epidemiology, risk factors, and evaluation. *UpToDate.* Retrieved from https://www.uptodate.com.

Simon, G. (2019). Unipolar depression in adults and initial treatment: General principles and prognosis. *UpToDate.* Retrieved from http://www.uptodate.com.

Skodol, A. (2021, February 18). Borderline personality disorder: Epidemiology, pathogenesis, clinical features, course, assessment, and diagnosis. *UpToDate.* Retrieved from https://www.uptodate.com.

Smith, J. P., & Randall, C. L. (2012). Anxiety and alcohol use disorders: Comorbidity and treatment considerations. *Alcohol Research, 34*(4), 414–431.

Snyder, P. J., & Rosen, R. C. (2020, January 11). Overview of male sexual dysfunction. *UpToDate.* Retrieved from https://www.uptodate.com.

Speer, K. E., Semple, S., Naumovski, N., D'Cunha, N. M., & McKune, A. J. (2019). HPA axis function and diurnal cortisol in post-traumatic stress disorder: A systematic review. *Neurobiology of Stress, 11,* 100180.

Stein, M. B. (2020a, February 4). Approach to treating posttraumatic stress disorder in adults. *UpToDate.* Retrieved from http://www.uptodate.com.

Stein, M. B. (2020b, April 16). Pharmacotherapy for social anxiety disorder in adults. *Uptodate.* Retrieved from http://www.uptodate.com.

Stein, M. B. (2021, March 16). Pharmacotherapy for posttraumatic stress disorder in adults. *UpToDate.* Retrieved from https://www.uptodate.com.

Stein, M. B., & Taylor, C. T. (2019, June 5). Approach to treating social anxiety disorder in adults. *UpToDate.* Retrieved from https://www.uptodate.com.

Stone, J., & Sharpe, M. (2020, January 7). Conversion disorder in adults: Clinical features, assessment, and comorbidity. *UpToDate*. Retrieved from https://www.uptodate.com.

Stovall, J. (2020, January 15). Bipolar disorder in adults: Epidemiology and pathogenesis. *UpToDate*. Retrieved from http://www.uptodate.com.

Stovall, J. (2021, April 11). Bipolar mania and hypomania in adults: Choosing pharmacotherapy. *UpToDate*. Retrieved from https://www.uptodate.com.

Strain, E. (2021a, July 28). Opioid use disorder: Epidemiology, pharmacology, clinical manifestations, course, screening, assessment, and diagnosis. *UpToDate*. Retrieved from https://www.uptodate.com.

Strain, E. (2021b, August 25). Pharmacotherapy for opioid use disorder. *UpToDate*. Retrieved from https://www.uptodate.com.

Stroup, T. S., & Marder, S. (2020, April 21). Pharmacotherapy for schizophrenia: Acute and maintenance phase treatment. *UpToDate*. Retrieved from https://www.uptodate.com.

Styles, M., Alsharshani, D., Samara, M., Alsharshani, M., Khattab, A., Qoronfleh, M. W., & Al-Dewik, N. I. (2020). Risk factors, diagnosis, prognosis and treatment of autism. *Frontiers in Bioscience (Landmark Edition), 25,* 1682–1717.

Su, L.-D., Xu, F.-X., Wang, X.-T., Cai, X.-Y., & Shen, Y. (2020, May 21). Cerebellar dysfunction, cerebro-cerebellar connectivity and autism spectrum disorders. *Neuroscience.* [Epub ahead of print]

Szechtman, H., Harvey, B. H., Woody, E. Z., & Hoffman, K. L. (2020). The psychopharmacology of obsessive-compulsive disorder: A preclinical roadmap. *Pharmacological Reviews, 72*(1), 80–151.

Tangpricha, V., & Safer, J. D. (2020, December 2). Transgender men: Evaluation and management. *UpToDate*. Retrieved from http://www.uptodate.com.

Tangpricha, V., & Safer, J. D. (2021, December 1). Transgender women: Evaluation and management. *UpToDate*. Retrieved from https://www.uptodate.com.

Taylor, S., Abramowitz, J. S., McKay, D., & Garner, L. E. (2020). Obsessive-compulsive and related disorders. In M. M. Antony & D. H. Barlow, *Handbook of assessment and treatment planning for psychological disorders* (3rd ed., Ch. 8). New York: Guilford Press.

Tenenbaum, R. B., Musser, E. D., Morris, S., Ward, A. R., Raiker, J. S., Coles, E. K., & Pelham, W. E. (2019). Response inhibition, response execution, and emotion regulation among children with attention-deficit/hyperactivity disorder. *Journal of Abnormal Child Psychology, 47,* 589–603.

Thomas, B. P., Tarumi, T., Sheng, M., Tseng, B., Womack, K. B., Cullum, C. M., . . . Lu, H. (2020). Brain perfusion change in patients with mild cognitive impairment after 12 months of aerobic exercise training. *Journal of Alzheimer's Disease: JAD, 75*(2), 617–631.

Thomas, S. (2020). *Alcohol and drug abuse statistics.* Brentwood, TN: American Addiction Centers.

Ting, I., Scott, N., & Palmer, A. (2020, February 2). Rough justice: How police are failing survivors of sexual assault. *ABC News* (Australia). Retrieved from https://www.abc.net.au.

Tong, P., Bo, P., Shi, Y., Dong, L., Sun, T., Gao, X., & Yang, Y. (2021). Clinical traits of patients with major depressive disorder with comorbid borderline personality disorder based on propensity score matching. *Depression and Anxiety, 38*(1), 100–106.

Tonge, N. A., Lim, M. H., Piccirillo, M. L., Fernandez, K. C., Langer, J. K., & Rodebaugh, T. L. (2020). Interpersonal problems in social anxiety disorder across different relational contexts. *Journal of Anxiety Disorders, 75,* 102275.

Tortella-Feliu, M., Fullana, M. A., Perez-Vigil, A., Torres, X., Chamorro, J., Littarelli, S. A., . . . de la Kruz, L. (2019). Risk factors for posttraumatic stress disorder: An umbrella review of systematic reviews and meta-analyses. *Neuroscience and Biobehavioral Reviews, 107,* 154–165.

Tremblay, M., Baydala, L., Khan, M., Currie, C., Morley, K., Burkholder, C., Davidson, R., & Stillar, A. (2020). Primary substance use prevention programs for children and youth: A systematic review. *Pediatrics, 146*(3), e20192747.

Tseng, A., Biagianti, B., Francis, S. M., Conelea, C. A., & Jacob, S. (2020). Social cognitive interventions for adolescents with autism spectrum disorders: A systematic review. *Journal of Affective Disorders, 274,* 199–204.

Usher, K., Durkin, J., & Bhullar, N. (2020). The COVID-19 pandemic and mental health impacts. *International Journal of Mental Health Nursing, 29*(3), 315–318.

Valinsky, J. (2020, April 29). Beer sales are soaring. These brands are winning the booze battle. *CNN Business*.

van den Brink, W., & Kiefer, F. (2020). Alcohol use disorder. In J. R. Geddes, N. C. Andreason, & G. M. Goodwin (Eds.), *New Oxford textbook of psychiatry* (3rd ed., Ch. 50). New York: Oxford University Press.

Vieta, E., Pacchiarotti, I., & Miklowitz, D. J. (2020). Management and treatment of bipolar disorder. In J. R. Geddes, N. C. Andreasen, & G. M. Goodwin (Eds.), *New Oxford textbook of psychiatry* (3rd ed., Ch. 72). New York: Oxford University Press.

von Greiff, N., & Skogens, L. (2020, April 2). Abstinence or controlled drinking: A five-year follow-up on Swedish clients reporting positive change after treatment for substance use disorders. *Drugs and Alcohol Today*.

Waldman, I. D., Rhee, S. H., LoParo, D., & Park, Y. (2019). Genetic and environmental influences on psychopathy and antisocial behavior. In C. J. Patrick (Ed.), *Handbook of psychopathy* (2nd ed., Ch. 14, pp. 335–353). New York: Guilford Press.

Walker, P., & Kulkarni, J. (2020). Re-framing borderline personality disorder. *Australasian Psychiatry: Bulletin of Royal Australian and New Zealand College of Psychiatrists, 28*(2), 237–238.

Wampler, K. S. (2020, October 12). *The handbook of systemic family therapy* (4 vols.). Hoboken, NJ: Wiley-Blackwell.

Wang, C., Pan, R., Wan, X., Tan, Y., Xu, L., Ho, C. S., & Ho, R. C. (2020). Immediate psychological responses and associated factors during the initial stage of the 2019 coronavirus disease (COVID-19) epidemic among the general population in China. *International Journal of Environmental Research and Public Health, 17*(5), 1729.

Wang, P. S., Lane, M., Olfson, M., Pincus, H. A., Wells, K. B., & Kessler, R. C. (2005). Twelve-month use of mental health services in the United States. *Archives of General Psychiatry, 62*, 629–640.

Wang, S.-P., Wang, J.-D., Chang, J.-H., Wu, B.-J., Wang, T.-J., & Sun, H.-J. (2020). Symptomatic remission affects employment outcomes in schizophrenia patients. *BMC Psychiatry, 20*(1), 219.

Watkins, E. R., & Roberts, H. (2020). Reflecting on rumination: Consequences, causes, mechanisms and treatment of rumination. *Behaviour Research and Therapy, 127*, 103573.

Watkins, M. (2021, November 11). *Alcoholism and family/marital problems.* Brentwood, TN: American Addiction Centers.

Wicklund, E. (2020, March 20). States move quickly to address coronavirus pandemic with telehealth. *mHealth Intelligence.* Retrieved from https://mhealthintelligence.com:news:states-move-quickly-to-address-coronavirus-pandemic-with-telehealth.

Williams, J., & Nieuwsma, J. (2020, June 26). Screening for depression in adults. *UpToDate.* Retrieved from http://www.uptodate.com.

Wolk, D. A., & Dickerson, B. C. (2020, December 11). Clinical features and diagnosis of Alzheimer disease. *UpToDate.* Retrieved from https://www.uptodate.com.

Worthington, M. A., Miklowitz, D. J., O'Brien, M., Addington, J., Bearden, C. E., Cadenhead, K. S., . . . Cannon, T. D. (2020). Selection for psychosocial treatment for youth at clinical high risk for psychosis based on the North American Prodrome Longitudinal Study individualized risk calculator. *Early Intervention in Psychiatry,* eip.12914.

Yager, J. (2019, April 29). Eating disorders: Overview of prevention and treatment. *UpToDate.* Retrieved from https://www.uptodate.com.

Yager, J. (2020). Managing patients with severe and enduring anorexia nervosa: When is enough, enough? *The Journal of Nervous and Mental Disease, 208*(4), 277–282.

Yang, Y., Song, Y., Lu, Y., Xu, Y., Liu, L., & Liu, X. (2019). Associations between erectile dysfunction and psychological disorders (depression and anxiety): A cross-sectional study in a Chinese population. *Andrologia, 51*(10).

Yıldız, E. (2020). The effects of acceptance and commitment therapy in psychosis treatment: A systematic review of randomized controlled trials. *Perspectives in Psychiatric Care, 56*(1), 149–167.

Yu, F., Vock, D. M., Zhang, L., Salisbury, D., Nelson, N. W., Chow, L. S., . . . Wyman, J. F. (2021, January 26). Cognitive effects of aerobic exercise in Alzheimer's disease: A pilot randomized controlled trial. *Journal of Alzheimer's Disease.* [Epub ahead of print]

van Gogh, V. (1889, April 21). Letter to Theo van Gogh.

Zakreski, E., & Pruessner, J. C. (2020). Psychophysiological models of stress. In K. L. Harkness & E. P. Hayden (Eds.), *The Oxford handbook of stress and mental health* (Ch. 22, pp. 487–518). New York: Oxford University Press.

Zeifman, R. J., Boritz, T., Barnhart, R., Labrish, C., & McMain, S. F. (2020). The independent roles of mindfulness and distress tolerance in treatment outcomes in dialectical behavior therapy skills training. *Personality Disorders, 11*(3), 181–190.

Zhang, T., Liu, N., Cao, H., Wei, W., Ma, L., & Li, H. (2020). Different doses of pharmacological treatments for mild to moderate Alzheimer's disease: A Bayesian network meta-analysis. *Frontiers in Pharmacology, 22*, 778.

Zhou, S.-J., Zhang, L.-G., Wang, L.-L., Guo, Z.-C., Wang, J.-Q., Chen, J.-C., . . . Chen, J.-X. (2020). Prevalence and socio-demographic correlates of psychological health problems in Chinese adolescents during the outbreak of COVID-19. *European Child & Adolescent Psychiatry, 29*(6), 749–758.

Zhu, J., Yang, Y., Touyz, S., Park, R., & Hay, P. (2020). Psychological treatments for people with severe and enduring anorexia nervosa: A mini review. *Frontiers in Psychiatry, 11*, 206.

Ziegelstein, R. C. (2018). Creating structured opportunities for social engagement to promote well-being and avoid burnout in medical students and residents: *Academic Medicine, 93*(4), 537–539.

Zurita Ona, P. E. (2021, January 28). *Living beyond OCD using acceptance and commitment therapy: A workbook for adults* (1st ed.). New York: Routledge.

Name Index

Subject Index